NETWORKED DISEASE

Studies in Urban and Social Change

NETWORKED DISEASE

EMERGING INFECTIONS IN THE GLOBAL CITY

Edited by

S. Harris Ali and Roger Keil

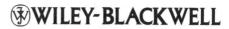

A John Wiley & Sons, Ltd., Publication

This edition first published 2008
© 2008 Blackwell Publishing Ltd

Blackwell Publishing was acquired by John Wiley & Sons in February 2007. Blackwell's publishing program has been merged with Wiley's global Scientific, Technical, and Medical business to form Wiley-Blackwell.

Registered Office
John Wiley & Sons Ltd, The Atrium, Southern Gate, Chichester, West Sussex, PO19 8SQ, United Kingdom

Editorial Offices
350 Main Street, Malden, MA 02148-5020, USA
9600 Garsington Road, Oxford, OX4 2DQ, UK
The Atrium, Southern Gate, Chichester, West Sussex, PO19 8SQ, UK

For details of our global editorial offices, for customer services, and for information about how to apply for permission to reuse the copyright material in this book please see our website at www.wiley.com/wiley-blackwell.

The right of S. Harris Ali and Roger Keil to be identified as the authors of the editorial material in this work has been asserted in accordance with the Copyright, Designs and Patents Act 1988.

Library of Congress Cataloging-in-Publication Data

Networked disease: emerging infections in the global city / [edited by] S. Harris Ali and Roger Keil.
    p.; cm.—(Studies in urban and social change)
    Includes bibliographical references and index.
    ISBN 978-1-4051-6133-6 (PLPC: alk. paper)—ISBN 978-1-4051-6134-3 (pbk.: alk. paper)
1. SARS (Disease)—Canada—Toronto. 2. SARS (Disease)—China—Hong Kong. 3. SARS (Disease) —Singapore. 4. Globalization—Health aspects. 5. Urban health. I. Ali, S. Harris. II. Keil, Roger, 1957- III. Series.
    [DNLM: 1. Severe Acute Respiratory Syndrome–prevention & control. 2. Communicable Diseases, Emerging–prevention & control. 3. Internationality. 4. Public Health Practice. 5. Urban Health. WC 505 N476 2008]
RA644.S17N48 2008
362.196'2–dc22

                                                            2008008194

A catalogue record for this book is available from the British Library.

Set in 10.5/12 pt Baskerville by SPi Publisher Services, Pondicherry, India.

1   2008

Contents

List of Figures

List of Tables

Notes on Contributors

S. Harris Ali is an Associate Professor in the Faculty of Environmental Studies at York University, Toronto. He holds a doctorate in Sociology and an undergraduate degree in Engineering, both from McMaster University. His research interests include the study of environmental health issues (including toxic contamination events and disease outbreaks) and the sociology of disasters and risk from an interdisciplinary perspective. He has published on this work in such journals as *Social Problems, Social Science and Medicine, The Canadian Review of Sociology and Anthropology, Urban Studies*, and the *Journal of Canadian Public Policy.*

Peter Baehr is a Professor and Head of the Department of Politics and Sociology at Lingnan University, Tuen Mun, Hong Kong. His research straddles politics and sociology. While continuing to write on the history of political and social thought, Baehr is now more actively engaged in the study of social and state responses to mass emergency. He is an Honorary Fellow of the University of Edinburgh, and a member of the Scientific Board of the IMT Institute of Advanced Studies, Lucca (Italy). Locally, Peter Baehr is a co-investigator in the Hong Kong Transition Project, and a member of the Hong Kong Forum (an affiliate of the Council on Foreign Relations, New York).

Nick Bingham is a Lecturer in the Geography Discipline at the Open University in the UK. He has published widely on the challenging geographies that emerge once the social is not assumed to be a solely human construction. His current empirical research on the making of biosecurities and the cosmopolitics of coexistence both feeds into and feeds off an ongoing concern to articulate the kind of bodies-in-the-midst-of-things and object-oriented politics that might be adequate to our sociotechnical condition.

Bruce Braun is a Professor in the Earth and Environmental Sciences Program at the City University of New York. He is the author of *The Intemperate Rainforest: Nature, Culture and Power on Canada's West Coast* (Minnesota, 2002) and the co-editor of *Remaking Reality: Nature at the Millennium* (Routledge, 1998) and *Social Nature: Theory, Practice, Politics* (Blackwell, 2001). His current research on post-human urbanism examines the city as a "more-than-human" assemblage, and explores what this means for our understanding of the spatio-temporal rhythms of urban life, the composition of human and non-human bodies within urban networks, the political technologies devised to regulate the exchange of properties between humans and non-humans, and the relation between science, democracy, and urban politics.

David Clifton is a doctoral candidate in the Joint Program in Communication and Culture program at York University. He has worked as a graduate researcher at the Robarts Center since 2003, where he coauthored a major study on the role of the media in the SARS crisis in Toronto. David's primary research area is the role of the media in democratic societies, with a focus on news production, public opinion polling and news broadcasting in Canada, the United Kingdom, and the United States. David has also done research on the interplay between technology and the public sphere, with a focus on the role of television and the Internet in shaping public discourse and public opinion.

Susan Craddock is an Associate Professor in the Institute for Global Studies and the Department of Gender, Women, and Sexuality Studies at the University of Minnesota. Her work focuses on the intersections of infectious disease, new biotechnologies, and globalizing medical practices that regulate access to medical therapies, reinvigorate debates over biosecurity and national borders, and introduce new modes of shaping and contesting meanings of biocitizenship. She is the author of *City of Plagues: Disease, Poverty, and Deviance in San Francisco* (Minnesota 2000), and co-editor of *HIV and AIDS in Africa: Beyond Epidemiology* (Blackwell 2004).

Daniel Drache is the Associate Director of the Robarts Centre for Canadian Studies and Professor of Political Economy at York University.

He has written extensively on globalization, North American economic integration, new state forms and practices, as well as on global dissent and cultural flows. His latest book is entitled *Borders Matter: Homeland Security and the Search for North America* (Fernwood, 2005). His research on global cultural flows, the WTO, and Counterpublics is available at www.robarts.yorku.ca. The report on SARS is funded by a SSHRC grant on new information technologies, of which he is the Principal Investigator.

Matthew Gandy completed his PhD at the London School of Economics in 1992. He is currently an ESRC research fellow with the project "Cyborg Urbanization: Theorizing Water and Urban Infrastructure" at University College London. His research into urbanization and public health has also been developed through collaborative work on the global resurgence of tuberculosis and infectious disease, as well as informed through his research on the theme of "urban metabolism," involving the development of sanitation, water supply, and urban environmental politics in Britain, France, Germany, India, Nigeria, and the United States. His book *Concrete and Clay: Reworking Nature in New York City* (The MIT Press, 2002) was awarded the 2003 Spiro Kostof award for the book within the previous two years "that has made the greatest contribution to our understanding of urbanism and its relationship with architecture."

Steve Hinchliffe is Senior Lecturer in Geography at the Open University. He is author of *Spaces for Nature* (Sage) and co-editor of, among others, *Understanding Environmental Issues* (Wiley) and *Environmental Responses* (Wiley). He has authored work on urban natures, zoonotic diseases, and environmental risk. His research lies at the interstices of geographical interests in space, life politics, and materialities. Its overarching aim is to demonstrate, through empirically and theoretically informed work, how social worlds are enacted in and through a variety of spatial practices. From public health and risk policies to urban redevelopment in areas of high socio-economic and environmental deprivation, the aim is to demonstrate the purchase that social, spatial, and political theory can have on socio-environmental issues and in turn contribute to theoretical debates through an ethnographically informed understanding of social practices.

Claire Hooker is a Senior Lecturer in Medical Humanities at the Centre for Values, Ethics and Law in Medicine at the University of Sydney, Australia. She has conducted research on community responses to health scare situations as well as completing extensive research in contemporary and historical public health, with a focus on acute risk issues. Her work has covered the evolution of tobacco control policy and legislation, community responses to epidemics, and disease control throughout the twentieth century, as well as the intellectual history of bacteriology and the history of science. She is the author of *Irresistible Forces: Women in Australian Science* (Melbourne University Press, 2005) and the co-editor of *Contagion: Cultural and Historical Studies* (Routledge, 2001).

Paul Jackson is a PhD student in Geography at the University of Toronto, whose research combines urban political ecology, disease, and the commodification of nature. Previous research, at York University in the Faculty of Environmental Studies, investigated the city/countryside divide with regards to agricultural land and farmers, ex-urban landscapes, conservation planning projects, and critical urban geography. He has recently co-authored an article in *City* with Gerda R. Wekerle, entitled "Urbanizing the Security Agenda: Anti-Terrorism, Urban Sprawl and Social Movements."

Roger Keil is the Director of the City Institute and a Professor of Environmental Studies at York University in Toronto. He is a co-editor of the *International Journal of Urban and Regional Research* and a founding member of the International Network of Urban Research and Action (http://www.inura.org). Among his recent publications are *Nature and the City* (2004, with Gene Desfor) and *The Global Cities Reader* (2006, with Neil Brenner).

Nicholas B. King is an Assistant Professor in the Biomedical Ethics Unit at McGill University's Faculty of Medicine in Montreal. He holds a PhD in the History of Science and an MA in Medical Anthropology from Harvard University; and from 2003 to 2005 he was a Robert Wood Johnson Health and Society Scholar in the Department of Epidemiology at the University of Michigan. At Case, he directs the Program in Genomics and Public Health, and co-directs the first block of the medical education curriculum. Dr King's research focuses on public health ethics and policy, including health inequalities, biodefense, surveillance, and emerging infectious diseases. He has published essays in *The American Journal of Public Health*, *The American Journal of Bioethics*, *Bioethics*, *Journal of the History of Medicine and the Allied Sciences*, and *Social Studies of Science*.

Mee Kam Ng is an Associate Professor at the Centre of Urban Planning and Environmental Management, the University of Hong Kong. She has published widely on urban planning and sustainability issues. She is a member of the Hong Kong Institute of Planners and the Royal Town Planning Institute. She was a founding vice-chairman of the Hong Kong People's Council for Sustainable Development and one of the founders of Citizen Envisioning@Harbour, which is concerned with the future planning and development of Victoria Harbour, in the heart of the city. In 2004, she

joined an international working group under the European Union spon-
sored Global Reporting Initiative to work on a public-sector supplement for
sustainability reporting. Currently, she is working on two major research
projects: sustainable world cities and sustainability impact assessments in
Hong Kong within the regional context. To learn more, please visit http://
www.hku.hk/cupem/home/Academic_staff_Mee.htm.

Shir Nee Ong is a Geography Lecturer at Hwa Chong Institution (College),
Singapore. Her current research interests are geographies of health and ill-
health, including AIDS and SARS. She has also co-authored a chapter on
HIV/AIDS in Singapore in a forthcoming book from World Scientific,
entitled *Population Dynamics and Infectious Disease in Asia*.

Victor G. Rodwin is a Professor of Health Policy and Management and
teaches courses on community health and medical care, comparative analysis of healthcare systems, and international perspectives on healthcare
reform. He is the recipient of a three-year Robert Wood Johnson Foundation
Health Policy Investigator Award on "Megacities and Health: New York,
London, Paris and Tokyo." He is the author of numerous articles and
books, including *The Health Planning Predicament: France, Quebec, England, and the
United States* (University of California, 1984); *The End of an Illusion: The Future
of Health Policy in Western Industrialized Nations* (with J. de Kervasdoué and
J. Kimberly; University of California, 1984); *Public Hospitals in New York and
Paris* (with C. Brecher, D. Jolly, and R. Baxter; New York University Press,
1992); and *Japan's Universal and Affordable Health Care: Lessons for the U.S.?*
(Japan Society, 1994). His most recent book, *Growing Older in Four World
Cities: New York, London, Paris and Tokyo* (edited with Michael Gusmano), will
be published by Vanderbilt University Press. Recent journal articles have
appeared in the *Journal of Urban Health*, *Indicators*, and the *American Journal of
Public Health*. Professor Rodwin directs the World Cities Project, a collaborative venture between the Wagner School and the International Longevity
Center-USA, which examines the impact of population aging and longevity on
New York, London, Paris, and Tokyo. He has consulted with the World Bank,
the UN, the French National Health Insurance Fund, and other international
organizations. Professor Rodwin earned his PhD in city and regional planning,
and his MPH in public health, University of California at Berkeley.

Philipp Sarasin is Professor for Modern History at the History Department
of the University of Zurich, Switzerland, and director of the centre "History
of Knowledge" (Zurich University and the Federal Institute of Technology,
Zurich). His recent books are *Anthrax: Bioterror as Fact and Fantasy* (Harvard
University Press, 2006) and *Michel Foucault zur Einführung* (Junius, 2005). He
has published on the history of the body and sexuality, on bourgeois culture

in the late nineteenth century, and on the theory of historiography. His current research on the history of popular science in the late twentieth century focuses on the impact of biology and sociobiology on European culture during the Cold War.

Peggy Teo is with the Department of Geography, National University of Singapore. Her research interests are in social gerontological issues and in tourism. Her work on older persons has focused on identity issues, health issues, policy, and the gendered experience of aging. She is the co-author of *Ageing in Singapore: Service Needs and the State* (Routledge, 2006) and co-editor of *Interconnected Worlds: Tourism in Southeast Asia* (Pergamon, 2001), *Changing Landscapes of Singapore* (McGraw Hill, 2004), and *Gender Politics in the Asia-Pacific Region* (Routledge, 2002). She has worked with NGOs such as the Tan and Tsao Foundations toward better services for older people, and with government departments such as the Department of Statistics and Ministry of Community Development and Sports.

Estair Van Wagner lives in Toronto, where she graduated from York University's joint Master of Environmental Studies and Bachelor of Laws program. She holds a BA from the University of Victoria in Political Science and Environmental Studies. Estair's research interests include global cities, urban politics and governance, democratic theory and public participation, and legal theory.

Brenda S.A. Yeoh is Professor, Department of Geography, as well as the Head of the Southeast Asian Studies Programme, National University of Singapore. She is also the Research Leader of the Asian Migration Research Cluster and Principal Investigator of the Asian MetaCentre at the University's Asia Research Institute. Her research interests include the politics of space in colonial and post-colonial cities; and gender, migration and transnational communities. Her first book was *Contesting Space: Power Relations and the Urban Built Environment in Colonial Singapore* (Oxford University Press, 1996; reissued Singapore University Press, 2003). On the area of migration and health issues, she has recently published *Migration and Health in Asia* (Routledge, 2005, with Santosh Jatrana and Mika Toyota) and *Population Dynamics and Infectious Diseases in Asia* (World Scientific, 2006, with Adrian Sleigh, Chee Heng Leng, Phua Kai Hong, and Rachel Safman).

Series Editors' Preface

The Blackwell *Studies in Urban and Social Change* series is published in association with the *International Journal of Urban and Regional Research*. It aims to advance theoretical debates and empirical analyses stimulated by changes in the fortunes of cities and regions across the world. Among topics taken up in past volumes and welcomed for future submissions are:

- Connections between economic restructuring and urban change
- Urban divisions, difference, and diversity
- Convergence and divergence among regions of the east and west, north, and south
- Urban and environmental movements
- International migration and capital flows
- Trends in urban political economy
- Patterns of urban-based consumption

The series is explicitly interdisciplinary; the editors judge books by their contribution to intellectual solutions rather than according to disciplinary origin. Proposals may be submitted to members of the series Editorial Committee:

Neil Brenner
Linda McDowell
Margit Mayer
Patrick Le Galès
Chris Pickvance
Jenny Robinson

Preface

Today public health challenges are no longer just local, national or regional. They are global.

Gro Harlem Brundtland, 2005

Infectious diseases are traveling around the world in humans, in insects, in animals, and in food and food products ... so we live in a world where globalization has permitted this interchange of humans and insects, meat, food products around the world.

David Heymann, the World Health Organization, 2005

Who is the WHO? They don't know what they're talking about. I don't know who this group is, I never heard of them before. I'd never seen them before.

Mel Lastman, Toronto Mayor, 1998–2003, on CNN, 2003

This book is the result of a cooperation that began five years ago in Toronto. As the academic term was winding down in April 2003, Severe Acute Respiratory Syndrome (SARS) had hit several urban regions in East Asia and then also in Canada. Many at our university of 50,000 people were grappling with the issue of how to respond to SARS, a mysterious virus that was causing "atypical pneumonia" as it was starting to make its way across Toronto hospitals, having already done so in cities such as Beijing, Guangzhou, Hong Kong, Singapore, and Hanoi. Would it be a good idea to make hundreds of young people literally sweat it out in gymnasia and lecture halls for their final exams, especially if some may have been traveling to and from those places that were suspected origins of the new disease? What, if any, actions should be taken under the circumstances? These were some of the practical challenges that were at the root of the original idea behind this edited volume. The two editors of the present book compared notes of their previous separate research on emerging infectious disease and global cities, and came to the conclusion that there might be value in combining these interests in a joint research project. S. Harris Ali had just completed work on a waterborne outbreak of *E. coli* O157:H7 in a rural community close to Toronto – the largest infectious disease outbreak of its kind in Canada. This particular pathogen was just one example of a series of "new and (re)emerging diseases" – such as cryptosporidiosis, legionellossis, the Ebola virus, Lyme disease, hepatitis C, HIV/AIDS, Hantavirus pulmonary syndrome, West Nile virus, antibiotic resistant tuberculosis, and avian flu – with which societies around the world now have to increasingly contend. Roger Keil, on his part, had studied global cities, their networked connectivity and local governance, as well as their political ecologies. Could the mysterious disease that Toronto now faced be, in part at least, explained in terms of such linkages between cities? And if so, what was the nature of these linkages? It seemed that the case of SARS could serve as the ideal project for the synergistic combination of our two different fields of expertise.

Both of us were interested in what social science could bring to the study of cities and infectious disease. In this light, our research has been informed by our overall contention that there was a connection between global city formation in Toronto, Hong Kong, and Singapore and the way in which SARS has affected and connected these cities. From this starting point, three related areas of inquiry were identified as worthy of attention. The first involved the relationship between the global city network and microbial traffic, with particular reference to the "clique" that was constituted by the three cities under investigation. Issues arising in this inquiry domain included, for example, questions such as: How has the global city network altered the worldwide distribution of pathogens? What did this mean for the fight against diseases such as SARS in particular global cities? The second inquiry domain related to institutional governance and regulation. Here, we would address issues of urban vulnerability and public health security in the context of the global city, including questions such as the following: How does the global city provide the social and environmental interactions necessary for the spread of an emerging disease? How do global cities provide microbes with a range of opportunities unavailable in other settings (particularly important with reference to hospitals in different urban settings)? How was this different from the past? The third area of research concerned the culture of civil society of the global city: How, for example, did the "racialization" of the SARS outbreak affect citizenship rights in Toronto, Hong Kong, and Singapore in general, and the multicultural fabric in Toronto, the city-state in Singapore, and the national question in Hong Kong in particular? This book details our attempts to answer such questions.

It was clear from the outset that the types of questions that we raised, due to the inherent complexity and multidimensionality involved, would need to draw upon the expertise of other social scientists. This had two implications. First, our research focus naturally expanded to consider the more general question of infectious disease and global cities (although we have retained our original focus on SARS as the exemplary illustration of an infectious disease in the era of globalization). Accordingly, we have included work on other infectious diseases, in particular those with a well-known association with cities (most notably, for example, tuberculosis, but others as well), as well as work dealing with other global cities (for instance, London, New York, Tokyo, and Cairo). Second, we enlisted the assistance of a number of our students and collaborators from the international academic community, many of whose works are included in this volume.

In the end, of course, many people have helped bring this project to fruition and we gratefully acknowledge them and hope that we have not left anyone out. We first need to thank the research students who have participated during the past five years in making our project a success: Claire Major, Catherine Huang, Ahmed Allahwala, Matthew Binstock, Joanna Bull, Ashley Burke, Mimi Cheung, Paul Jackson, Sabiha Merali, Kirk Reid, Fernando Rouaux, Roxana Salehi, Sarah Sanford, and Estair Van Wagner. Heather McLean has edited the manuscript, Ahmed Allahwala translated a key chapter from German to English (Sarasin), and Krystina Faria helped with the bibliography.

Thanks also need to be extended to our international collaborators and participants in our SARS project workshop in 2004. Besides those who ended up as authors in this book – Bruce Braun, Mee Kam Ng, and Victor Rodwin – Ute Lehrer also contributed with her work to our project, as did Roxana Salehi, and Sarah Sanford.

We also wish to thank Drs Ortrud and Wolfgang Sonnabend in St Gallen, who have provided us with advice on the general medical questions related to infectious disease, and have generously left us their issues of the invaluable journal *Emerging Infectious Diseases*.

At York University, we would like to thank research officer Pat Laceby, who gave us more than reasonable amounts of time to support our project.

In the larger community, we would like to thank the public health officials, emergency management officials, nurses, civil society representatives, politicians, teachers, WHO officials, and others who we interviewed, and who gave us their time and insights.

We are also grateful to Harvey Molotch and Neil Brenner, as well as the editorial board of the SUSC series, our editor at Blackwell, Jacqueline Scott, and Geoffrey Palmer. We are extremely appreciative of the wisdom of John Hannigan and Neil Brenner, who commented extensively on a previous draft of our manuscript.

We have had the opportunity to present some of the work collected in this book at university seminars and in public lectures in Asia, Europe, and North America. Some of the ideas and some of the writing found in this book has appeared in journals such as *TOPIA, Urban Studies, Antipode, Canadian Public Policy, Social Theory and Health,* and *Area.*

The book would have been impossible without a generous standard research grant from the Social Sciences and Humanities Research Council of Canada, through which this project has been funded.

Finally, the photographs used on the part and chapter titles were taken by Roger Keil, with the exception of Chapter 15 (Ute Lehrer) and Chapter 16 (S. Harris Ali).

Roger Keil and S. Harris Ali

Introduction: Networked Disease

S. Harris Ali and Roger Keil

Speculation about the coming pandemic, some form of infectious disease, most likely a respiratory illness that will reach epidemic proportions, has become part of the global vernacular. While there is much focus in this global public debate on the readiness of national healthcare systems to deal with the expected fallout of the new "plague," not much specific work has been published on the urban aspects of emerging infectious diseases, particularly in the increasingly significant context of globalizing cities and the global cities network. This book will begin to address this gap in the current literature by focusing on certain relevant and broad questions that will serve as springboards for discussion.

First, we use the empirical case of SARS to investigate in what ways processes of globalization have affected the transmission and response to this disease within and between global cities such as Toronto, Hong Kong, and Singapore. SARS represents one of the most recent examples of how a new and emerging disease can spread under contemporary conditions of globalization, and the consideration of this case, as we shall see, offers considerable insight into the practical issues related to global cities and disease. Second, we seek to situate the issues raised by the first question into a more appropriate theoretical context; that is, we wish to move toward the development of a conceptual framework that is better suited to study the myriad issues involving the very complex relationship between urban settings and infectious disease. It is our contention that such a framework would be negligent if it does not emphasize the dynamic role of the urban–global dialectic in the analysis of the spread and reaction to infectious disease in today's world. Third, because we are dealing with infectious disease, whether in the form of viruses, bacteria, or parasites, we are by definition dealing with a biophysical phenomenon. However, the spread of infectious disease could only occur if certain social practices, conditions, and circumstances were in place, as HIV/AIDS most dramatically reveals, but so too does the contemporary spread of tuberculosis in inner-city areas. We will therefore be dealing with a second dialectic; namely, one involving nature and society (which, it should be noted, is sometimes expressed in terms of another dialectic – that is, between the rural and urban). Consequently, the inherent complexity involved in our project involves a consideration of various scales of action and impact, from the local/municipal all the way through to the regional, national, international, and global; noting that each of these scales themselves have various biophysical, social, political, cultural, and economic aspects associated with them. The resultant matrix of factors to consider in studying the relationship between cities and disease leads to an encompassing project. Accordingly, we have organized our presentation in specific parts, each related to different dimensions of the city–infectious disease problematic. We will elaborate upon these toward the end of our introductory remarks. At this point though, we begin by presenting some background information and description necessary for understanding the point of entry into our analysis.

The SARS Outbreaks

In March 2003, a single traveler from Hong Kong arrived in Toronto, and with her a virus. She had previously stayed in the Metropole Hotel in "Asia's World City," where she had acquired the virus that causes the disease – later referred to as Severe Acute Respiratory Syndrome (SARS). This disease, which had come to Hong Kong by way of a physician who had treated patients in Guangdong province in southern China, eventually affected 29 countries in the world and infected 8,427 people, of whom 813 died. A typical Emerging Infectious Disease (EID), it was caused by a previously unknown coronavirus, that family of viruses that also cause the common cold (CDC 2003). When the virus had burnt itself out in the summer of 2003 – the WHO declared the pandemic over on July 5 – it had wreaked havoc in many urban and rural communities around the world.

Rural China, where a virus based in animals crossed the species boundary into humans through live animal markets, is now only an airplane ride away from distant places on the globe, such as the Toronto region. In turn, a healthcare worker, who may have become infected in Toronto, is only a plane trip away from a wedding party in the Philippines, where she may infect an entirely unrelated group of people. Both people and viruses were breaking down traditional boundaries of time, space, and the human everyday. Further, the infection of a member of a tightly knit Toronto religious community, whose very existence appeared as the epitome of insularity, had now become part of a health crisis of global proportions. Microbes no longer remain confined to remote ecosystems or rare reservoir species, for them, the Earth has truly become a Global Village.

Clearly, the damage done to human life and well-being had economic, social, ecological, and political dimensions. Globally, it is estimated that SARS resulted in financial losses of at least $US 54 billion as many sectors, but particularly the travel, hospitality, and retail sectors, bore the brunt of the impacts in the affected global cities throughout the world (Lee and McKibben 2004). Social bonds were tested in communities in affected cities as the disease strained engrained relationships of class, ethnicity, and gender, and posed rarely known stress on the public health and hospital based healthcare systems of major urban centers from Beijing to Toronto. Politically, the SARS outbreak lead to major legitimacy crises for governments as different as those of the Province of Ontario and the Special Administrative Region of Hong Kong. Ecologically speaking, SARS severed the metabolic exchange between the urban and rural as live animal markets were banned, or at least forced to temporarily suspend operations. Cross-species transfer (zoonosis) played an important role in the biological origins of SARS. Crossover of the virus from the animal to the human host was thought to have occurred in the live animal markets of southern China, where the civet cat was sold for human consumption, as a culinary delicacy, to the country's rapidly growing economic elite. Thousands of animals, civet cats in particular, were culled, as it was suspected that this animal species served as the host reservoir for the SARS virus. The live animal market therefore served as an interface between the rural and the urban, where animals captured in the rural wild were sold to relatively affluent urban dwellers (Bell et al. 2005). In sum, global forces and networked relations of all types (e.g., economic, cultural, political, and spatial) now need to be taken into account when investigating questions related to the spatial diffusion of a virus under contemporary conditions. This is the concern of this book.

Cities and Disease

This book is about the non-medical aftermath of the SARS pandemic. Such an analytic emphasis is, of course, not new and in this regard we share the view of a whole host of prominent thinkers who have pointed to the socially produced, regulated, and negotiated aspects of health and disease – as demonstrated, for example, in the work of Paul Farmer (1999), Nancy Krieger

(1994, 2001), A.J. McMichael (1993), and Laurie Garrett (1994, 2000), and the seminal writings of Rudolf Virchow (1848/1985) over a century and half ago. Locating ourselves in this analytic orientation, we wish to emphasize, however, the fundamentally important role that cities may play in these socially informed processes of health, particularly under the uniquely contemporary conditions brought about by globalization. We will examine the fallout of the SARS crisis in the context of re-emerging infectious diseases (including, for example, HIV/AIDS, TB, and pandemic flu), particularly in the centers of a rapidly urbanizing world. The association of cities with health and disease is, of course, obviously not a novel phenomenon unique to our era. It has a history going as far back as the time when cities first became formally established as a distinct human settlement pattern, as different from hunter–gatherer and agricultural societies. McMichael (2001) notes that accompanying each historical transition in the relationships of human beings with nature, there have been profound changes in the pattern of infectious disease distribution. The development of the city is one such transitional pivot. Infectious disease pathogens require a certain population density of hosts to sustain themselves; without a sufficient number of these, the pathogen will kill off its host before it can be transferred to another host to ensure its own perpetuation. Cities provide pathogens with exactly that which they need to survive – a large number of human beings in close proximity to each other, thus ensuring a sustainable chain of transmission. In response to these conditions, city-dwellers have a long tradition of implementing measures to combat infectious disease, from the enforced 40-day quarantine of ships arriving at European ports to deal with bubonic plague in the fourteenth century (Banta 2001) to the development of the engineered sanitary infrastructure and embryonic public health system of the "bacteriological city" of the twentieth century (Gandy 2006c). Today, in the age of globalization, rapid travel and increased population movements, particularly between the major urban centers of the world, pose particular challenges in responding to infectious diseases. SARS brought these challenges to the fore. By situating disease outbreaks in the context of the historical relationship of cities with health and illness, this book will emphasize the specific processes triggered by the SARS crisis of 2003. And throughout all this, we should not forget that the relationship between the city and infectious disease intrinsically implicates the nature–society dialectic. In this light, it is not surprising to learn that, of the six factors identified in the influential report of the Institute of Medicine (IOM 1992) as contributing to the emergence of infectious disease, five of them are explicitly social in nature: human demographics and behavior, technology and industry, economic development and land use, international travel and commerce, and breakdown in public health; while the sixth, microbial adaptation and change, is partly the result of social behavior and social change (Mayer 2006).

Global Cities and Disease

Globalization and cities have been linked conceptually for a generation now. Peter Hall's 1996 publication *The World Cities* (see, e.g., Hall 1984) opened a neo-urbanist discourse on the role of metropolitan centers in the world economy, which has now developed into a lively subfield of urban studies (Knox and Taylor 1995; Marcuse and Van Kempen 2000; Taylor 2004; Brenner and Keil 2006). The work of John Friedmann (1986) and Saskia Sassen (1991, 1998) has created a strong basis on which a small cottage industry of global cities research has been erected. We knew before SARS that cities in the world economy have been connected through material and information flows (Castells 2000), labor market and investment cycles (Scott 2001), knowledge and policy transfers, cultural exchange (Flusty 2004), and the transnational movement of people (Smith 2000). What was not so clear was that the global cities network could also potentially serve as a network for disease transmission. This is a direct consequence of the rather obvious fact that the flows of human beings and pathogens are intimately linked. It has now become glaringly evident that, as patterns in human travel changed with globalization, so too did the patterns of pathogen distribution – and at lightening speed. Cities, now more than ever, play an important role in the distribution of disease, because under the conditions of globalization, they serve as ever-dynamic hubs in the intensified flow of people. In point of fact, cities can serve as the sites of convergence of many of the types of the global flows described above, and this has profound implications not only for the way we think about the city, but the way pathogens may flow through the city and between cities.

The relationship of cities and infectious disease was redefined once more through SARS. Some complacency was likely experienced with the historical success of institutionalized public health systems based on such interventions as: the collection of vital statistics, mass vaccination programs, the pasteurization of milk, ensuring less hazardous workplaces, less crowded living conditions, and the promise of antibiotics and antiviral drugs in the fight against infectious disease. It was against this backdrop that the SARS pandemic marked a historical change as cities, as bulwarks of disease control, have become once again places of heightened vulnerability. As the scaled hierarchy of global cities becomes the conduit of disease transmission, another reality becomes readily visible: the global cities hierarchy is really a complex network of topological relations both externally (cities among one another) and internally (the capillary system of the globalized metropolis). What is central to such conceptualizations of both the relationship amongst global cities, and within global cities, are the notions of mobility, flow, and dynamism, and the consideration of such factors is perhaps best understood through more networked and topological understandings of the city. It is toward the qualitative explication of these understandings that we proceed.

The Organization of This Book

This book is divided into five parts. The first three parts contain substantive works that reflect the main investigative foci of our project: global networks, urban health governance in a globalized world, and the cultural challenges of emerging infectious diseases in globalizing cities. This is followed by a part containing chapters that deal with issues of global health and biosecurity in an age of re-emerging infectious disease. The book's final part provides some broader theoretical implications that may be derived from the preceding parts. We end with some concluding remarks and directions for future research.

Part I, "Infectious Disease and Globalized Urbanization," includes contributions that introduce our main theoretical starting points and important concepts and definitions – such as what is a global city, and how are global cities connected? Part I also contains a chapter that, while not specifically focusing on SARS, provides important background and current research on some of the issues that stem directly from the study of global cities and health. Written by authors residing in those cities in which SARS spread, the chapters in Part II, on "SARS and Health Governance in the Global City: Toronto, Hong Kong, and Singapore," direct attention to the impacts this disease has had on social and political life, especially as they relate to the governance of public health within each of these three major metropolises. The contributions in Part III, "The Cultural Construction of Disease in the Global City," discuss the impacts of SARS on urban culture (and vice versa). They do so by considering the various defining facets of the culture of global cities, including multiculturalism, the mass media, and aspects of everyday urban life and popular culture. The issue of public health governance is taken up more generally and expanded upon Part IV, "Re-emerging Infectious Disease, Urban Public Health, and Global Biosecurity." The set of readings in this part consider the broader implications that directly result from the way in which public health institutions deal with infectious disease. Two broad and interrelated sets of implications can be discerned from these chapters. The first pertains to questions of health inequalities and injustice, while the second deals with the exercise of biopower and the "securitization" of public health. It is perhaps self-evident that global cities are as widely recognized for their dynamic cultural qualities as they are for their political and economic functions. It is therefore clear that culture forms an important foundation of life in the global city. In this light, the critical question arises – How did SARS shake this foundation? Picking up on the empirical findings presented in the preceding substantive parts, the contributions in Part V, "Networked Disease: Theoretical Approaches," identify and explore in greater detail some of the main theoretical themes that have been implicitly raised throughout this book, and include a discussion of some of the conceptual implications that naturally follow from our work. Notably, these chapters make the case that under the present social and political circumstances brought on by urbanization and globalization, there is a need for theoretical reconceptualizations of various sorts when dealing with the analysis of infectious disease. These include, for example, the reconceptualization of the relationships of infectious disease with: the city and the body; animals and food; responses to human migration patterns within globalization; and the various emergent and particular configurations of people and technologies (i.e., "actor-networks").

We hope that the collection of readings in this volume will stimulate discussion in new and exciting ways – especially in relation to questions of how pathogens interact with economic, political, and social factors in an increasingly globalized and uniquely defined urbanized world. Furthermore, it is hoped that such knowledge will help ensure that detection, monitoring, and response efforts to emerging disease outbreaks will be compatible with the current political, social, economic, and ecological developments unfolding within our global cities and beyond.

Part I

Infectious Disease and Globalized Urbanization

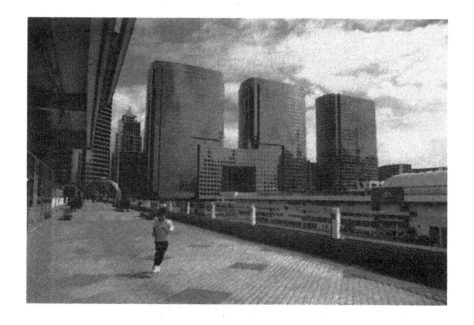

Introduction

S. Harris Ali and Roger Keil

It has been noted that, for the first time in history, more than half of the world's population is now living in urban areas (United Nations Population Fund 2007). This outcome – the result of intensified urbanization – has coincided with a second large-scale development, namely globalization. Globalization has been conceptualized in various ways, but most definitions include the following elements as identified by Held et al. (2002): extensivity – a widening reach of social activity and power; intensity – an increase in the number of interconnections between places of the world as patterns and flows begin to transcend particular localities; velocity – an overall increase in the speed with which ideas, goods, information, capital, and people travel; and impact propensity – the fact that the impact of distant events is magnified at the local level, while at the same time, localized events have magnified impacts on distant locales.

The repercussions of the dialectical interaction of these two master processes of urbanization and globalization are both numerous and wide-ranging, but perhaps one of the most vivid manifestations of the urban–global dialectic is the emergence of the "global city." The research group on Global and World Cities (GaWC) defines a global city in terms of various indicators such as: population size (typically several million); an active influence and participation in international events and world affairs; the presence of an international airport that serves as a hub for international carriers; the existence of an advanced transportation and communications/information infrastructure; a strong presence of international communities and cultures; a vibrant sports and cultural scene, with world-renowned cultural institutions and festivals; and the presence of influential international financial, legal, and corporate firms and headquarters, as well as the tendency for translocal economic forces to have more weight than local policies in shaping urban economies (GaWC 2004). Through the performance of their institutional structures and processes, global cities articulate the local economy with the world economy by providing a space for capital accumulation while serving as nodes for global communication and population migration, thus resulting in sites of intense economic and social interaction (Friedmann 1986).

Global cities around the world are linked through flows of various sorts – capital, people, commodities, transportation vehicles (planes, ships, cars, trains, trucks, etc.), as well as information and communications (Friedmann 1986; Sassen 1991, 2000; Knox and Taylor 1995; Smith and Timberlake 2002; Taylor 2004; Brenner and Keil 2006). A natural consequence of these linked flows is that global cities serve as nodes of connection within an emergent network; that is, the global cities network. It is important to note that because the flows that essentially constitute both the global city and the global cities network are always in motion – they are, in essence, in a constant state of flux – for this reason global cities should no longer be thought of as static, bounded entities (Thrift 1996, 2000b). Consonant with this reasoning, one of the central objectives of this book is to draw attention to the networked, yet fluid, nature of global cities and the networks to which they belong, in order to emphasize the role that these characteristics have not only for the contemporary spread of infectious disease, but for understanding the social and political reactions to disease spread under the conditions of intensified urbanization and globalization – that is, under the influence of the urban–global dialectic.

The changes generated by the urban–global dialectic provide windows of opportunity for altering the microbial traffic of pathogens by changing the social and biophysical conditions required for disease emergence and spread. Thus, the noted virologist Richard Krause (1993, p. vii) remarks that: "Microbes thrive in these 'undercurrents of opportunity' that arise through social economic change, changes in human behaviour, and catastrophic events ... They may fan a minor outbreak into a widespread epidemic" (cited by Davis 2005, p. 55). Second, analysts have noted that we may be heading toward a single global disease ecology (McNeill, 1976; Barrett et al. 1998), wherein previously localized and bounded disease ecologies have undergone a process of convergence due to factors such as the revolutionary changes in transportation technology (Cossar 1994), and the increasing permeability of geopolitical boundaries (Farmer 1996) – factors that are integral elements of the urban–global dialectic that undergirds the global cities network. Consequently, any event can have unexpected, disproportionate, and emergent effects that are often distant in time and space from when and where they originally occurred (Smith 2003, p. 566). The case of SARS, as we shall discuss at various points throughout this volume, illustrates this point well. The spread of SARS can be viewed as a "borderless" phenomenon, as evidenced by the fact that the virus spread across nations and regions but within the global cities network. The SARS virus represented another flow type that connected global cities. The spread of SARS in this manner therefore underscores the fact that today infectious diseases cannot simply be considered as a public health issue that is exclusively confined to the developing world or pegged to a particular level of scale (whether it be the local, regional, or national).

The two chapters in this part introduce us to various aspects and implications of the themes outlined above. Building on the previous work of Ali and Keil (2006), Estair Van Wagner explores how we can begin to move toward the development of a theoretical framework that will help us grapple with the problem of simultaneously elucidating the fluid pathways of urban connectivity while analyzing the role of spatially fixed sites in the spread of new and emerging diseases such as SARS. The theoretical precepts involved in the work concerning the spread of infectious diseases within the urban–global dialectic introduce practical challenges for policy-makers within the global city. Victor Rodwin draws out and discusses some of these challenges in terms of how health and disease, public health infrastructure, and the health system may be compared among New York, London, Paris, and Tokyo. He highlights the convergent health risks and contrasting views of urban health in the literature and calls attention to the notable neglect of poor and vulnerable populations within high-risk areas of global cities.

1

Toward a Dialectical Understanding of Networked Disease in the Global City: Vulnerability, Connectivity, Topologies

Estair Van Wagner

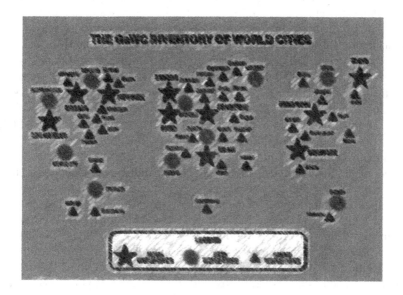

Globalization means that if someone in China sneezes, someone in Toronto may one day catch a cold. Or something worse − if, in Guangdong province, 80 million people live cheek by jowl with chickens, pigs and ducks, so, in effect, do we all. Global village indeed.

Editorial Comment, Globe and Mail, *March 29, 2003*

The rapid global spread of SARS between cities in Canada and Asia in 2003 exposed the unanticipated vulnerability of global urban centers, linked to each other through networked and complex flows of people, capital, and commodities across the globe, to the spread of emerging infectious diseases.[1] While SARS claimed lives and wreaked havoc on economies and health systems globally, sites of contemporary globalization and urbanization were unexpectedly exposed as environments in which infectious diseases can thrive and prosper. Whether we consider the SARS case, the anticipated avian influenza pandemic, or the re-emergence of tuberculosis in recent years, the need to understand how and why infectious diseases are emerging (and re-emerging) and spreading is clear and increasingly urgent.

Assertions of a "human victory" over the forces of illness and disease, and notions of geographical containment, are being disproved with increasing frequency and force (Garrett 1996). After SARS, we are coming to terms with the realization that the networked relationships of cities in contemporary globalization are more than the pathways of global capital and human mobility – they are also the pathways of rapid and undetected viral transmission. While the emergence and spread of infectious diseases is more than an academic problem to which clever theoretical solutions can be applied, building a theoretical framework through which we can understand the relationship(s) between globalization, urbanization, and emerging infectious diseases is fundamental to the development of informed and ultimately successful practical responses to future, and potentially more devastating, outbreaks of infectious disease. The focus of this chapter is to explore how the evolving body of research known as the literature on "global cities" (Sassen 2000, 2002; Brenner and Keil 2006) or "world cities" (Friedmann and Wolff 1982; Friedmann 1986; Knox and Taylor 1995; Taylor 2004) can assist us in this project of simultaneously elucidating the fluid pathways of urban connectivity and analyzing the role of spatially fixed sites in contemporary globalization.

Global cities research offers important insights into the trajectory of SARS, which David Fidler has referred to as the "first post-Westphalian pathogen" (2003, p. 486). Building on Ali and Keil's (2006) analysis of SARS, I propose that we must combine insights from both more traditional global cities perspective of relationships between nodes in a hierarchical network (Sassen 2000, 2002; Knox and Taylor 1995; Taylor 2004) as well recent topological approaches (Amin and Thrift 2002; Smith 2003b). While I contend that global cities research can make an important contribution to our understanding of emerging infectious disease in the global city, I also point to a number of ways in which approaches to understanding urbanization and contemporary globalization are challenged by the gaps, problems, and questions exposed by the experience of SARS.

Contemporary Globalization and Urbanization: The Renewed Potential for Disease

A deepening of global connectivity, in which aspects of our lives traditionally understood to occur primarily at the local or national level are increasingly embedded in broader global processes (Appadurai 1996; Hall 1991a,b), is occurring simultaneously as more and more of us are living in cities. Already over 50 percent of the global population are urban dwellers, with UN projections showing that 67 percent of the world's population will be by 2030 (UN-HABITAT 2006). A number of significant features of both global cities and of contemporary neoliberal globalization indicate a renewed potential for the emergence and re-emergence of infectious diseases: the speed and ease of global travel; flows of international migration; rapid and uneven urbanization; increasing population density; ecological changes ranging from global climate change to dam building; war and displacement; poverty; malnutrition; inadequate access to basic infrastructure and services; and the breakdown of public health and medical systems and aging populations (Lines et al. 1994; Louria 2000).

As Jonathan Mayer (2000) suggests, truly understanding disease causality in an era of intensification of both urbanization and globalization requires moving beyond the biomedical model of causation. He calls on us to examine how relationships of political and economic power define all levels of human–environment interaction, shaping our social, physical, and spatial reality. The impact of human interactions with our environment and each other is clearly visible in the globalized urban environment as populations expand and migration to urban centers increasingly overwhelms infrastructure and services of cities, particularly those of the global South.

While cities have often been associated with the development of public health systems and advanced medical care, they have also been sites of some of the most devastating epidemics, due to poverty, inequality, and lack of infrastructure. The case of SARS and its rapid and undetected spread between global cities illustrates how the globalized urban environment may be a particularly hospitable environment for emerging infectious diseases. Recent outbreaks of emerging infectious disease appear to be strongly related to features of contemporary urbanization (Vlahov and Galea 2003), as a brief overview of the experience of Toronto in the 2003 SARS crisis will demonstrate.

Toronto and SARS: Global Citiness as Vulnerability

Toronto is Canada's global city, through which the national economy is articulated into the global economic system (Todd 1995; Sassen 2000; Kipfer and Keil 2002). Taking it as an example, it becomes clear that many of its global city qualities are the very relations that made it most vulnerable to the SARS outbreak. Toronto is home to the busiest airport in the country with 30,000–40,000 passengers taking off to international destinations every day (St. John et al. 2003). As no two airports in the world are more than 36 hours apart (Gould 1999, p. 203), airports become "interchanges" in disease transmission and spread (Ali and Keil 2006), with the time between Toronto and any other city likely much less than the incubation period of any emerging infectious disease. The time-space of air travel contrasts with that of the body (Dodge and Kitchin 2004) and of viruses such as SARS, which has an incubation period of between two and ten days, during which a traveler could be across the world with no signs of illness (WHO 2003a).

A destination for large-scale international immigration and home to a number of different diasporic communities, Toronto is often called one of the most "multicultural" cities in the world (Driedger 2003; Ali and Keil 2006). This indicates a connectivity extending beyond economics to cultural and social links with global reach involving relationships across geographical distance facilitated by communication technologies, but also face-to-face contact and physical travel, which becomes critically important in understanding the spread of infectious disease (Urry 2004; Ali and Keil 2006).

Toronto's vulnerability cannot be understood only in relation to the movement of the virus through individual people. There are a number of other subtle and long-term ways in which "global citiness" shaped Toronto's experience with SARS, particularly in regards to public health and health governance. While federal funding and legislation provides an overall framework for health care in Canada, provinces have authority in regards to where and how money is spent. However, despite this provincial jurisdiction, health care is administered and experienced primarily at the local level. Hospitals are subject to standards set by the province that funds them, but they are locally controlled by community level boards that are only loosely coordinated and the approach to care is marked by discontinuity between institutions (Armstrong and Armstrong 2003). Also, arguably the most important branch of the health system for the prevention of infectious diseases, public health in Canada falls to the level of government with the least power, resources, and autonomy at its disposal. As a statutory 'creature' of the province, the municipal government of Toronto had very limited ability to deal with the SARS outbreak, given that the scale of prevention had as much to do with the global as it did with the local. As Warren Magnusson points out, for a local government to "… deal with questions of public health, it would have to project its authority far beyond its immediate boundaries. In a sense, it would have to follow its particular connections throughout the world" (1996, p. 291). During SARS, the problematic nature of an uncoordinated and geographically fixed approach to health governance and administration were made blatantly clear:

> We were not prepared for SARS, nor did we have a system wide critical care communication strategy in place. From a critical care perspective, the most important limitation in the response to SARS was the absence of a coordinated leadership and communication infrastructure. (Booth and Stewart 2005, p. S58)

In recent decades, the drive to build globally "competitive" cities has become a dominant force in Toronto's urban restructuring (Kipfer and Keil 2002). Pressure for Canadian cities to be efficient and management oriented has been accompanied by the downloading of significant costs and responsibility from federal and provincial governments, who at the same time have decreased funding to municipalities. Shifts toward neoliberal public administration models such as New Public Management (NPM), coupled with the decreased capacity of the local government to satisfy the needs and desires of the public, has resulted in the increasing privatization and contracting out of public services. Guided by the imperative of attracting transnational business and elites, local governments are shifting their focus from redistribution to the creation of wealth (Porter 1995). As Rodwin and Gusmano's (2002) research on health governance and infrastructure has revealed, rising inequality between social groups and barriers in access to health care, particularly for the poor and ethnic minorities, are "onerous health risks" faced by global cities (2002, p. 449).

In Canadian cities these risks have been exacerbated by neoliberal restructuring that continues to dismantle Canada's universal public healthcare system and push social services into the private sector. Like entrepreneurial models of urban governance emerging in Canada, health reform has been driven by the private sector, emphasizing speed and efficiency (defined in market terms), leading to an increased reliance on outpatient services. This kind of assembly line medicine makes the diagnosis of a disease such as SARS, with subtle and non-specific symptoms, increasingly difficult and unlikely. As well, basic sanitation services have been drastically cut in recent years and hospitals increasingly rely on contracting-out for cleaning and laundry services, eliminating full-time and unionized staff as a way to cut costs. Hospital environments, and particularly emergency rooms, are increasingly dirty, making them highly vulnerable to the spread of infectious diseases such as SARS. Neoliberal discourses of efficiency minimize these aspects of health care, focusing on treatment instead of prevention (Armstrong and Armstrong 2003; Keil and Ali 2007).

Re-Reading Global Cities: "The Dialectic of Mobility and Fixity"

Understanding the complexity of emerging infectious diseases in the age of global cities calls for more than a straightforward collaboration between medical or epidemiological research and global cities perspectives. Building an appropriately complex and flexible theoretical framework requires more than adding a "health" or "disease" perspective to our understanding of global cities, or including an "urban" perspective in the study of health and disease. Rather, it calls for an innovative reading of global cities research; one that questions fundamental assumptions about how and why global city networks are formed and produced, and for what purposes we should attempt to understand them. We can, and should, simultaneously consider what the emergence and development of a "global cities network" means for emerging infectious diseases, and what emerging infectious diseases mean for a global cities network.

The relationship between cities and infectious diseases challenges us to consider both the fixed nature of spaces in which diseases are experienced and health is governed *and* the fluid mobility of microbes that thrive in the connectivity of globalized urban environments. As Ali and Keil (2006) have noted, "[I]t is the dialectic of mobility and fixity that is truly characteristic of the urban condition under globalised circumstances." Following from this, I suggest that an appropriate theoretical framework accounts for the ways in which cities are fixed nodes in networks bound by specific contexts – historical, social, and political developments within socio-spatial structures of local, national, and regional scales that are further embedded in the global economic system. At the same time, this context demands a conception of time and space through which we can see the city as fluid and hybrid, constantly in the process of change and transformation, populated by a multiplicity of actors, themselves constantly emergent.

"Global Cities," "World Cities": Situating the Urban in Globalization

Since the early 1980s, scholars have linked their treatment of the urban to explorations of the relationship between global forces and cities (Brenner and Keil 2006). "Global cities" research has highlighted the role of the cities as critical sites in contemporary globalization, breaking with traditional approaches to economic and political analysis that have tended to ignore the local actors, emphasizing the role of the nation-state (Keil 1998a). Important contributions by scholars such as John Friedmann, Saskia Sassen, Michael Peter Smith, Michael Timberlake, and Manuel Castells have helped to define the relationship between globalization and urbanization as a critical agenda for urban scholars (Brenner and Keil 2006).

Global cities, hierarchy, and vulnerability

A significant amount of global cities research has focused on the way in which specific cities have emerged in the post-Fordist era as central nodes in a global urban network, functioning as the capitals of finance and advanced producer services, and as the headquarters of transnational corporations (TNCs), which produce the global economy (Friedmann and Wolff 1982; Zukin 1991; Friedmann 1986; Sassen 2002). Efforts to map the hierarchical organization of cities within contemporary global capitalism have tended to focus on a select group of "global" cities that act as "command and control" centers in the various geographical regions of the global economy (Friedmann 1986; Sassen 2000, 2002; Taylor 2004). In *The Global City* (2002), Saskia

Sassen used New York, London, and Tokyo to illustrate the emergence of a global urban system in which a few "core" cities, supported by a larger network of "peripheral" cities, articulate the global economy.

Work by Taylor (2004) and others as part of the GaWC (Globalization and World Cities) research at Loughborough University (see research bulletins at http: www.lboro.ac.uk/gawc/; Beaverstock et al. 2000) has attempted to show how global cities are organized hierarchically according to the importance and influence that they exert internationally. Although variations in the hierarchy do emerge, depending on exactly what kind of firm or service is being analyzed, generally similar configurations are found, with the same players emerging on the top: London, New York, Hong Kong, Paris, Los Angeles, Tokyo, and Singapore (Beaverstock et al. 2000). Efforts to map this hierarchical organization, such as those undertaken by the GaWC researchers in the "Inventory of World Cities" (2004), are important, as they reveal a "skeleton of the new world economy" (Ali and Keil 2006) that can help us to uncover aspects of vulnerability and resilience.

The hierarchical representations that global cities researchers have offered thus far are centered primarily on economic and political functions, but this concept of hierarchical configurations amongst cities could be extended to consider what alternative orderings might emerge when patterns of health and disease are considered: Are particular cities central nodes in the flows of health and disease? Do different patterns of hierarchical influence and importance emerge in respect to health governance and disease control? The notion that certain cities emerge as disproportionately influential and connected is important and should be expanded upon, to look at configurations that emerge in relation to these other aspects of contemporary globalization, particularly in relation to the increasing threat of emerging infectious diseases.

After SARS, it becomes impossible to think about infectious disease as a local or contained problem (Ali and Keil 2006), and the structures and patterns of hierarchical organization and influence depicted by global cities research can provide important clues as to the link between global citiness and vulnerability to infectious disease. Connection to the network of international travel and trade between these nodes is an essential aspect of what makes a particular city "global" – the more critical to the flows moving through the network, the more global the city is. Understanding precisely what kinds of flows and relationships makes a city "global" can help us to understand how patterns of disease are affected by the nature of these globalized and globalizing spaces (Ali and Keil 2006).

One of the most important lessons of SARS is that this prized status as a "global city" may facilitate the movement of microbes and disease as much as that of capital, commodities, or people. Changes in urban development and technology greatly enhance the ability of microbes to rapidly move from animal to human, rural to urban, and local to global. With effects on health systems, economies, political chains of command, and social perceptions of diversity and multiculturalism, SARS became lethal not just to the individual human in the globalized urban environment, but to the status quo of the global city network of contemporary capitalist globalization. SARS unsettled the assumption that it was possible to guarantee safe travel, healthy environments, and access to medical treatment for the global elite, everywhere in the world.

The Global Cities Network: Articulating the Global Economy

Global cities are conceptualized as linked together through networks of flows of capital, people, information, and commodities, which have predominantly been analyzed in terms of the relationships of corporate firms spatially located in different cities (Friedmann 1986; Knox and Taylor 1995; Smith and Timberlake 2002; Taylor 2004). In this "network society" (Castells 2000), the increase in mobility for people and things, particularly through air travel between global cities, has made connections between cities more fluid than traditional links between port cities. This notion of a fluid network is one of the aspects of contemporary globalization that sets it apart from former stages of international travel, trade, and colonization (Ali and Keil 2006). While global cities are understood to be fundamentally shaped by these interconnections and the flows moving through them, they are also seen as having an active role in defining the global economy through particular historical and socio-political contexts (Keil 1998a). Through the organization and management of these flows, global cities provide spatial articulation to facilitate the processes of global capitalism.

Despite considerable interest in the networks of flows between cities, there is still relatively little known about precisely how cities are actually connected and what the consequences are for the everyday lives of people who live in them (Derudder 2003). While much of the case-study based work on individual cities has been rich and detailed (see Sassen 2000, 2002), Short et al. (1996) have pointed out the lack of empirical data detailing how the connectivity of global network of world cities is formed and maintained by the flows between and through them (for an example of wide-ranging empirical work, see Beaverstock et al. 2000; Taylor 2004).

The case of SARS exposes the difficulty of adequately understanding other kinds of connectivity, such as the flows of infectious disease between particular cities, through such an approach. The relationships illuminated by the path of the SARS virus between cities such as Toronto and Hong Kong or Singapore, which are otherwise seen as loosely connected, are not easily explained by data available through conventional global cities analysis. Much of the empirical basis for connectivity between global cities remains speculative, particularly for relationships involving "second-tier cities" such as Toronto. Derudder et al. (2004) have stressed the many obstacles to the use of air travel data, noting that it is particularly problematic with respect to Canadian and Chinese cities due to the bias of airline data to direct connections, which are less likely between second-tier cities and are not clearly linked to origin and destination information. This gap in the data is surprising, considering Short's (2004) research placing Hong Kong, Toronto, and Singapore amongst the most globally connected cities. It is also particularly problematic in the context of the growing economic networks of trade between Canada and Asia and the large South Asian and Chinese diasporic communities in Toronto (Statistics Canada 2005b; Ali and Keil 2006).

Cliques: The "Tangible Relational Patterns" of the Global City Network

Understanding the relationship between these SARS-affected cities means that we have to ask different questions about the relationships and connectivity between cities. As Smith points out: "… what is needed are new approaches that help us to go beyond counting; to go through those doors to find out precisely how networks work and are maintained over long-distances" (Smith 2003a, p. 31). While we must indeed find ways to go beyond counting, we must also critically consider what we are counting and why. What else we might we be counting in order to grapple with basic questions about how and why global city networks are formed? Emerging and spreading infectious disease can offer "a new entry point for the already lively debate on connectedness in the global city universe" (Ali and Keil 2006, p. 3).

Derudder and Taylor (2005) employ the concept of the clique to explore relationships within the global cities network with greater precision. They define a clique as "a maximal set of actors in which every actor is connected to every other actor" (ibid., p. 77). According to their research on "The Cliquishness of World Cities," membership in a clique indicates a cohesive relationship to other members and a weak relationship to those outside, helping us to break down the concept of the global city network into "tangible relational patterns" (ibid., p. 75). By looking at world cities on the basis of political economic data, such as the number of corporate headquarters, their research clusters global cities into smaller relational groups, giving us more specific information about how, where, and what kinds of flows are traveling between places. Clique analysis reveals sub-levels of network connectivity, which Derudder and Taylor argue represent "regional–global nexuses within contemporary globalization" (ibid., p. 85).

Like the tools used by researchers in hierarchical mapping, clique analysis has focused largely on *economic* relationships between global cities; however, as Derudder and Taylor themselves propose, clique analysis is a tool that can be extended to consider other kinds of relationships in the global city network (ibid., p. 85). Therefore while current clique analysis, focused largely on corporate headquarters and business elites, reveals little about the kinds of relationships that exist between the SARS-affected cities, looking at relationships between the specific subgroup of the SARS cities within the global city network, may yield important lessons. A clique analysis informed by some of the critiques discussed below and recent topological perspectives on cities and networks may provide unique insight into why SARS was able to emerge in particular places and not others.

Expanding the Global City Network: Which Cities Count, Which Flows Matter?

While the work of global cities research, which has centered on a small group of elite cities, has revealed central aspects of contemporary urbanization and economic globalization, critiques of this narrow focus and of the emphasis of global cities research on quantitative analysis have led to a number of innovative attempts to broaden fundamental understandings of how "global citiness" can, and should, be understood and measured. A number of authors have attempted to counter the exclusion of major portions of the globe from global city analysis, particularly the global South, as well as de-industrializing cities in Europe and North America, (Simon 1995; Shatkin 1998; Robinson 2002; Ley 2004). This extension of global cities perspectives to reflect "the experiences of a much wider range of cities" (Robinson 2002, p. 532) has resulted not just in the inclusion of locations previously "off the map" (ibid.), but has also informed new under-standings of what globalization is and how it interacts with particular historical, social, political, and economic contexts in different places (Shatkin 1998; Marcuse and van Kempen 2000). SARS showed us that the connectivity that matters in relation to the global spread of disease does not necessarily parallel the relationships that are most obvious from global cities maps.

As well, important interventions have pointed to the wide range of actors and practices that are part of global city formation on the ground, actively resisting and shaping dynamics of globalization (Keil 1998b; Abu-Lughod 1999; Smith 2001). Recent work linking urban studies and questions of scale has revealed how static conceptions of the global cities network fail to account for the constantly changing and emergent nature of cities (Thrift 1996, 2000b; Brenner 2000). These approaches suggest that the messiness of urban life, populated by a multiplicity of actors operating in various scaled and networked relationships, requires a more complex understanding of time and place through which the fluidity and hybridity of global cities can be conceptualized, acknowledging that "space is also rather messy, complex, juxtaposed, or perhaps that there are many kinds of space" (Smith 2003b).

The introduction of insights from post-structuralist and actor-network theory (ANT) (see Ali, Chapter 14) into the field of urban studies is a critical development in efforts to expand the focus of global cities research beyond the confines of a strict political economy approach limited by a spatial and temporal fixidity (Smith 2003b). Topological approaches, such as the work of R.G. Smith (2003a,b), introduce a more complex picture of everyday life in the city, populated by intricate networks of humans and non-humans to produce "a liquid theatre alive with the unruly times of urban practices." Smith pushes our understanding of the city beyond rigid portrayals of cities as discrete units and their relationships as fixed and linear, by emphasizing the ways in which they are "in constant movement, undergoing a series of transformations, translations and traductions" (Smith 2003b, p. 575).

The example of SARS calls on us to question assumptions in global cities research about what is meaningful about connectivity, and how we conceptualize it. The speed at which this newly emerged disease was able to spread indicates that there are significant human and non-human aspects of connectivity that are not adequately confronted by our images of network connectivity. Understanding infectious diseases in the global city network demands not only that we acknowledge overlooked flows, but also work toward understanding how these relate to and transform/are transformed by the more traditionally understood flows, such as capital and information. As Smith argues, "globalization and world cities are too intermingled through scattered lines of humans and non-humans to be delimited in any meaningful sense" (2003, p. 570). The limitations of a fixed notion of geographical scale are exposed in the face of emerging infectious diseases such as SARS, which "jump-scales" (Brenner 2000) easily, operating simultaneously at purportedly distinct local and global levels (see Ali and Keil 2007). The need to expand our understanding of the urban beyond the activities of transnational corporations and the movements of a small transnational elite is made urgent in the face of undetected actors with lethal potential to travel in the global city network. The case of SARS suggests that the network linkages detected by economically focused analysis create a limited picture of the global cities network that is not adequate for an analysis of emerging infectious diseases. As Danny Dorling (2004) suggests, we must turn our attention to the pathways and flows that determine the production of health and disease in particular places.

"Unexpected, Disproportionate, and Emergent Effects"

With globalization, any event can have unexpected, disproportionate and emergent effects that are often distant in time and space from when and where they occurred.
R.G. Smith (2003b, p. 569)

Emerging infectious diseases complicate the relationship between globalization and urbanization, with unpredictable and unexpected consequences, of which the emergence and spread SARS is a perfect example. Such "unexpected, disproportionate and emergent effects" (Smith 2003b, p. 566) challenge the ways in which global cities have traditionally been understood, and how the global city network has been conceptualized (Ali and Keil 2006). Infectious diseases appear as one of the first agents with material potential to unravel the global city network – in both theory *and* practice. SARS has made it impossible to guarantee that the borderless enclave of the identical hotels, condos, office buildings, and convention centers that facilitate the mobility of the transnational elite is disease free. In the face of a possible avian influenza outbreak, which is predicted to be much worse in scale than SARS, and is likely to appear suddenly without effective vaccines or treatments prepared, the presumption that our governance and health infrastructure have either the knowledge or the power to control infectious diseases is no longer tenable and appears dangerously arrogant.

While I have noted the importance of locating urban development within a broader context of the global economy, emerging infectious diseases indicate the need for a more messy and complex picture of the urban, one that sees "life in all of its sticky and slack human/nonhuman, inorganic/incorporeal, phenomenal/epiphenomenal, and banal/intense everydayness" (Seigworth 2000, p. 246, quoted in Amin and Thrift 2002, p. 9).

The work of R.G. Smith (2003b), Amin and Thrift (2002), and Thrift (1996, 2000b) builds on post-structural and actor-network theories (ANT) to construct a non-scalar, non-linear representation of space and time in the global city. This multidimensional and "messy" perspective, accounting for the multiplicity of actors and the constant of change, points to alternative explanatory possibilities for how cities and their relationships work. Rejecting the limitations of dominant quantitative approaches and modern assumptions of linear space and time, and the human/nature dualism, these approaches see cities as more than platforms for economic and structural forces. Instead, globalization is produced in the everyday of the streets and neighborhoods of the global city (Keil 1998a; Flusty 2003; Smith 2003b). Rather than conceiving cities as "command and control" centers (Sassen 2000, 2002), Smith complicates network connectivity and the role of global cities, describing them as "'switches', 'intermediaries', 'middles', in a continuum," who exercise their power through "their ability to enroll and mobilize others to perform in 'their' network" (2003b, p. 576).

The appearance of SARS in a wealthy city, in a developed Northern nation, contests Dorling's (2004) assertions that the cities populated by the wealthy transnational elite will be the healthiest; and, debunks notions that vulnerability to infectious disease is a problem of a distant "other" on the side of the world. Such a view relies on the fixed and rigid depictions of the global city network and its portrayal as a seamlessly integrated web of built environments and transport systems operating a non-stop, 24-hour network of capital that transcends nature, moving "with ease from space to space and time to time" (Smith 2003b, p. 576). In contrast, Amin and Thrift (2002) depict the city as a porous space; even those parts that have attempted to shut themselves off are vulnerable to flows and movements. Fixed notions of the polarization of the city into a "core" and "periphery," "human" and "natural," hides the "trails of mobility" that connect spaces within and between cities (2002, p. 22). Just as elites cannot ever really seal themselves from the complexity of urban life, those on the margins are not immune to unintended effects of the transnational mobility of a select group of elites. Infectious diseases are not contained by office buildings or gated communities; they coexist with their human and animal host – as of yet undetected by the architects and analysts of the global cities network.

The vulnerability of global cities is usually depicted in relation to things humanly created and controlled in economic or technological terms, such as stock market crashes and technological failures. SARS demonstrated that the vulnerability of the global cities network might lie outside all of these modern constructions, in the non-human realm rarely considered by global cities research. Assumed to be subdued and controlled by the human built and controlled urban environment, socio-nature relationships are invisible in boosterist discourses of the global city – neither a threat nor a benefit to the elite spaces of the global city (Kaika and Swyngedouw 2000). The notion of the global city network as a space of flows of capital, people, and commodities appears to assume that viruses (nature) can be killed or controlled to maintain the functioning of global capitalism; and that cities and their human residents exist above, or outside, of "nature." Accounts centered on the de-territorialized spaces of airports, chains of identical hotels, and convention centers worldwide not only leave out vital spaces and human actors that make these places function, from streetscapes to markets to taxi drivers and janitorial staff, but also the non-humans that inhabit urban spaces, from animals to machines to microbes.

From a topological perspective, the study of the flows within and between global cities becomes much more complex (Smith 2003b) through conceptual tools by means of which we can move our analysis beyond connectivity as defined exclusively in terms of human environments and human actions. Cities as particular nodes are made from the "traffic" that moves through them, and this "traffic" is understood to be made from multiple and interconnected entities. The "human/nonhuman, inorganic/incorporeal, phenomenal/epiphenomenal" are constantly encountering each other in new and different ways, to produce unexpected and unpredictable effects (Seigworth 2000, p. 246, quoted in Amin and Thrift 2002, p. 9).

Drawing on Latour's actor-network theory (ANT) (see Ali, Chapter 14), Smith calls on "world cities researchers to consider networks as being constantly made by *both human and nonhuman actors*" (Smith 2003b, p. 36). Diseases have to be understood not as alien visitors to otherwise safe and sanitized global cities; they are both products and producers of the city themselves, often fundamentally shaped by their urban existence: "in the process of 'adapting' nonhumans to contemporary social settings, management policies and practices often transform the object of concern into a distinct and different entity" (Lulka 2004, p. 443). In many ways, emerging infectious disease are what they are *because* of cities, not despite them.

Infectious Disease and Global Cities: Building a Theoretical Framework

The (re-)emergence of infectious disease in the context of contemporary globalization challenges scholars and practitioners alike to consider the complexity of globalized urban spaces, and to turn our attention to the multiplicity of flows and pathways of connectivity in which they are embedded. Rather than treating emerging infectious disease as an isolated matter of biology and epidemiology contained by the modern city in which nature is killed or controlled, SARS forces us to consider the "[a]ntagonistic relations that emerge from this juxtaposition of trenchant modern social structures and transient actors [which] have yet to be resolved in any satisfactory fashion" (Lulka 2004, p. 443). As I have demonstrated above, an approach to understanding global cities that more adequately considers the role of emerging infectious diseases requires both the insight of global cities research into processes of urban (re)development in contemporary globalization and the innovative and "messy" understanding of urban life that topological approaches provide. The experience of SARS made clear the limitations of our modern understandings of the relationship between cities and disease. I suggest that a creative reading of global cities research reveals concepts and tools with which we can begin to build a new and innovative "dialectical" (Ali and Keil 2006) approach to understanding the relationship between infectious diseases and the global city network, one which can better equip us to face the challenges of vulnerability and the threat of infection that lies ahead.

NOTE

1   For the purposes of this chapter, we have adopted Feldmann et al.'s (2002) definition of emerging infectious diseases: "those in which incidences have increased in the past decade as a result of the introduction of a new agent, recognition of an existing disease that has previously gone undetected, a reappearance (re-emergence) of a known disease after a decline in incidences or an extension of the geographic range of a disease."

2

Health and Disease in Global Cities: A Neglected Dimension of National Health Policy

Victor G. Rodwin

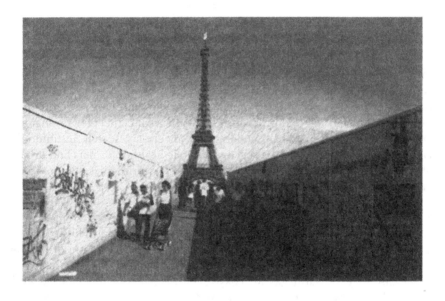

Richard Horton (1998), editor of *The Lancet*, once noted, "... for all of its rational efficiency and benevolent intent, the city is likely to be the death of us." Will global or world cities (terms I use interchangeably here) evolve into socially infected breeding grounds for the rapid transmission of disease? Or can they become critical spatial entities for the protection and promotion of population health (Freudenberg 2000)? The presumption of this book is that the inhabitants of global cities are increasingly vulnerable to infectious diseases, particularly those that may spread rapidly across global city networks (Ali and Keil 2006). In an age of SARS, and increasing concern about the possibility of an avian flu pandemic, can global cities take effective measures to protect themselves against emerging threats to population health, or will these vulnerable giants increasingly be viewed as risky places to live? However one might answer this question, it seems evident that the problem of disease transmission across global cities is a neglected dimension of health policy among nations around the world.

I examine the four largest cities among some of the wealthiest nations in the world: New York, London, Paris, and Tokyo. I begin by highlighting the health risks faced by these cities and summarize, more generally, two contrasting views of urban health. Next, I provide an overview of population health status, the health system and public health infrastructure in these cities.[1] Finally, I suggest that despite the differences, there is an emerging and noteworthy form of public health intervention in all four of these cities – the attention to geographical concentrations of poor and vulnerable populations that pose disproportionate health risks.

Health Risks and Contrasting Views of Urban Health

In a rapidly urbanizing world, New York, London, Paris, and Tokyo – in contrast to most megacities of the global South – have a recent history of relative success in assuring their population's health and share in common a range of characteristics and problems. They are great centers for prestigious university hospitals, medical schools, and medical research institutions. Despite these resources and the success of public health reformers and urban planners in improving their quality of life, these world cities still confront onerous health risks for at least four problems:

1 The return of infectious diseases (e.g., tuberculosis) and the emergence of new ones – AIDS, SARS, and perhaps one day Avian Flu (H5N1).
2 Terrorism, including bioterrorism, and emergencies stemming from climate change; for example, heatwaves (Cadot et al. 2007). Since the release of toxic sarin gas in Tokyo's subway, bombs in the Paris and London subways, and 9/11 followed by anthrax in New York and beyond, there has been an acute awareness of these risks.
3 Barriers in access to medical services for ethnic minorities and/or the poor. This has been recognized as a problem not just in New York City, but also in London and Paris. Only in Tokyo is there less public discussion of this issue.
4 Rising inequalities among social groups. This is reflected in the simultaneous growth of homelessness, poverty, and wealth in all four cities.

These problems will challenge any big city to develop a solid public health infrastructure. With or without such investments, there is already a widespread belief that urban health is not as good as that of the population as a whole. This belief is supported by a substantial body of work. But those who disagree point to contrary evidence.

The sick city

Since the city is, by definition, the place where human density is greatest, it is hardly surprising that it is a vector for the transmission of infectious disease. The Chicago Department of Health collected data on basic measures of population health for 46 large cities across the United States (Benbow et al. 1998) Such measures – for example, average incidence rates for infectious diseases such as tuberculosis, AIDS, and syphilis – are much higher in these cities than for the United States as a whole. More striking, however, are the mortality data reported by these cities for the leading causes of death from non-communicable diseases; for example, heart disease and cancer (Table 2.1). Another important source on urban health in the United States, a compendium of data on the 100 largest cities (NAPH 1995), also reveals a greater prevalence of a large number of health problems in cities than in suburbs and rural areas (Table 2.1), which suggests that there is an urban health penalty (Andrulis 1997).

In Europe, a valuable source of information on urban health, among capital cities, comes from *Project Megapoles*, which has compared age-specific mortality for most European capitals to their respective national rates (Bardsley 1999). Once again, this comparison provides supporting evidence for the "sick city hypothesis." For example, on average, mortality rates for infants (0–4 years) are 7 percent higher in European capital cities than in their respective nations. In five cities, however – Helsinki (–18 percent), Lisbon (–9 percent), Lazio (–12 percent), Madrid (–20 percent), and Lyon (–25 percent) – these rates are lower than the national average. This raises

Table 2.1 Population health status in the largest US cities and in the United States as a whole (1997)

Health status measures	Largest cities[a]	United States
Average age-adjusted mortality		
Heart disease[b]	164	145
Cancer[b]	153	132
All causes[b]	654	507
Years of potential life lost (YPLL)	75	54
Gonorrhea (25 largest cities, 1995)	434	172
Infant mortality (100 largest cities)	12.2	9.8

[a] Forty-six largest cities.
[b] Per 1,000 population aged 45 years and over.

Sources: Data for the 46 largest cities are from Benbow et al. (1998). Data on mortality rates and YPLL are from Chicago Department of Health. Data on gonorrhea and infant mortality rates are from NAPH (1995).

Table 2.2 Infant mortality and life expectancy (LE) in world cities and their nations (2000–4)

		Infant mortality	LE at birth, males	LE at birth, females	LE at age 65, males	LE at age 65, females
2002–4	New York City	6.2	74.5 (2000)	80.2 (2000)	17.0 (2000)	20.1 (2000)
	United States	7.0 (2002)	74.3 (2000)	79.7 (2000)	16.3 (2000)	19.2 (2000)
2000–2	Greater London	5.4	76.1 (2000–4)	80.9 (2000–4)	15.6 (1997–9)	19.2 (1997–9)
	England and Wales	5.3 (2003)	76.3[a] (2000–4)	80.8[a] (2000–4)	15.7 (1999–2001)	18.9 (1997–9)
2002	Paris	4.0[b]	77.6[c] (2002)	83.1[c] (2002)	17.7 (1999)	21.7 (1999)
	France	4.1	77.1 (2002)	83.4 (2002)	16.5 (1999)	21.0 (1999)
	Tokyo: 23 wards	2.8 (2001–4)			17.7 (2000)	22.2 (2000)
	Japan	3.2 (2000)	78.0 (2000)	84.4 (2000)	17.5 (2000)	22.5 (2000)

[a] For England only;
[b] for Paris and First Ring;
[c] for Paris only.

Sources: US – National Center for Health Statistics/Centers for Disease Control (CDC); London and England – Office of National Statistics, London Health Observatory; Paris and France – INSEE, Observatoire Régional de la Santé de l'Île de France.

second thoughts about the hypothesis that urban health is necessarily worse than national averages.

What about world cities such as New York, London, Paris, and Tokyo? With respect to infant mortality and life expectancy, available data indicate that there is no urban health penalty and perhaps even a qualified advantage for their residents (Table 2.2). This advantage appears to be decisive across all four cities with respect to life expectancy at the age of 65. Such findings – however intriguing – do not refute the hypothesis that cities are unhealthy, for the strongest case has yet to be made. It is that these wealthy world cities, along with all other megacities, are places where flagrant inequalities exist among neighborhoods and subpopulation groups. All of the averages we have considered mask pockets of poverty with disadvantaged groups that suffer disproportionately poor health status.

The healthy city

The case for the healthy city is typically grounded in economic arguments, or celebrations of its vitality and innovation in such diverse realms as architecture, urban design, culture, technology, and more. For example, President Clinton's State of the Union message in 1998 refers to American cities as the "vibrant hubs of great metropolitan regions" (HUD 1998). Indeed, between 1982 and 1998, metropolitan areas in the United States generated 85 percent of all jobs and 86 percent of the nation's total economic growth (HUD 1998). This economic power is concentrated among some regional giants that dwarf not only their own states but most of the world's nations. Metropolitan New York's economic output, for example, is greater than that of 45 of the 50 states (HUD 1998).

Claims for the enduring power of cities, including big cities, often come from the literature on urban planning and do not typically invoke measures of population health. But there is also some evidence from public health in support of the hypothesis that urban health compares favorably to that of the nation as a whole. The National Health Interview Survey (NHIS), for example, is one of the most reliable indicators of perceived functional health in the United States. In contrast to the *Big Cities Health Inventory* (Benbow et al. 1998), which relies on outcome measures of health, NHIS suggests that most indicators of self-assessed health status are better in major metropolitan areas than for the country as a whole (Table 2.3).

Beyond these comparisons of metropolitan areas, there is also evidence, from the literature on urban and rural differences, in support of the urban advantage hypothesis (Liff et al. 1991; Mainous and Kohrs 1995; Alexey et al. 1997). We can conclude, then, that while there is clearly evidence of an "urban penalty" in the United States, there is also evidence of an "urban advantage" in terms of self-assessed health status, health habits, and with

Table 2.3 Selected health characteristics (1988–9)

	All large CMSAs and MSAs[a]	Rest of the country
Health characteristics		
Percent limited in activity	12.4	13.7
Percent with fair or poor respondent-assessed health	8.7	9.4
Disability days		
Restricted activity days per 100 persons	1,389.8	1,470
Chronic conditions per 1,000 persons per year		
Arthritis	113.1	129.9
Deafness	71	90.8
Deformities or orthopedic impairments	121.6	111.6
Heart disease	71.6	84.1
High blood pressure	108.2	121.5
Hemorrhoids	43.6	45.8
Chronic bronchitis	46.2	49.4
Asthma	44	41.2
Hay fever	88.6	93
Chronic sinusitis	114.2	139.7

[a] MSAs are metropolitan statistical areas. The NHIS report contains data for 18 Consolidated Metropolitan Statistical Areas (CMSAs) and 15 MSAs. The total population represented in the survey is 117,211,000. The definition and titles of MSAs are established by the US Office of Management and Budget (OMB), with the advice of the Federal Committee on Metropolitan Statistical Areas.

Sources: US data from *Current Estimates from National Health Interview Survey 1988, Series 10, #173*; MSA and CMSA data from *Health Characteristics of Large Metropolitan Statistical Areas: US, 1988–1989.*

respect to quality cancer screening services. What is more, among the four world cities, there appears to be an urban advantage with respect to persons 65 years and older. The reasons why the evidence reviewed here is mixed and possibly confusing are two-fold. (1) There are many ways to define and measure health, ranging from disease prevalence, infant mortality, and life expectancy at birth to life expectancy at 65 years, age-specific mortality rates, and indicators of self-assessed health. (2) There are many ways to define and measure cities. For example, some United Nations' publications equate New York City with the entire metropolitan region, while many Europeans view New York as the borough of Manhattan. Likewise, definitions of London, Paris, and Tokyo range as widely in population size and spatial dimensions (Rodwin and Gusmano 2006).

A selective review of evidence can support the urban advantage hypothesis. There is insufficient evidence, however, to provide strong support for either the urban health penalty or the urban health advantage hypothesis. The reason why we have so little solid evidence is that there are no routine information systems for monitoring the health of populations living in cities. While institutions responsible for disease surveillance – at the international, national, and local authority levels – collect vital statistics and epidemiological data by geographical location, national health policy in most nations is typically made without systematic analysis of information for monitoring health status, public health infrastructure, and the performance of health systems in cities.

The rationale for comparing New York, London, Paris, and Tokyo is to illustrate the extent of variation in health status, health systems, and public health infrastructure among cities that share important characteristics and problems in so many other respects (Rodwin and Gusmano 2002). Although this analysis also illustrates many of the difficulties of finding comparable data across relevant spatial units and time periods, it is nevertheless a good starting point, because these cities have some of the most extensive databases available anywhere.

An Overview of Health and Health Systems in Four World Cities

New York, London, Paris, and Tokyo are not only the largest urban centers of the wealthy nations belonging to the Organization for Economic Cooperation and Development (OECD) nations; they also play a special political and social role as the "cultural capital of a wide orbit, generally heir to a long history, and always … (belonging) to the entire world as much as to … (their) own country" (Gottmann 1979). These world cities exercise a dominant influence over other cities, worldwide, and serve as models that range from best practices to interesting failures across different policy sectors. Although these cities have been compared along multiple dimensions – their architecture and transportation systems (Focas 1988), their economic development strategies (DOE 1996), and more – with respect to the health sector, there is no readily available database akin to those of the UN, the WHO, or the OECD for comparing cities.

New York, London, Paris, and Tokyo have survived devastating disease epidemics. In response, they developed systems of public health infrastructure, reflecting their distinctive institutional and cultural characteristics, which have resulted in a history of relative success in assuring their population's health and averting potential catastrophes. It is difficult, however, due to the difficulties of obtaining comparable data, noted above, to assess their population health and health systems. Moreover, their public heath infrastructure has never been described systematically, let alone compared. I shall therefore summarize some of what we have learned to date about population health and the health systems of these cities, based on research from the World Cities Project (WCP – see http://www.ilcusa.org), and conclude by pointing to some common directions in which these cities are moving to meet the public health challenges that they face.

Comparable spatial units of analysis

The first task of any comparative inquiry is to define the relevant units of analysis, and this is not self-evident in comparing these four world cities, because there is no agreement in the literature on what spatial boundaries make up the relevant units. I therefore begin by summarizing how the WCP distinguishes their urban cores from their surrounding first rings (Figure 2.1).

The definition of their urban core was guided by five criteria: (1) historic patterns of urban development; (2) large populations; (3) high population

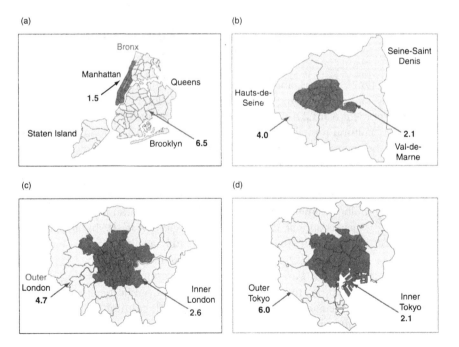

Figure 2.1   Four world cities: urban core and first ring populations (millions). (a) New York City; (b) Paris and First Ring; (c) Greater London; (d) Central Tokyo

density; (4) a mix of high- and low-income populations; and (5) functions as central bubs for employment and healthcare resources.

First, with respect to urban development, Manhattan, Inner London, and Paris represent the historic centers from which these metropolitan regions grew. In Tokyo, the same can be said of its 11 inner wards within the surrounding Yamanote railway line. Second, in terms of population size, Manhattan, Inner London, and Paris range from 1.5 to 2.7 million. Third, in terms of density, Manhattan and Paris are similar: 66,000 versus 53,000 inhabitants per square mile. Both Manhattan and Paris have almost twice the population density of Inner London. Likewise, however, one might define an urban core in Tokyo: the density is much closer to that of London than to Manhattan or Paris. Fourth, the urban cores of these cities combine a mix of high- and low-income populations. Finally, a number of criteria related to their functions as central hubs – what geographers call "central place theory" – suggest two striking parallels among Manhattan, Inner London, Paris, and Inner Tokyo (Berry 1961; King 1984):

- *Concentrated employment centers.* They function as employment centers that attract large numbers of commuters. Approximately one third of the first ring's employed labor force commutes to Manhattan, Inner London, Paris, and Inner Tokyo every day.
- *Concentrated healthcare resources.* The urban core as a unit of analysis provides a frame within which to focus cross-national comparisons on a more coherent and discernable set of health system characteristics. For example, with respect to the concentration of medical resources, Manhattan, Paris, and Inner Tokyo are characterized by a high density of teaching hospitals, medical schools, acute hospital beds, and physicians (Table 2.4).

In summary, Paris – the city of 2.1 million inhabitants all living within its nineteenth-century walls and the peripheral freeway that surrounds its 20 *arrondissements* – is the "urban core" against which a comparable urban core for New York, London, and Tokyo can be defined. The Paris population and area (105 square kilometers) is miniscule in comparison to Greater London's 7.1 million people and 1,590 square kilometers; New York City's 8 million people and 826 square kilometers; and Central Tokyo's 7.9 million people and 616 square kilometers. Paris is comparable to the urban core of these cities (Figure 2.1). For New York City, this is Manhattan; for London, it is the 14 boroughs known as "Inner London." For Tokyo, since there is no conventional definition of an urban core, we rely on the five criteria noted earlier and define an urban core comprised of 11 inner wards that cover an area of 67 square miles (roughly 173 square kilometers) and have a population of 2 million.

Table 2.4 Healthcare resources: Manhattan, Inner London, Paris, and Inner Tokyo (1995–2000)

	Manhattan	Inner London	Paris	Inner Tokyo
Number of teaching hospitals	19	13	25	9
Number of medical schools	5	4	7	7
Acute hospital beds per 1,000 population	5.5 (2002)	4.1 (1990)	7.0 (2002)	12.8[a] (2000)
Physicians per 10,000 Population	85.5 (2004)	36.9 (2000)	84.6 (2002)	70.0 (2000)

[a] This figure is an estimate derived by reducing the number of general hospital beds by 30 percent so as not to include beds in which length of stay is over 30 days.

Sources: Manhattan – New York State Department of Health (NYSDOH), 1998. London – UK Department of Health and Health of Londoners Project. Paris – physicians, Ministère de l'Emploi et de la Solidarité, Direction de la Recherche, des Etudes, de l'Evaluation et des Statistiques (DREES) repertoire ADELI, January 1. 2002: hospitals, DRESS, SAE, 2001. Tokyo – "Report on Survey of Physicians, Dentists and Pharmacists 1998," Tokyo Metropolitan Government, Bureau of Public Health, 2000.

Health status and access to health care

Where is population health status the best? Drawing on the spatial units defined above, Table 2.5 compares infant mortality rates among the urban cores and broader spatial areas of these cities. Table 2.6 compares life expectancy at birth (LEB) and life expectancy (LE) at 65 years for the broader spatial areas only. Beginning with infant mortality, a well-accepted indicator of social conditions, New York City and Greater London stand out – both for their urban cores and first rings – as having higher rates than Tokyo and Paris. Among their urban cores, over the 2000–4 period, Manhattan has lower rates than Inner London. Among the broader areas, Greater London does better than New York City. This reflects the greater extent of concentrated poverty within Inner London in comparison to outer London, a condition well documented with respect to older persons as well (Evandrou 2006). In Manhattan, infant mortality rates have dropped below those for Inner London since the decade of the 1990s, when Manhattan had the highest rates. What continues to distinguish Manhattan, however, are the greater disparities among its neighborhoods than those found in the other urban cores (Neuberg and Rodwin 2002). These disparities reflect Manhattan's greater income disparities, among other factors, for in stark contrast to Tokyo, Paris, and London, there is a statistically significant association between infant mortality rates and income in Manhattan (Rodwin and Neuberg 2005).

Table 2.5 Infant mortality rates: Manhattan, Paris, and London (2001–4)

	Rate[a] (N)
Urban core	
Manhattan[b] (2002–4)	4.4
Inner London[b] (2002–4)	5.9
Paris (2003)	3.6
Inner Tokyo (2001–4)	2.8
Urban core and first ring	
New York City[b] (2002–4)	6.2
Greater London[b] (2002–4)	5.4
Paris and First Ring (2002)	4.0
Central Tokyo (23 wards)	2.8

[a] Per 1,000 live births.
[b] Three-year average.

Table 2.6 Life expectancy at birth and at age 65: New York, London, Paris, and Tokyo

	Life expectancy at birth		Life expectancy at age 65 years	
	Male	Female	Male	Female
New York City[a] (2000)	74.5	80.2	17	20.1
Greater London[a] (2000–2)	76.1 (2000–4)	80.9 (2000–4)	15.6 (1997–9)	19.2 (1997–9)
Paris and First Ring (2002)	76.4	83.1	17.7 (1999)	21.7 (1999)
Central Tokyo (23 wards)			17.7 (2000)	22.2 (2000)

[a] Three-year average.

Turning from infant mortality to life expectancy comparisons among these cities, once again, Tokyo comes out on top with the longest LEB as well as LE at 65 years of age (Table 2.6). The evidence is not consistent with regard to Greater London and the broader Paris agglomeration, but New York City and London, respectively, do worse for LEB and LE at 65 years than Paris and Tokyo (Table 2.6). Consistent with these patterns, a comparison of mortality from heart attacks ranks Tokyo as number one, followed

Table 2.7 Age-adjusted mortality rates from acute myocardial infarction for people aged 65 years and over:[a] New York, London, Paris, and Tokyo (1998–2000)[b]

	Men (N)	Women (N)
New York	485.3 (1,735)	415.8 (2,492)
London	654.0 (2,302)	366.3 (2,171)
Paris and First Ring	244.2 (746)	147.2 (811)
Central Tokyo (23 wards)	176.2 (933)	127.0 (961)

[a] Per 100,000 population.
[b] All rates for New York, London, and Paris are standardized by a direct method using age-adjustment weights based on the 2000 US population aged ≥65 years. These were previously published by Weisz and Gusmano (2004).

by Paris, New York, and London (Table 2.7). This ranking is consistent at all levels of aggregation – the urban core, the broader city agglomeration, as well as the national level. With respect to cumulative cases of AIDS, New York bears the highest burden of this disease, followed by Paris, London, and Tokyo (Rodwin and Gusmano 2002).

In contrast to these rankings, however, there are two indicators for which New York City ranks number one. The first is with respect to age-specific mortality rates at 85 years and over, where Tokyo has the highest rates, followed by London, Paris, and New York. The second is with respect to case incidence rates of tuberculosis, where Tokyo, once again, has the highest rates, followed by Paris, London, and New York (Table 2.8). The case of TB is notable because in contrast to the previous indicators, all of which reflect social determinants of health, the TB rates tell us something about the health system's capacity to contain an infectious disease. New York City's aggressive and well-financed program of directly observed therapy made an extraordinary dent in TB rates in the decade of the 1990s, and has drawn delegations from each of the other cities to learn about this program.

Another more general way to gauge the health system's capacity is to compare a measure of mortality amenable to medical care, often referred to as "avoidable mortality" (Nolte and McKee 2004; Weisz et al. 2007). At the city-wide level, Tokyo drops to number two, after Paris (number one), London is number three, and New York returns to the bottom of the gradient (Table 2.9). Still another measure of the health system's capacity is to rely on a well-recognized measure of access to primary care – population-based hospital admissions, by area of residence, for discharge diagnoses that could most probably be avoided if patients had received timely and compe-

Table 2.8 Tuberculosis case incidence rates:[a] New York, London, Paris, and Tokyo (1996–2000)

	Year	Urban core	First ring
New York	2000	24.3	17.3
London	1999	36.0	33.4
Paris	1999	48.6	29.8
Tokyo	1998	53.9	

[a] Per 100,000 population.

Sources: New York – NYCDOH, 2001, Tuberculosis Control Program, "Information Summary: 2000"; London – UK Department of Health, 1999, Centre for Public Health Monitoring, Compendium of Clinical and Health Indicators; Paris – Observatoire Régional de la Santé de l'Île-de-France, 1999, "La Tuberculose en Île-de-France"; Tokyo – Tokyo Metropolitan Government, Bureau of Public Health, 2000, "Tuberculosis in Tokyo, 1998."

Table 2.9 Avoidable mortality (AM) and hospital conditions (AHCs): four world cities (1998–2001)

	Mortality rate, all causes[a]	AM rate[b]	AHC[c] admission rate
Manhattan	3.69	0.91	27.6
Inner London	4.32	1.07	9.3
Paris	2.94	0.58	10.4
Central Tokyo[d] (23 wards)	2.76	0.8	NA

[a] Calculated for ages 1–74 years, per 1,000 population.
[b] Calculated for ages 1–74 years, per 1,000 population. Causes of death amenable to health care include cerebrovascular disease, hypertension, maternal death, a range of malignancies, and all infectious diseases, and are based on the work of Nolte and McKee (2004). These rates exclude ischemic heart disease, because its prevalence ranges so widely among these cities.
[c] Calculated as a three-year average (1998–2000) for ages 45 and over, per 1,000 population.
[d] AHC data are not available for Inner Tokyo.

tent primary care. These discharge diagnoses are known in the literature as avoidable hospital conditions (AHCs). Discharge rates for these conditions are two and a half times less in Paris than in Manhattan (Gusmano et al. 2006). Data for calculating AHCs are not available for Tokyo, but calculations for Inner London place it closer to Manhattan than to Paris, despite the presumption of good access to primary care under the National Health Service (Table 2.9).

What, then, can one conclude from such comparisons of health status and access to health care? To be sure, it is difficult to draw definitive conclusions – even for cities that are relatively well endowed with data for a range of comparable indicators. It is even more difficult to make comparisons and monitor health status for the 20 megacities of the world, let alone all cities with a population of a million or more inhabitants. Yet surveillance of this kind, as well as careful monitoring of disease outbreaks in large cities, is an important function of public health infrastructure, and the capacity to conduct it will increasingly become recognized as an important component of national health policy.

Public Health Infrastructure across Four World Cities

Differences among world cities – for example, patterns of income inequalities and family structure – may reflect national patterns and policies with regard to income maintenance and immigration. Other differences – patterns of infant mortality and AHCs – may reflect distinctive urban characteristics, such as the striking contrasts between exceedingly high- and low-income subpopulations and neighborhoods. London, Paris, and Tokyo are capital cities in strong unitary states that have more power and willingness than the federal government in the United States to intervene in the life of their capital. But in all four cities the organization of public health functions involves important links between local, regional, national, as well as global health authorities. In what follows, I sketch, in pointillistic fashion, some of the distinguishing characteristics of public health in each of these cities.

New York City (NYC): a strategic local role in health

New York City has the greatest local authority and responsibility for managing its local public health infrastructure. Its Department of Health and Mental Hygiene (DHMH) has exercised this authority in containing tuberculosis, regulating smoking, and more generally integrating its public health surveillance system and developing community health profiles that have led to targeting high-risk areas of the city.

In comparison to other big cities in the United States, NYC is exceptional (Bellush and Netzer 1990). It is the largest city in the nation, with the oldest and most autonomous health department, and has twice the national average rate of uninsured Americans, children living below the poverty line, and recent immigrants. The DHMH was established in the 1860s in response to a cholera epidemic. Although much has changed about New York City and the DHMH, its mission to protect New Yorkers against infectious disease remains strong in light of the recent AIDS and TB epidemics, the West Nile and SARS scare, and post-9/11 concerns about the risks of terrorism, bioterrorism, and, more generally, emergency preparedness.

Having recognized the need to improve public health infrastructure at the local level in 1999, the CDC awarded grant funding to the DHMH to improve the city's public health surveillance activities, including the capacity to develop community health profiles across the city's neighborhoods. Reinforced by the post-9/11 world, these activities led the DHMH to integrate its public health surveillance programs, especially the nature of its collaboration and organizational relationships with the New York State DOH, the CDC, and other local agencies: the municipal Health and Hospitals Corporation (HHC), the city's Office of Emergency Management (OEM), and, of course, the fire and police departments. Also, the DHMH developed improved relations with the physician community so that 80 percent of NYC physicians now communicate reportable diseases directly to the Department. Finally, DHMH developed a system of syndromic surveillance in which 60 percent of hospital department emergency departments participate.

London: strategies to improve the health of Londoners

London's health institutions are paradoxically more fragmented, even though many of them are part of the centralized National Health Service and Department of Health and Social Security. For example, with regard to the regulation of restaurants, each of the 33 local authorities (the boroughs of Greater London) exercises this function independently, whereas in Paris it is handled by the prefecture for all of Paris, and in NYC by the DHMH.

Since 2000, the Greater London Authority has had an elected mayor. There were some notable health-promoting efforts associated with this change in city-wide governance, which were highlighted by the city government in an attempt to secure "healthy city" status from the WHO. To begin with, the new mayor, Ken Livingstone, was given a powerful mandate to develop a public health agenda for Greater London. He placed significant emphasis on intersectoral interventions to improve health, which included a strategy affecting transportation, a biodiversity action plan, a municipal waste management strategy, an air quality strategy, and an ambient noise strategy.

To implement this new approach, the new mayor emphasized partnerships with the London Development Agency, the government health agencies, and the city's voluntary sector. There is currently more public health monitoring and epidemiological surveillance than ever before. Also, given the growing gap, in London, between a well-off majority and a poor minority, and the fact that nearly a quarter of the capital's population are ethnic minorities (Bellush and Netzer 1997), much attention was placed in thinking about what policy interventions, programs, and monitoring activities should be developed to make Londoners more healthy.

Paris – a strategic local health role in a centralized state

Despite a long tradition of French centralization, Paris illustrates the critical role of local authorities in assuming safety-net responsibilities that have eluded its system of universal coverage under national health insurance. Although there are relatively minor financial barriers to health care in comparison to NYC, where 28 percent of the population is uninsured, the Paris Department of Health and Social Action nevertheless plays an important role in the organization and financing of health centers and social services. With a slew of new public health agencies (for AIDS, food safety, and public health surveillance), however, the central government continues to play the dominant role in health.

The Paris authorities have taken strong measures, since the Middle Ages, to protect their citizens from health risks, including bubonic plague. Following the French Revolution, local responsibility for public health was explicitly defined. Despite its national commitment to the public hygiene movement in the nineteenth century, and its identity as a strong centralized state, until recently the central government has played a limited role in public health. At the time of the cholera epidemic (1837) and the outbreak of Spanish influenza (1918–19), the Paris Health Council was largely responsible for addressing the public response. Since World War II, three public agencies have shared responsibility for the public health of Parisians: the public hospital system, *Assistance Publique*, the Directorate for Sanitary Action, and the Bureau of Social Aid.

Following the crisis over contaminated blood in the 1990s, concern about AIDS and drug-resistant TB, and new awareness about the dangers of food poisoning, many new national agencies were established to safeguard public health. At the same time, the Paris Department of Health and Social Action, the *Assistance Publique*, and the voluntary sector have forged new alliances to protect public health and confront the rise of social inequalities, homelessness, delinquency among youth, and social exclusion.

With respect to disease surveillance, Paris resembles London, in that both would quickly come under the direction of national institutions. For example, in France, the *Institut de Veille Sanitaire* (the French equivalent of the US CDC) has established local agencies (*CIRE*), including one for the greater Paris metropolitan region (the Île de France) whose charge is to coordinate epidemiological surveillance for the region. In the event of an emergency – for example, an avian flu pandemic – key decisions would be taken by the French Department of Homeland Security (the *Ministère de la Défense*) and Paris would come under the responsibility of a designated zone connected to the Prefecture for the Police.

Tokyo – a healthy city with emerging problems

Tokyo is the city with the most even income distribution and interesting forms of social cohesion (Bestor 1989). Since it is the healthiest city of these four giants, by traditional health indicators (Tables 2.5, 2.6, and 2.9), and a WHO-sponsored "healthy city," it makes an intriguing standard of comparison. The problem, however, in studying Tokyo is that disaggregated health and social data, by local administrative wards, is often unavailable.

Tokyo suffered the devastation of the Great Kanto Earthquake, in 1923, and significant population evacuation, damage, and near famine during World War II. In the early 1990s, Tokyo was the richest city in the world. It may no longer be the richest; but it is the largest metropolitan area of these four world cities. It is the only one that has an active WHO-sponsored healthy cities movement and research team (Takano 1991; Takeuchi et al. 1995). The Tokyo Metropolitan Government (TMG), which includes Central Tokyo's 23 wards, is one of Japan's 47 prefectures. TMG has a Bureau of Public Health that exercises supervisory responsibilities over the entire Prefecture. In the event of an emergency – for example, an earthquake – TMG would exercise key control functions. But each of the wards of Central Tokyo is a semi-independent municipality, with its own elected mayor and council nation (Takeuchi et al. 1995), and each is responsible for making its own city health plan within the context of a unitary, centralized state that provides strong guidelines for the entire nation.

Just as Japan is number one, in comparison to OECD nations, with respect to infant mortality and life expectancy, Central Tokyo, in comparison to New York, Greater London, and Paris, has the lowest infant mortality rates and the longest LEB. Despite these impressive achievements, however, Tokyo must now face new public health problems – congestion and road traffic noise, the risks of more subway terrorism, AIDS, and homelessness (not to mention water and air pollution, mental disorders, iatrogenic disease due to enormous consumption of drugs, and more).

Will neighborhoods within Tokyo's wards maintain their past ability to promote solidarity and social cohesion in a relatively homogeneous society? Will the information that is routinely collected for disease surveillance be sufficient to address the threats that face global cities today? I have not found these questions easy to answer. But there are nonetheless some convergent patterns that seem to unite all of these cities in their efforts to protect themselves from disease.

Convergent Trends in Public Health Intervention

New York City stands out, in contrast to London, Paris, and Tokyo, because it has the largest share of its population not covered under a national system that eliminates financial barriers to healthcare access. Likewise, it stands out in comparison to the other cities with respect to its electronic surveillance systems, because it probably has one of the most sophisticated ones, particularly with respect to syndromic surveillance. It is, indeed, paradoxical that the health system characterized by the most severe access barriers to basic primary health care should be the one that is most prepared – from the perspective of surveillance – to move decisively in the event of an infectious disease epidemic.

Beyond these differences, however, and the contrasts in terms of public health organization, what is perhaps most striking is the emergence of convergent trends in public health intervention. Among all four cities, there is increasing awareness, among public health leaders, that the neighborhood is a critical spatial unit for targeted interventions to protect against risk factors for disease and to promote health. All four cities are characterized by significant spatial disparities among income, unemployment, educational attainment, housing, environmental conditions, and crime. These factors exercise profound effects on differential population health status measures across city neighborhoods. They have important implications not only for how to target health protection and promotion programs, but also for how to improve emergency preparedness and communication with diverse urban populations.

Broader forces of globalization have, no doubt, reduced somewhat the contrast between New York and the other cities over the past few decades. Consider an example of this phenomenon – the disparities in infant mortality rates among neighborhoods of these cities across two five-year periods in the 1990s (Figure 2.2). There is a slight diminution of disparities within Manhattan and an increase in Paris, London, and Tokyo, which suggests a possible Manhattanization of global cities. Another way of interpreting these data and many more of the health indicators compared is to distinguish between hard and softer global cities (Body-Gendrot 1996). The softer ones tend to implement national programs that protect their most vulnerable populations from some of the forces of globalization. Thus, London and New York come out on the harder end and Paris and Tokyo are distinctly softer. Beyond such a taxonomy, however, it is important to elaborate on the convergent trends in public health intervention, which are increasingly targeted to "high-risk" neighborhoods (Figure 2.3).

New York City's DHMH has embarked on a decisive strategy to place disproportionate emphasis on the city's highest-risk neighborhoods in the south Bronx, east Brooklyn, and central Harlem. It has even engaged in a

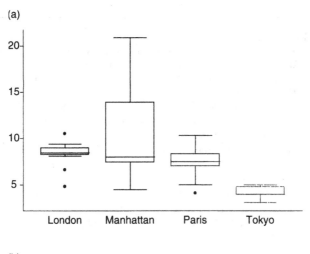

(a)

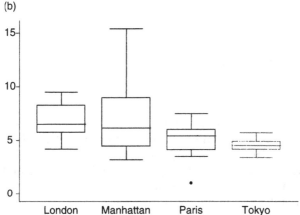

(b)

Figure 2.2 Box plots of neighborhood infant mortality rate distributions: London, Manhattan, Paris, and Tokyo: (a)1988–92; (b) 1993–7. These box plots show differences in spread and symmetry in the distribution of neighborhood infant mortality rates for the four cities. The common vertical axis is the neighborhood infant mortality rate. The thick middle horizontal line across the full rectangle is at the median neighborhood rate on the vertical axis. The upper and lower horizontal lines of the full rectangle are at the 75th and 25th percentile rates, respectively. The remaining two horizontal lines, the whiskers, are at the largest and smallest rate of the distribution on the vertical axis, unless there are rates a substantial distance from the others. Such rates are outliers, and a box plot represents them as dots

For Inner London, we included each of the 14 boroughs (Camden, City of London, Hackney, Hammersmith and Fulham, Haringay, Islington, Kensington and Chelsea, Lambeth, Lewisham, Newham, Southwark, Tower Hamlets, Wandsworth, and Westminster); for Manhattan, each of the ten sub-borough units used by the HVS (Greenwich Village/Financial District, Lower East Side, Chinatown, Stuyvesant Town/ Turtle Bay, Upper West Side, Upper East Side, Morningside Heights/Hamilton

Caption for Figure 2.2 (cont.)
Heights, Central Harlem, East Harlem, Washington Heights, and Inwood); for Paris, each of the well-known 20 *arrondissements* (I^c–XX^c); and for Inner Tokyo each of the 11 *ku* (wards): Chiyoda, Chuo, Minato, Shinjuku, Bunkyo, Taito, Sumida, Koto, Shibuya, Toshima, and Arakawa.
Sources: The birth and death data on which these rates are based may be found in our Data Appendix, online at http://www.ilcusa.org/media/pdfs/ajph.dataappendix.pdf. We obtained them from the following sources:

London – Office of National Statistics, birth registration and linked mortality files: number of live births (1990–7); population below one year of age and number of infant deaths (1988–97).

Manhattan – data were extracted from birth and death files, Division of Vital Statistics, Department of Health and Mental Hygiene.

Paris – the number of live births and infant deaths for 1988–92 are from "La santé de la mere et de l'Enfant à Paris," Department des Affaires Sanitaires et Sociales, Ville de Paris, July 2000. For the period 1993–7, these data were provided by Eric Jougla, Institut Nationale Scientifique d'Etudes et de Recherches Medicales (INSERM).

Tokyo – data for 1988–92 are from Tokyo Eiseikyoku (1993), "Annual Report on Health in Tokyo." Data for 1993–7 are from Fiscal Year 2000 Report of the Bureau of Public Health, Tokyo Metropolitan Government, 2000.

form of bureaucratic decentralization by opening up three DHMH offices in each of these areas. In addition to establishing a DHMH presence in these areas, the mission of these health department branch offices is to coordinate a range of formerly vertical public health programs and serve as advocates for improving community health.

In London and Paris, the highest-risk areas tend to be located along an east–west divide, although the extent of residential segregation and social polarization is less severe than in New York. Both cities are also engaged in some targeting of higher-risk areas, but their approach is more influenced by national policies. In London, health "inequalities" have been the subject of many reports by the Department of Health and Social Security. As part of the effort to target health action zones (HAZs) at the national level, areas such as Tower Hamlets, Newham, Hackney, Camden–Islington, Lambeth, Southwark, and Lewisham have been selected for special attention. This involves borough-wide efforts to promote neighborhood "regeneration" through partnerships with social service agencies, housing improvement programs, and a variety of players ranging from local government, chambers of commerce, the police, and other voluntary organizations.

In Paris, the national urban targeting program (the *politique de ville*) identified 11 neighborhoods based mostly on such criteria as high unemployment rates, for special targeting of resources for community development. In contrast to London, efforts in these neighborhoods involve less explicit

(a) (b)

(c) (d)

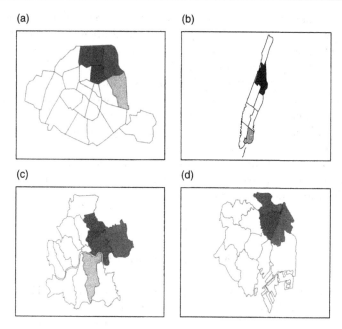

Figure 2.3 Poor areas in four world cities. (a) Paris (X^e, XVIIIe, XIXe, and XXe *arrondissements* highlighted); (b) Manhattan (Lower East Side, Morningside Heights, Central Harlem, and East Harlem highlighted); (c) London (Hackney, Newham, Southwark, and Tower Hamlets highlighted); (d) Inner Tokyo (Taito-ku; Sumida-ku, and Arakawa-ku highlighted)

and active participation of the public health community. Rather than formulating explicit health improvement programs from which relations to other agencies radiate, this approach subsumes public health concerns within the broader net of social prevention, inclusion, and renewal programs. But, increasingly, there are discussions among city authorities about how to target limited resources to areas of the city in the greatest need. The areas selected by the *politique de ville* are spread out across all of Paris, but five out of the 11 projects are concentrated in the VIIIe and XXe *arrondissements*, in neighborhoods such as the Goutte-d'Or, Barbes, Belleville, and Chateau Rouge, in the north-east of Paris, and parts of the XIIIe *arrondissement*, in the south-east.

In Tokyo, although it is generally assumed that the city is one with great uniformity compared to other world cities, analysis of socio-economic conditions and health status reveals considerable differences among wards. Beyond the affluence of the most central wards such as Chiyoda, Chuo, and Minato, some of the northeastern wards of the city – for example, Arakawa, Sumida, and Taito – have far lower per capita incomes and larger shares of their population receiving public assistance. In comparison to New York City, London, and Paris, there appears to be less targeting of these areas for city-wide public health interventions. Perhaps this reflects a greater local discretion for individual wards, with respect to social services, as among local authorities in London. Nonetheless, as Tokyo responds to the threats of emergent infectious disease, its health authorities may well become more interested in what can be learned from the experience of other world cities in targeting "high-risk" areas.

In conclusion, all global cities are increasingly exposed to similar health risks, as well as to speculation about how the coming pandemic alluded to in the introduction of this book might be transmitted across the global cities network. We would do well to begin systematic comparative analyses of how global cities are addressing these risks and how they may learn from their respective successes and failures.

ACKNOWLEDGMENTS

The research for this chapter was funded, in part, from a Health Policy Investigator Award, Robert Wood Johnson Foundation. I also thank Michael K. Gusmano and Daniel Weisz (World Cities Project, a joint venture of the International Longevity Center – USA, New York University's Wagner School, and Columbia University's Mailman School), whose collaboration I treasure.

NOTE

1 By "public health infrastructure," I mean the capacity of local officials to perform what Roper et al. (1992) call the core functions of public health: (a) assessment, "The regular, systematic collection, assembly, analysis, and dissemination of information on the health of the community;" (b) policy development, "The development of ... health policies (on the basis of) scientific knowledge ..."; and (c) assurance, "The assurance to constituents that ... necessary (services) ... are provided ..." The capacity of local officials to perform these functions will depend, in part, on the size and quality of their workforce; their information systems for epidemiological surveillance; and the organizational links that they can forge to implement regulations and deliver public health services.

Part II

SARS and Health Governance in the Global City: Toronto, Hong Kong, and Singapore

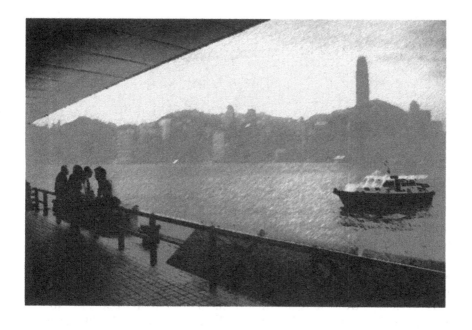

Introduction

S. Harris Ali and Roger Keil

Although public health policy delivery has always been an intensely local process, the "Westphalian" state system had defined health policies in national containers ordered and segmented among others by the World Health Organization (WHO) guidelines, but mostly under the sovereign jurisdiction of nation-states.[1] Public health was defined as *national* health and health policy was *national* health policy under this regime. WHO interventions had to occur within the framework of national sovereignties, whose concern was with both popular health and economic welfare – not necessarily in this order (Fidler 2004; Heymann 2005; interview with David Heymann, 2005). When SARS hit major metropolitan regions in Asia and North America, the need to rethink both global and sub-national health governance was exposed. The process of revising the outdated International Health Regulations (IHR), which was well under way when SARS struck, was momentarily put on hold and ultimately received a boost from the experience gained from that global outbreak in 2003 (interview with WHO infectious disease expert, 2005). The reliance on the hierarchical and hermetic system of nationally based health policy was put to the test as the WHO attempted to carve out a novel activist role in protecting global health beyond national interests, and as sub-national governments, economic, and civil society players moved to react to a localized global health crisis with coordinated action of their own (Abraham 2004; Fidler 2004). At both ends of the redefinition of international health governance – the local and the global – an "institutional void" (Hajer 2003) existed that could not be filled automatically by traditional, national health governance institutions and their international affiliates:

> [M]ore than before, solutions for pressing problems cannot be found within the boundaries of sovereign polities. As established institutional arrangements often lack the power to deliver the required or requested policy results on their own, they take part in transnational, polycentric networks of governance in which power is dispersed. The weakening of the state here goes hand in hand with the international growth of civil society, the emergence of new citizen-actors and new forms of mobilization. (2003, p. 175)

In this part, we discuss the consequences of these shifts, with particular attention to the level of urban health governance. Under the contemporary conditions of intensified globalization, there is an urgent need for urban governance to be prepared to deal with infectious disease. If today, the local is global and the global is local, then there will be important consequences for the manner in which health governance institutions at different scales are structured, and how the different scales of health governance relate to each other. Such factors will clearly influence the ability to respond to EID. From this perspective, it is important to recognize that global health governance overall may be improved by realizing the opportunities that rest in metropolitan governance.

As major metropolitan centers, global cities possess a wealth of health resources (e.g., healthcare facilities, hospitals, and staff – see Rodwin, Chapter 2), which suggests that compared to other places, global cities would be better prepared to respond to an infectious disease outbreak – or, for that matter, any other type of medical emergency. Despite this mostly accurate generalization, the authors in this part report on significant problems during the SARS outbreak response in three cities which were among the hardest hit by the disease in 2003: Toronto, Hong Kong, and Singapore. Such problems involved limitations in resource mobilization, accessibility, and even availability, and these were critical factors in the public health responses that unfolded in those three cities in the wake of SARS. The contributions in this part also highlight the fact that there were notable similarities and differences in the specific types of problems each city faced, as well as in the nature of the responses that unfolded. For example, both Toronto and Hong Kong shared similar problems associated with inadequate communication linkages and information-sharing capabilities, which thwarted a more expedient response to SARS, at least during the earlier stages of their respective outbreaks. In contrast, although the Singapore response has garnered praise from the World Health Organization in terms of information and resource mobilization, it was criticized on other fronts, most notably in regard to possible civil and privacy rights violations during the outbreak response.

At the core, resource availability and mobilization are political issues, because they deal with resource distribution and investment decisions by those in power. This is no different in the domain of public health. All authors explicitly acknowledge that the political economic context within which global cities function had significant implications for understanding the manner in which the respective government and public responses to SARS took place. The question is how exactly? To address this question we would need, at the very least, to consider the particular political economic history of each of these cities, and all three chapters pay some attention to this dimension in the respective analyses. Second, aside from the historical influences, the current state of the global city will also influence the response. In this light, all three readings implicitly underline the fact that today global cities must first ensure that infrastructure and security features are in place so as to maintain their embeddedness within the global circuits of capital, information, people, and resources. For example, they must provide a suitable communication and information infrastructure, as well as a safe and secure environment for business and everyday life (Friedmann 1986; Castells 2000). For this reason, local governments will often refashion their policies, programs, and development projects with the aim of integrating their metropolitan area in the global space of flows in both material and discursive realms. Such actions, however, may also have consequences for the manner in which a government is able to respond to local health crises. Many specific examples of these are given in the chapters of this part.

Perhaps one way to gain an overall understanding of the specific actions taken and issues faced in each of the cities is to draw upon the work of Olds and Yeung (2004), who discern three types of global cities on the basis of the nature and type of integration each has in the world economy. Such a classification may be useful in understanding the nature of the SARS responses in each city. The first type is the "hyper global city," which refers to cities such as New York or London that are well integrated into the global economy through both the inward and outward flows of capital and resources. In contrast, global cities such as Toronto, that have not yet reached this high level of integration, tend to have a greater reliance on inward flows from the global economy and are referred to as "emerging global cities." These types of cities in essence dominate the regional economy and help articulate this regional economy with the global economy. What is notable about emerging global cities are that they are dependent upon on the endowments of institutional resources from higher levels of government, particularly from the national level. A certain level of national resource support ensures that the emerging global city is able to play a critical role within the country, especially in terms of ensuring that key actors and institutions are engaged with the global flows (Olds and

Yeung 2004, p. 506). The importance of fund transfers from the national to municipal level is revealed most explicitly in the chapter by Roger Keil and S. Harris Ali, in their account of how Toronto's response to SARS was very' much hampered by neoliberal-inspired cuts to public health. The consequences of these were seen, for example, in terms of a resultant lack of surge capacity, problems with information handling and communications, and difficulties related to disease surveillance, case management, contact tracing, and quarantine.

In contrast to Toronto, Hong Kong and Singapore are "global city-states" that have a unique governance structure but nevertheless are very well integrated into the global economy. The uniqueness of the governance structure stems from a much greater integration of the national and urban levels of government. As a result, global city-states have the political capacity and legitimacy to mobilize strategic resources to achieve (national) objectives that are otherwise unimaginable in non-city-state global cities. This likely accounted for the ability of Singapore to quickly mount an effective response to SARS. That is, unfettered global city-state capabilities enabled national and urban resources to be quickly mobilized and directed with limited bureaucratic hurdles that were, for example, faced in Toronto. Furthermore, as Peggy Teo, Brenda Yeoh, and Shir Nee Ong note in their chapter, adding to the effectiveness of Singapore's response was that the particular historical and political trajectory of this city-state led to the presence of a citizenry more likely to be trusting, and therefore more compliant with government directives during an emergency situation such as SARS.

While Hong Kong is a city-state similar to Singapore, it is also part of China, and its "One Country, Two Systems" reality posed considerable problems during the SARS crisis. As outlined in the chapter by Mee Kam Ng, many of the problems faced in Hong Kong's response to SARS were due to poor communication, inadequate information sharing, as well as a total lack of coordination involving the various public health agencies. Most of these problems could be traced to a recent historical event; namely, the 1997 British handover of Hong Kong back to China. But as Ng notes, it also had to do with the Asian financial crisis, the ensuing property and stock slump in the city resulting in budget cuts in the health sector and beyond. The economic crisis clearly accounted for reduced resources for the health sector. The lack of coordination between the central government in China and the government in Hong Kong resulted in bureaucratic obstacles in epidemiological data sharing that severely hindered the public health response. Consequently, those political efficiencies characteristic to the city-state that served to benefit Singapore were not existent during the SARS response in Hong Kong. Although Hong Kong was also a global city-state, it was one in political transition, and as such, it was put in circumstances similar to those faced in an emerging global city such as Toronto – as dramatically illustrated by the fact that Toronto and Hong Kong faced remarkably similar obstacles during SARS.

NOTE

1 "'Westphalian' refers to the governance framework that defined international public health activities from the mid-nineteenth century," based on the political logic of sovereign nation-states that had come into existence after the Thirty Years War (Fidler 2003, pp. 485–6).

3

SARS and the Restructuring of Health Governance in Toronto

Roger Keil and S. Harris Ali

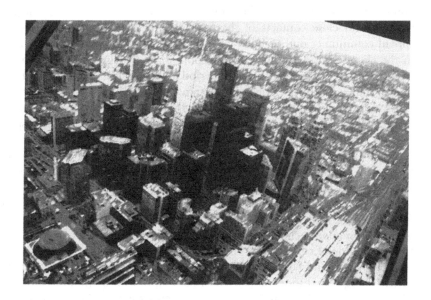

Introduction

If SARS was practice for the pandemic, Toronto was the practice field. It was the Western focus for the disease, the perfect host. But why? Why not Chicago or Vancouver or Jacksonville? Toronto's vaunted multiculturalism ensures regular traffic with hundreds of nations, and it's a travel hub; 26 million passengers came through Pearson [the city's international airport] in 2002. Globalization is a factor: an exotic animal market in Guandong Province is only hours away. And our medical system has been in a state of underfunded decline for many years, poorly prepared for any outbreak.

(Gillmor 2004, p. 64)

SARS in Toronto

The Canadian SARS index case was an elderly woman who returned from the Metropole Hotel in Hong Kong on February 23, 2003, but died at home shortly thereafter. Her son (the primary case) became infected and was admitted to a Toronto hospital two days later. As the disease was not yet identified as a public health threat, many patients and staff were inadvertently exposed to the primary case before he was eventually placed in isolation. Partly due to hospital overcrowding, this individual remained in the emergency department long after doctors had authorized a hospital admission. The spread of the disease was largely limited to healthcare workers and close contacts of the infected, but the possibility of a wider spread community outbreak revealed itself when a cluster of 31 cases arose in the closely knit Toronto religious community (Naylor 2003). As no new cases occurred during the two-week period following this, the SARS outbreak in Toronto was officially declared as having ended, and the WHO travel advisory imposed on the city was lifted. Shortly thereafter, however, in late May 2003, a second smaller outbreak occurred in a Toronto area hospital, but was quickly contained.

Over the duration of the outbreaks, approximately 250 people in the Greater Toronto Area (GTA) were infected with SARS and 44 died, while patients were treated in over 20 GTA hospitals (Basrur et al. 2004). Five schools were temporarily closed and there was one reported case of an employee who defied a quarantine order by returning to his place of work at an information technologies firm – infecting a co-worker and leading to the quarantine of close to 200 employees (Naylor 2003). The overall degree of cooperation and compliance was extremely high, with only 27 isolation orders being issued to those who did not comply with quarantine directives (Basrur et al. 2004). During the outbreak, approximately 2,000 case investigations were conducted, each taking an average of nine hours to complete (Basrur et al. 2004). In the end, over 23,300 people were identified as contacts, of whom 13,374 were placed in quarantine.

What were the main issues Toronto faced in the fight against SARS? How did the specific conditions of health governance in the federal system of Canada intersect with the new disease that ravaged the healthcare sector of its major city? There were basically three related problems that highlighted the frictions of multi-level governance in an urban setting. First, there was the general flow of information, of which risk communication between healthcare professionals, politicians and bureaucrats on one hand, and the general public on the other was the most important one; in addition, communication inside the complex and uneven Toronto health sector was highly fragmented and hardly able to cope with the rush of data generated through contact tracing, monitoring, and the flood of global information, the results of which had to be integrated daily into healthcare practice. Second, SARS constituted a real test to the institutional architecture of Canadian public health in a reframed post-Westphalian political ecology. And third, SARS produced a new arena for urban governance, as the region has begun to integrate the lessons learned from SARS in bracing itself for the impending flu pandemic. We will work through the three issues using the three SARS reports and expert interviews as the basis for our analysis. But before that, let us briefly look at Toronto as a globalizing urban region.

Global City Toronto

It is important to understand the 2003 developments in the context of global city formation. Toronto is an urban region of 5.5 million in the industrial heartland of Canada. Its core city is home to the highest concentration of financial and producer service industries in the country. Articulating Canada's economy into the world economy, the Greater Toronto Area has developed into a dynamic and diversified workbench from which regional elites are pursuing their ambitious goals in international inter-urban competition (Boudreau et al. 2006, 2007). Following Olds and Yeung (2004), Toronto can be understood as an Emerging Global City in terms of drawing significant amounts of resources and inputs from across the country, thus serving as a site to channel more inward rather than outward flows. Because of the net inward flow into the city, at this point Toronto does not fully act as a global city on the stage of the world economy; rather, its influence is mostly on the regional economy, as the resultant regional economy takes measures to become more engaged with the global economy. The Toronto situation signifies clearly the increasing vulnerability of places in the global economy to two contravening dynamics: the accelerated opening of the urban region to flows of capital, people, and now increasingly also viruses and the enhanced turbulence in the governance structures set up to address these vulnerabilities (Parker 2004, p. 111). SARS hit Toronto as a consequence of the city's close interconnectivity with other global cities, and in this case, particularly the 'clique' it forms with Singapore and Hong Kong (Van Wagner, Chapter 1). Open to the shipment of goods, bodies, and cultures from these places and connected through business and personal ties with large groups of residents there, Toronto became a logical, if not inevitable, branch in the tree of SARS transmission in the spring of 2003. The two consecutive outbreaks in Toronto occurred at a time when the city was slowly emerging, bruised, from eight years of conservative public-sector restructuring, which had seen the city's civic institutions redefined, its boundaries redrawn, and its coffers raided by waves of provincial and federal austerity measures and provincial downloading. In addition, the federal political architecture was in a state of flux, as politicians at all scales entered a lively debate on a new role for sub-national levels of government, with a New Deal for Cities carrying most of the discursive weight (Boudreau et al. forthcoming). Toronto was at once subject to institutional shifts in healthcare governance in Canada overall and the arena for a new governmentality of health. Responsibilities for subjects and objects of healthcare measures, both public and private, collective and personal, were reassigned, a process strongly reinforced through the SARS crisis. Concretely, this meant that as the potential expansion of local health responsibilities beyond the scale of the city was demonstrated in the SARS case, previously sealed boundaries of healthcare provision and disease management were perforated extensively. This posed the question more generally whether the city "worked" for its residents and visitors when it comes to protection from infectious disease. This question can, ultimately, only be answered through practice in future outbreaks (such as the impending flu pandemic, for which Toronto is currently seeking an institutional and procedural prophylactic). But analytically, already, we can use the SARS case to begin to understand the more general challenges faced by the city's healthcare system and the intersections it faces with global city formation.

As an urban phenomenon in Toronto, the spread and reactions to SARS were directly linked to the emergence of new modes of social regulation, new technologies of power, and new coercive measures often identified with the neoliberal state. The "new normal" was the situation, in which the local state (in the broader sense of the word) played an important role in the reorientation of social practices in an increasingly more insecure world. As local states have limited autonomy and no sovereignty, their strategies of control and regulation are limited to a range of options. One of these strategies is the imposition of spatial controls, which aim predominantly at the control of individuals: the bodies of specific urban inhabitants – for example, tourists, workers, hospital patients, and immigrants. Let us now turn specifically to the three areas in which governance in Toronto was put to the test.

*Fragmented Health Care and Risk Communication
in the Fight against SARS*

Emerging Global Cities such as Toronto (see Olds and Yeung 2004) are to large degree supported by higher levels of government. If the amount of support offered by these higher governmental levels is diminished, this will of course have an impact on the ability of the city to carry out its functions, such as the protection of local public health.

Three investigative reports in the SARS outbreak carried out by different levels of government were in agreement that budget restrictions imposed on public health care within Ontario and Toronto had several important repercussions for the SARS response (Naylor 2003; Campbell 2004; Walker 2004). First, limitations in facilities and hospital resources not only meant crowded conditions in hospital waiting areas and an inadequate number of isolation rooms, but they also limited the ability to pursue proper infection control procedures, such as ensuring that N95 masks were properly fitted on healthcare workers. This so-called "lack of surge capacity" was further exacerbated by a trend toward the casualization of nursing staff. As part of the cost-saving measures, nurses in Ontario were commonly not hired on a full-time basis and as such did not receive any workplace benefits or a full-time wage. Consequently, many nurses worked at multiple hospitals to obtain an adequate income. With SARS, the possibility of transfer of the virus through infected nurses traveling from one hospital to the next was a real possibility and, as such, nurses were banned from working at more than one location (Affonso et al. 2004). Notably, as the pool of available nurses became reduced during the outbreak because of self-quarantine, the remaining nurses were forced to work longer shifts under conditions of fatigue.

Another series of factors identified by the inquiry commission related to a lack of financial investment in the health communications systems. In particular, this led to significant problems in the sharing of information during the outbreak. For example, it was noted by the municipal medical officer of health[1] that the information systems needed to conduct disease surveillance, case management, contact tracing, and quarantine were very out of date and that investment was required to update the systems. At the time of SARS, the information system used – referred to as the Canadian Integrated Public Health system (CIPHS) – did not have the capability to share information across any sort of boundaries. Consequently, data from one hospital could not be directly shared with the provincial ministry of health or other hospitals in the GTA – a problem that was compounded by the fact that Ontario has the only healthcare system that is not regionalized; that is, each hospital works in an autonomous fashion.[2]

Information difficulties were also faced during the very early stages of the outbreaks, when decisions had to be made on the basis of incomplete data. For example, during the convening of a meeting of the emergency management and public health officials in the downtown operations center, where it was decided that a state of provincial emergency would be called and where directives were being established for hospitals as to restricted access, closings, cancellations of certain procedures, and so on, it was noted by one Toronto hospital official that:

> So what would happen is that policies would be written in this war room with all of this expertise, and then they would go up and they would start to get scrutinized by another level, which was more the bureaucratic aspect of things, and

things were starting to get slowed down. Information was not coming in, because [the provincial medical officer of health] was not providing the information openly, he wanted it sort of filtered through his group before it came to our [local Toronto] group, and we needed that information to make decisions about what kind of precautions to be using, the length of incubation, how long somebody should be in isolation. And that started to become a real issue, and people were just getting spread too thin. (Interview, November 11, 2005)

On the ground in Toronto, communication inside hospitals and among various actors in the fight against SARS was extremely disjointed. As one infectious disease official put it, "work was being done in silos," with various activities going on without cooperation in a networked fashion or through coordination by the ministry.[3] Some of this disjointedness was a direct consequence of the idiosyncratic situation in Ontario, which lacked regional coordination among healthcare providers such as hospitals and with public health units at various government scales. In particular, the autonomy of hospitals in the regional healthcare system proved to be a major obstacle to coordinated response when SARS struck.[4]

A leading public health official, then with the City of Toronto, confirmed that the flaws of the communication infrastructure were dramatic as information systems were out of date "using 1980's computer technology." It turned out to be extremely challenging under these circumstances "to conduct disease surveillance, case management contact tracing and management, and then quarantine. And it's relevant because that was, that ought to have been our primary mechanism for just surely counting the number of cases we had on a day-by-day, hour-by-hour basis. And reporting [from] there on to the [provincial] Ministry of Health, and through them to the national and international public health bodies," was clearly hampered by this situation and this expert notes that the outdated technology

would still be the technology if it hadn't been for SARS I can guarantee you that. Absolutely, there was no money, there was no will, there was no time, there was no nothing to replace it, cause it wasn't a priority until it all fell apart in the public eye, and that, those systems were totally inadequate to do this kind of function on the scale that was required, when the World Health Organization issued their travel advisory it was in part based on the lack of confidence in the case number, and thus the adequacy of control measures that Health Canada was able to convey to the World Health Organization, so you can literally boil it down to a whole number of factors, people, and place, and systems and what not, and part of that was just sheer information systems. (Interview, April 10, 2006)

Throughout the SARS crisis, the relationships between Toronto, a city larger than some provinces, and the provincial and federal governments remained a perennial issue, and the governance of theses intergovernmental relationships has become contentious in itself. This leads us to broader considerations on the political pathology of the SARS crisis in the Canadian federal system.

A Post-Westphalian Political Pathology: The Toronto Context

The Institute on Governance defines health governance in Canada as follows:

> In Canada, the governance of health care is built on intergovernmental coop-eration, reflecting a formal division of powers regarding health care as out-lined in the Canadian Constitution and the Charter of Rights and Freedoms. In addition, governance of health care also takes place outside the govern-mental sphere. This complexity requires organizations, sectors, regions, First Nations communities and governments to forge capacities to govern. (http:// www.iog.ca/knowledge_areas.asp?pageID=23, accessed November 1, 2005)

Despite the complexity and multi-scalarity of health governance, the role of cities in health governance is usually considered secondary. There is, on one hand, the traditional obscurity that municipal politics suffers in the Canadian state architecture (Boudreau et al. forthcoming); on the other hand, there is a more general eclipse at work here that disregards or even dismisses the role of urban governance in the management of societal mat-ters in a post-Westphalian world. We believe, though, that urban public health authorities and their associates in local hospitals, urban non-state actors in the health field as well as workers in urban medical settings have played important roles in the detection, identification, monitoring, and fight against EIDs in particular.[5] They have provided the core responsibilities of public health – assessment, policy development, and assurance – often with-out support and sometimes in conflict and contradistinction to higher-level health authorities (Rodwin and Gusmano 2002, p. 446 fn). Lim et al. (2004, p. 697) have said about the Ontario situation during SARS that "The prov-ince of Ontario was ill-prepared to deal with an infectious disease threat on such a scale. In Canada, the provision of health care, including public health, is a provincial responsibility. However, *the financial and operational responsibility for public health had increasingly been shifted to municipalities* such that, at the time of the SARS outbreak, funding was shared equally between the two levels of government. This funding shift created a decentralised public-health system, with the province's 37 public-health units operating quite independently of each other" (emphasis added).

Urban health governance is embedded in a larger system of urban governance with its vertical and horizontal ties to other levels of government and into civil society and the private sector. Urban governance in Toronto had been characterized by the city's forced amalgamation in 1997. Politically, the old core city of Toronto had been a power base for left-liberal municipal reform policies since the late 1960s, which had expanded, under the pressure of an ever active and mobilized local civil society, the rights of citizens in education, housing, the environment, health, and other policy fields directly of importance to local citizens. This seemed to change when Toronto was swallowed up jurisdictionally by the larger "megacity" formed after 1997. The five suburbs (Etobicoke, York, North York, East York, and Scarborough), which were consolidated with Toronto and the Municipality of Metropolitan Toronto into the new City of Toronto, were less progressive in outlook and political practice and they became more influential after 1998. The new major of the megacity, Mel Lastman, symbolized the small-townish and provincial attitude that began to take hold of Toronto politics after amalgamation. While the new suburban hegemony with its preferences and concern for fiscal conservatism, small government, family lifestyles, and property values took hold, the city entered a period of tremendous economic expansion of exploding condominium development and accelerated immigration. Toronto elites rallied around several emphatic projects of urban growth and development: waterfront regeneration, a failed Olympic bid, a new official plan, arts mega-projects, and so on. Whereas homelessness soared, squeegee kids[6] were harassed by the police under the pretext of provincial legislation against panhandling, and while poverty continued to grow, the bravado of the city's elites continued to dazzle outsiders and local populations alike. All this coincided with fundamental changes to municipal politics and internal governance processes as the city has been trying to establish a sense of harmonized "good government" and civic engagement after amalgamation. The outcome of these processes was contradictory: on the one hand, hardcore neoliberal reforms were rolled out and downloaded by the Tory provincial government between 1995 and 2003, and often followed through by a conservative and boosterist mayor Mel Lastman, who was unapologetically the spokesperson of an aggressive business lobby, and particularly the development industry; on the other hand, progressive politicians operated effectively at the municipal level with the support of a continuously active social and environmental movement sector, the public-sector unions, and an electorate that had not forgiven the Tories for their attack on Toronto political traditions. The outcome of these contradictions was that urban governance in Toronto at the time of the SARS outbreak was split as a result of continued reform in the municipal administration, and certain "forgotten" policy areas such as food, homelessness, the environment – and public health – competed with the neoliberal development mantra of a business elite that began to use the newly amalgamated city as their strategic terrain for inter-urban competition. Inside the City proper, departmental restructuring and harmonization had led to insecurity, at least temporarily, as to the procedures and substance of urban policy when political cultures of suburban jurisdictions were melded with the downtown's more progress-ive, democratic traditions, which had led to more sustained rights claims of more diverse populations. This progressive city/conservative suburb split in the geography of Toronto's urban governance was challenged by the new immigration and settlement patterns, which made suburbs more diverse than the inner city and the inner city potentially less dynamic politically than the multiculturally invigorated suburbs. During the time of the SARS outbreak, this complicated matters significantly, as the crisis was played out in geo-graphical and social areas of the city – Scarborough and North York – that remained largely *terra incognita* to the old Toronto elite.

The SARS outbreak intersected with business as usual in urban governance in as far as it was recast quickly from a health crisis to an economic crisis once the worst of the infection was over (see Drache and Clifton, Chapter 6). The worry among Toronto politicians and business people over lost business in tourism and entertainment fell in line with the usual propensity of urban officials and civic leaders to heave their city above its competitors in economic development, cultural creation, and tourist attraction. In this sense, the SARS crisis interfered with the strategic goals of the governing regime of Toronto and the governing institutions that had created their success. The peculiar balance of social, economic, environmental, and state interests in elite and popular circles that made up the governing coalition of the urban region was threatened by SARS, which was contextualized in a series of losses to the region's economic progress and civic self-esteem, and the defeat of the bid for the 2008 Olympic Games by Beijing in particular.

Finally, Toronto is tied into an increasingly diverse global network of diaspora and migrant cultures at the base of the city's hybrid globality (Goonewardena and Kipfer 2005). The connection between the globalizing political economy and the cultural and demographic changes that it brings with it is crucial to understanding the everyday practices and socio-cultural interactions that characterize today's world, and more specifically the everydayness of global cities. Toronto – like other cities in the global city network and elsewhere – has taken on far-reaching responsibilities for the settlement of immigrants. This has become a central concern of metropolitan governance now. As in past waves of immigration, cities have become the actual border points for new immigrants, which in turn has significant implications for societal reactions to infectious diseases in urban centers, particularly those prejudicial associations of disease with race (see, for example, discussion concerning the "racialization of SARS" in Keil and Ali, Chapter 9).

Learning the Lessons from SARS: Urban Planning and Governance
Prepares for the Avian Flu

The outbreak of SARS in Toronto sparked a period of reconceptualization of risk through infectious disease and its mitigation at various Canadian governance levels. One influential new federal document, *The Canadian Pandemic Influenza Plan for the Health Sector* (Public Health Agency of Canada 2006), makes repeated reference to SARS and its lessons for the management of future outbreaks (p. 52). The experience is cited as instrumental in highlighting "the importance of preparatory planning and establishing a surveillance infrastructure capacity for the detection and monitoring of emerging respiratory infections" (ibid., p. 560). Viewed immediately as a "dress-rehearsal" for pandemic influenza, SARS was very much considered a national crisis despite, as we have argued here, its concentration in the global city core of Toronto (ibid., p. 78). The establishment of a Health Emergency Communications Network (HECN) was seen as direct response to the communications problems experienced in 2003 between various actors at different government and healthcare levels (ibid., p. 70). Technical as well as rights aspects of the crisis were taken into account as references to the technicalities of disease control stood side by side with discussions of "justifiable, temporary limitation of personal autonomy in the interests of limiting the spread of a specific communicable disease" (ibid., p. 46). The 2003 crisis provided the opportunity to reassess the role of emergency planning with regards to the containment and treatment of infectious disease in cities. It was registered along the same lines as the terrorist attacks of September 11 and the 1998 ice storm, as an event that helped shape a better understanding of multi-level government-based emergency preparedness.

One consequence of the SARS experience was a localization of emergency planning. An infectious disease official in a Toronto hospital admitted:

> we realized that self-reliance is a good thing and if we actually had a bad pandemic, we could not expect the ministry nor Toronto public health to sort of come to our rescue. And so there's a very concrete example of where we actually are ... taking it much more local than we would expect. Nobody wants to get directives from the ministry any more without having a lot of say in terms of what those directives are going to say. We all ... post SARS ... I got a lot more involved in work the ministry was doing because I never wanted to be on the receiving end of that again, without having a say in what was going on and the hospital very much supports that. So I'd say absolutely there's been a lot more local ... local way of thinking about these things. You know, the Provincial Government doesn't necessarily believe Health Canada's going to have its Tamiflu stock pile ready. We don't really believe the ministry's going to have its Tamiflu stock pile ready, which is why we are purchasing it ourselves. (Interview, November 4, 2005)

Urban governance had traditionally played a major role in devising, implementing and monitoring strategies of urban public health. Planning remains an important practice in this process. But in contrast to traditional notions of top-down, military-style disaster management planning, which often subordinated community and civic concerns to functional considerations, planning needs to respond to growing public awareness and attention to the maintenance of civil rights even in crisis situations as well as issues related to the unequal distribution and experience of risk (namely the aftermath of Katrina). Planning for emergencies occurs less in the arcane backroom conversations of public agencies but increasingly in the public domain, as citizens express their concerns about which measures to take and which strategies to pursue.

In this vein, the City of Toronto has been undertaking a consultative process with its own Pandemic Flu Plan. This process has incorporated a large number of private and civic organizations, whose individual emergency preparedness plans are considered an important foundation for the overall municipal plan. Consultative practices may not be news for progressive municipal planners, especially in the rather politicized and democratically minded civic bureaucracy of Toronto. But for disaster managers, traditionally trained in the hierarchical Command–Control–Communicate model of emergency management, a deliberative, democratic mode of operation may appear alien. Public health officials, municipal planners, and emergency managers were thus forced into a continuing dialogue regarding the changing societal demands and procedures to be followed as a consequence. In particular, it will have to be seen how the discourse on individual civil rights may mesh with the traditionally perceived need by emergency decision-makers to temporarily suspend certain rights in order for public authorities to arrive at an effective collective response to the emergency.

In the case of a disease outbreak, these issues are even more pressing because of the imposition of such measures as surveillance and quarantine on the public to contain the spread. Public health, as part of the medical establishment, has well-established protocols such as patient confidentiality to protect individual rights. The protection of sensitive data may not exist in other sectors. In planning for a future infectious disease pandemic, officials may need to access data from various sectors and organizations. The need to gather such information ought to be questioned publicly, and if emergency planners opt to use such data they should be tightly protected, with measures taken to prevent abuse of these data. One concern here is to ensure that data for "public health security" is not appropriated by other political interests in the name of "security" – a real concern in today's "new normal" and geopolitical climate predicated on the "war on terrorism" (Wekerle and Jackson 2005).

The SARS outbreak in Toronto has begun to change, for the time being, the relationships of the urban collective to the larger issue of infectious disease. A heightened awareness among business and civil society leaders for the issue of pandemic preparedness would have been improbable or even impossible before 2003, when such matters were seen to be ensconced in an arcane biopolitical arena of experts, largely hidden away from public view, if not made outright redundant in periods of aggressive neoliberal cutbacks that had ravaged the non-frontline public health system of Ontario and Toronto since the 1990s.[7] In the years after SARS, it is not unusual at all to fill City Hall with dozens of public service providers who come to learn from municipal public health officials about the plans they will have to devise to prepare for avian flu, or to witness public officials and Toronto Board of Trade representatives receive flu-shots in front of 70 media people. Dealing with emerging infectious disease has become a prime topic in this global city, and it has become a subject of public discourse and urban governance.

Conclusion

The Toronto urban health governance system experienced a very specific set of pressures, which spoke to the kinds of fundamental decisions that have to be made by urban-scaled and municipal authorities in a moment of epidemic disease. Affonso et al. (2004, pp. 573–4) have perceptively identified three sets of paradoxes that led to three sets of dilemmas in the governance of the SARS outbreak. These paradoxes/dilemmas were as follows: (1) Healthcare workers became sources of transmission and active sustainers of the SARS case matrix, leading to the dilemma of forcing to decide whose safety gets priority – patients or caregivers? (2) Hospitals were sources of SARS infection in the community, breaking down the boundaries of medical care and community in threatening ways – How far do providers of health care have to go to provide safe spaces? (3) A culturally and ethnically diverse city may be particularly vulnerable to infectious diseases, thus prompting the question about the relationship of civil liberties and disease control. In terms of urban governance, these three couples of paradoxes and dilemmas denote spatio-institutional uncertainties of a new kind, which challenge traditional modes of integration and regulation of economic institutions (labor markets/ workplaces), specialized functional spaces (hospitals), public institutions (public health agencies), codified private behaviors (patient versus citizen rights), and so on. In an urban governance model, questions need to be directed at the particular ways through which state action (public health; security, etc.), private-sector involvement (providers of masks, medical equipment, drugs, etc.), civic organizations (ethnic initiatives against racism, protection of workers' rights, etc.) and individual civil rights claims (patients, quarantined individuals, travelers, etc.) are coordinated by whom at what scale, and with what procedural democratic means (Affonso 2004, pp. 574–7).

It is important to note, in the context of the question of urban governance before us, that each of these intended measures would have a tangible impact on the day-to-day business of governing cities through democratic political rather than managerial–administrative processes at the municipal level. The core dilemmas that these processes would face in the reality of current Canadian municipalism are, first, the lack of autonomy that local agencies have in the face of an unreformed federalism, which sees cities (and their institutions) as mere units of the administrative state (of the province and Canada) and not as political decision-makers on their own terms; and, second, the tremendous weakening of lower state and governance structures – often despite rhetorical statements to the contrary to the effect of devolution and subsidiarity – in the face of the globalization and neoliberalization of the Canadian state, including the increasing porosity toward supra-national institutions such as the WHO.

We have some evidence on how the local state institutions in Toronto themselves saw the crisis and what lessons they suggested to draw from it. The former provincial medical officer of health, Colin D'Cunha (2004), detailed the various lessons learned from the outbreak mostly through the lens of health reporting.[8] The provincial scale is extremely important in the Canadian system, where municipalities are dependent on upper-level policy frameworks and financing, without much autonomy for local agencies and institutions. Urban governance is severely constricted and clearly defined by this situation. While the municipal state may also be the most politicized of the three levels of government, it remains under the tight supervision of the province in particular, and while state expenditures have risen consistently since the 1950s in the federal and provincial governments, municipal funds have not kept pace with the demands placed on them through decades of downloading and devolution (Villeneuve and Séguin 2000). D'Cunha, whose agency was responsible for 37 local health units in Ontario, notes in particular that the Reportable Disease Information System in place when SARS hit had been introduced in the 1980s. A new system of reporting, the Integrated Public Health Information System (PHIS), though available since early in the twenty-first century, was only to be implemented in the spring of 2003 and was further delayed through SARS. The provincial level system of surveillance was tied in with the Global Public Health Intelligence Network (GPHIN). The provincial Health Protection and Promotion Act (HPPA) makes disease reporting and control mandatory. It was amended after the SARS crisis to empower the province to facilitate isolation of infected individuals (D'Cunha 2004). D'Cunha's office was also left in dire straits in the wake of serious de-funding of public health institutions at the provincial level under a Tory government after 1995. The provincial health authority appeared very much like an empty shell, which had the coordinating functions of a local authority, but could not muster the resources to do a good job in giving direction and providing credible leadership to municipal and regional agencies.[9]

In the context of this legal and institutional framework, local-scale health agencies do their work. Sheela Basrur, the former municipal officer of health, and co-authors have noted that the main roles of Toronto public health during the outbreak were case investigation and management, identification and quarantine of contacts, disease surveillance and reporting, health risk assessment, and infection control advice to health institutions and other community settings (Basrur et al. 2004, p. 22). The SARS crisis posed a significant stress on the already severely compromised public health system of Toronto, as other public health services were cut or reduced to "essential services only" (ibid., pp. 23–4). The kinds of measures under the responsibility of the municipal public health hegemony reflect the temporally layered and overlapping traditions stemming from the "bacteriological city," updated and redefined through more recent developments. The point to note in this respect is the often-confusing unevenness in measures from various periods, phases, and moments of urban governance, which were haphazardly regrouped into a recombinant mix of place-specific sets of trials and errors. While the coercive and enabling qualities of an existing municipal public health system were tested daily, with unexpected twists in the proliferation of the disease, a new administrative reality emerged in the shadow of the successes and failures of an iterative policy process. Cases of temporal unevenness were, for example, the deployment of quarantine and isolation orders for the first time in 50 years (with no living administrative memory of, and hence no experiential knowledge with, such measures in the system) and the much younger (but failing) 14-year-old provincially authorized surveillance system (which had not kept pace with both technological advances and procedural necessities that had occurred since its inception: Basrur et al. 2004). The unevenness here related in both cases to the fact that two measures at two ends of a developmental scale in public health measures – the rather traditional and rather blunt tool of the quarantine and the biopolitical, yet informationalized surveillance – were potentially at odds with the constituencies and clienteles that they were meant to protect (and whose general rights sensibilities were a far cry from the mid-twentieth century[10]) and, in the case of the failed surveillance, certainly not up to the challenge that the SARS outbreak posed.

NOTES

1   In an interview conducted on April 12, 2006.
2   Interview with the director of infection prevention and control in a GTA hospital, November 4, 2005.

3 Ibid.

4 Ibid.

5 Interviews with various municipal and provincial public health officials and nursing association administrators.

6 Young people who clean car windows at intersections for change with so-called "squeegees," a T-shaped implement edged with rubber for the cleaning of windows.

7 Interview with the municipal medical officer of health during SARS, April 10, 2006.

8 D'Cunha was removed from the position he held during the crisis, because many considered his performance during the crisis as incompetent and insufficient. He was replaced on January 19, 2004 by Sheela Basrur (the former Toronto Medical Officer of Health).

9 Interview with the director of infection prevention and control in a GTA hospital, November 4, 2006.

10 It must be noted, however, that Canadians on the whole are less civil liberties conscious than most Americans. Collective necessity and public security often trumps concerns over individual freedoms in Canada. Whether it was the War Measures Act during the October crisis of the 1970s, when tanks rolled in Montreal, or in current public opinion about stricter security measures in the "war on terrorism," Canadian pollsters have consistently found strong support for "stability and security" (Clark 2005).

4

Globalization of SARS and Health Governance in Hong Kong under "One Country, Two Systems"

Mee Kam Ng

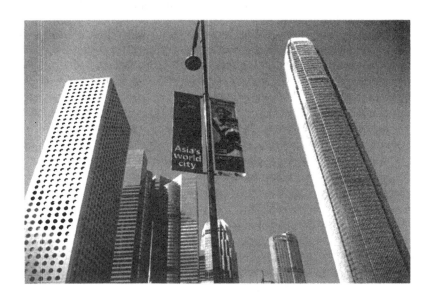

Introduction

In 2003, Hong Kong was hard hit by the Severe Acute Respiratory Syndrome (SARS), a deadly coronavirus that belongs to a family of viruses that cause the common cold. The following chapter discusses how the battle against SARS exposed problems in Hong Kong's healthcare system that are related to the unique modes of regional and local governance under the concept of "One Country, Two Systems." The "globalization" of SARS has not only laid bare major health governance issues in the city; it has also highlighted the fundamental importance of appropriate regional and local modes of health governance for the international community to fight against the next epidemic. Let us first examine the city's mode of health governance.

Health Governance in Hong Kong: Compartmentalized with Minimal Regional Integration

After 1842, when Hong Kong became a British colony, the city pursued a road not traveled by the mainland (Ng 2005). The two socio-economic and political entities had minimal, if any, formal interactions until the 1980s, when China carried out dynamic urban reforms and when the "1997 Question" had to be tackled. The "1997 Question" was eventually settled under the "One Country, Two Systems" formula, the corollary of which is that except for foreign and military affairs, Hong Kong would be a highly autonomous Special Administrative Region (SAR). Hence, the political unification in 1997 did not result in formal institutional integration of the two systems. Indeed, the arrangement has deterred cross-boundary cooperation.

Since becoming a SAR in 1997, Hong Kong has remained a non-democratic liberal city with a state-centered mode of governance. The bureaucrats in the administration continue to play a quasi-political role in formulating policies. In July 2002, the first Chief Executive implemented the Principal Officials Accountability System. The three most senior civil service positions – those of the Chief Secretary, the Financial Secretary, and the Justice Secretary – were converted to "political" appointments and 11 political appointees were added to run the 11 policy bureaus. The official reason for the introduction of this system is to make government more responsive to public concerns, but since these political appointees are all accountable to the Chief Executive, many considered such an arrangement a convenient means for the then first Chief Executive, who came from the business sector, to better harness an all-powerful and long-serving bureaucracy (Ng 2006).

The Legislative Council in Hong Kong consists of 60 members, half returned from geographical constituencies and half returned from functional constituencies. Although citizens in Hong Kong have never enjoyed full democratic rights, the city is a liberal society that respects basic human rights for its citizens. In a largely economics-oriented society, people in Hong Kong are known for their generosity in sharing with those who are less fortunate. Activities undertaken by the civil society organizations during SARS were further testimonies to this unique culture of Hong Kong (Loh and Welker 2004; Thomson and Yow 2004).

Public health policies in Hong Kong at that time were the domain of the Health, Welfare, and Food Bureau (now renamed as Food and Health Bureau – henceforth Health Bureau, HB), which is one of the 11 policy bureaus in the city that are also responsible for social welfare, food and

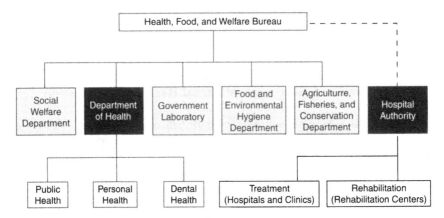

Figure 4.1 The organization structure of the healthcare delivery system in the public sector
Source: SARS Expert Committee (2003, p. 9).

environmental hygiene, and women's interests. As can be seen in Figure 4.1, the Department of Health (DH) is the executive arm of the HB in policy execution. DH is at the same time the health adviser to the government and a health advocate to the lay public. Another important body in the health scene in Hong Kong is the Hospital Authority (HA), which is a statutory and independent body established in 1990 under the Hospital Authority Ordinance to manage all public hospitals, and is responsible for the provision of all public hospital services in Hong Kong. Funded by the HB, the HA manages 43 hospitals and institutions with a total capacity of 29,500 beds and employs some 53,000 staff (LegCo 2004, p. 233). Currently, public hospitals receive 82 percent of all hospital admissions and are also responsible for some (15 percent) primary care services (SARS Expert Committee 2003, p. 5). The HA is governed by the Hospital Authority Board (21 members), which formulated the policies and monitors the performance of the HA management.

The high staff costs and a low staff turnover rate together with an increasing demand for medical services have squeezed the financial position of the HA. This problem was formidable in Hong Kong then, because the city, hard hit by the Asian financial crisis in 1997, had five consecutive years of fiscal deficit. For the HA alone, its budget deficit in 2001/2 was HK$2 billion (US$256 million) (Shek 2002). Government funding to the HA was cut by 5 percent for three consecutive financial years, starting from 2000/1 (Hospital Authority of Hong Kong 2002). In order to solve the financial problem, the HA adopted a series of measures, including the implementation of a cluster management system from 2001, to improve the cost-effectiveness of the public medical services. Under the cluster system, all public hospitals are divided geographically into three mega and four intermediate clusters. The chief executive of a major hospital within the same group is appointed as the cluster chief executive, taking charge of the management, planning, development, and operation of medical services as well as resources allocation of all hospitals of his or her cluster (Hospital Authority of Hong Kong 2002). All the Cluster Chief Executives are directly under the supervision of the Chief Executive of the HA. There have been mixed reviews of the cluster management system. Major concerns include the legitimacy and accountability of the clusters and cooperation between clusters. Frontline health workers also worry that their concerns and complaints cannot reach the HA's top management (Chou 2003). Besides cluster management, the HA has been downsizing its establishment, which has resulted in a heavier workload for the remaining staff. Hence when the SARS epidemic hit, the establishment of the HA was stretched to its utmost limit.

SARS: Global, Regional, and Local Nexus

Referred to by the World Health Organization on March 15, 2003 as SARS, the epidemic infected 8,422 patients in 32 countries and claimed 916 lives worldwide (SARS Expert Committee 2003, p. 79). Hong Kong, Taiwan, the Chinese mainland, and Macau together accounted for 91.9 percent and 90.5 percent of the respective numbers of patients and deaths. In Hong Kong, 1,755 people were infected and, among them, 300 died (ibid., p. 79). About 22 percent (386) of those infected were healthcare workers, eight of whom died. The epidemic left a permanent imprint on many families, and 75 children lost one or both of their parents (LegCo 2004, p. 1). According to the Asian Development Bank, SARS cost the Asian economies a total of US$18 billion (Leu 2003, p. EDT5). The China mainland alone lost US$6.1 billion, about 0.5 percent of GDP. Hong Kong lost US$4.6 billion, about 2.9 percent of GDP (ibid. 2003, p. EDT5). Another estimate of total economic loss in the Far East was US$30 billion (Mingpao 2003).

As argued by the SARS Expert Committee (2003, p. 3), "[t]he SARS epidemic in Hong Kong must be seen in geographical, socio-economic, political and organisation context." In fact, the SARS epidemic needs to be appreciated with a historical perspective as well. Not only was the SARS epidemic something new – and hence it was difficult for medical professionals to understand its properties and bring it under control – but the challenge was related to the fact that Hong Kong and the China mainland have had little experience in coordinating urban growth and management for over half a century. In fact, China's incessant reforms to cope with a rapidly globalizing economy mean that the social infrastructure, both at the central and local levels, has been unsettled and hence not really prepared for the SARS outbreak, whereas Hong Kong's fragmented governance structure and a government budget that was in deficit in the early 2000s had hindered a concerted front to fight the SARS battle, at least in the first few months when the city was besieged by the epidemic.

On the other hand, China as a socialist country has tight control over the media, which remain the mouthpiece of the Communist Party and the government (Zheng and Lye 2003, p. 49). As a result, very little was known about the rumored outbreak of atypical pneumonia in Guangdong in late 2002. A worst-case scenario was indeed put forward by Luk (2003): China might not have the necessary information to share with Hong Kong. A major component of China's heroic economic reforms is decentralization of administrative and urban management functions, which include health services. As a result, the central or even provincial governments are often left in the dark when something bad happens at the local level. As local governments have little experience in managing urban growth and development in a socialist market economy, human resources and the institutional set-up leave a lot to be desired. The situation had probably been worse in secondary cities. Similarly, the central government has to learn to adjust its changing role. Under these conditions, it is understandable that China simply did not have the spare capacity to work together with Hong Kong in fighting SARS.

The development of the epidemic to a "global" scale has much to do with Hong Kong as an international city. Hong Kong has performed the role as a major bridge between China and the rest of the world ever since the mainland's Open Door Policy in late 1978. Such a role has allowed Hong Kong to thrive through epochs of economic restructuring in the latter part of its colonial days and after its political reunification with the mainland. The downside of being a major bridge between a reforming socialist country groping to integrate market mechanisms, with a Party-led top-down political and administrative framework, and a "globalized" world with well-developed protocols in the economic, social, and political arena cannot be better illustrated than in the SARS disaster. The world as a whole and Hong Kong in particular have learned an expensive lesson in the episode.

Figure 4.2 tries to capture, within the constraint of published information, the linkages of the global and local SARS epidemic in Hong Kong. Since it is difficult to trace all the SARS cases in Hong Kong, let alone the whole world, the figure is incomplete. It is generally believed that the 64-year-old retired medical professor Liu Jianlun from Guangzhou, who checked into the Metropole Hotel in Mongkok on February 21, 2003, was an index patient, infecting many overseas tourists who had stayed on the ninth floor of the hotel, which consequently led to the global epidemic in different parts of the world. It was reported that Professor Liu had been feeling unwell

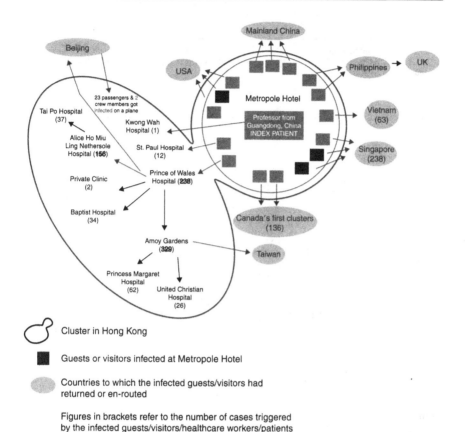

Figure 4.2 The SARS epidemic: the global and local impacts of the index patient in the Metropole Hotel

Source: Modified and synthesized from SARS Expert Committee (2003, pp. 35–52) and various newspaper reports.

since February 15, 2003 when he was in Guangzhou, but he still chose to come to Hong Kong because he and his family had to attend a wedding ceremony on February 21, 2003. When Professor Liu was admitted to the Kwong Wah Hospital on February 22, 2003, he had told the medical staff there that he had a virulent disease and so precautious measures were taken and no healthcare worker was infected there.

As shown in Figure 4.2, guests staying on or visiting the ninth floor of the hotel had led to seven clusters of infection in different parts of the world. The major ones involved a Chinese-American businessman who had stayed in the Metropole Hotel and then went to Vietnam, where he infected over 60 people. The businessman was sent back to the Princess Margaret

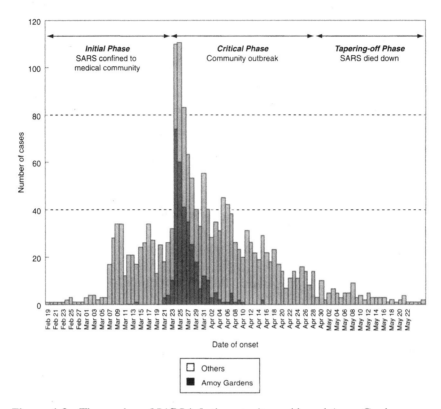

Figure 4.3 The number of SARS infections: territory-wide and Amoy Gardens
Source: Extracted from a PowerPoint pdf file presented by the then Secretary for Health, Welfare and Food on June 17, 2003 but according to SARS Expert Review (2003, p. 24), the date of onset was adjusted.

Hospital and eventually died. In Singapore, the return of the three visitors to the Metropole Hotel had caused an outbreak involving 238 infections, including 33 deaths. Two Canadians of mother and son relationship also died of SARS when they returned to Canada after staying in the Metropole Hotel. They led to the first cluster of 136 infections in Canada. The largest cluster of infection happened within Hong Kong. A visitor to the ninth floor of the hotel had eventually become an index patient for the unexpected outbreak in the Prince of Wales Hospital, which started on March 8, 2003 (Figure 4.3). One of the infected patients became an index patient in the infamous Amoy Gardens outbreak, where 329 people were infected, resulting in 42 deaths.

The SARS Outbreak in Hong Kong

The development of SARS in Hong Kong can be broadly divided into three phases: the initial, critical, and tapering off phases (Figure 4.3). This initial phase started with reports of atypical pneumonia outbreaks in Guangdong province in November 2002 and ended with the outbreak of this infectious disease in various medical establishments within Hong Kong in March 2003. Among all the healthcare institutes, the Prince of Wales Hospital received the hardest blow of all, since it admitted a SARS patient in early March. There were a total of 238 infections, involving 87 of the medical staff. During this stage, Hong Kong was identified as the origin of infections for Vietnam, Singapore, and Canada. On March 15, 2003, the WHO officially named the disease Severe Acute Respiratory Syndrome, and issued a travel advisory and specified the disease's main syndromes and signs. The government of Hong Kong had insisted that there was no community outbreak of SARS and had refrained from aggressive and dramatic actions to contain the epidemic. A critical turning point came on March 19, 2003, when the government confirmed the need to investigate the Metropole Hotel, more than three weeks after Professor Liu, the index patient who caused the global outbreak, first checked in. This initial phase ended when the Chief Executive of the HA was admitted to hospital with SARS symptoms.

As reflected in the epidemic curve in Figure 4.3, there was a clear community outbreak by late March 2003, by which time over 200 residents in Amoy Gardens had come down with SARS. The increased number of patients had led to numerous hospital outbreaks during this stage. The WHO revised its travel advisory to international travelers, recommending postponement of all but essential trips to Hong Kong and Guangdong province. To contain the epidemic, the Chief Executive set up and convened the first meeting of the Chief Executive's Steering Committee (CESC) on March 25, 2003 to take over the HB Task Force's role as the overall commanding body, and initiated a number of stringent and important measures: the introduction of a home confinement policy; the enhancement of health check measures at the boundary; dissemination of information to the public and the international community; the enhancement of investigation work and liaison with the Mainland authorities and protection of the elderly; and so on (LegCo 2004, p. 238).

During this period, the then Director of Health (Dr Margaret Chan, now Director-General of the WHO) designated medical centers for the early detection of cases in the community (from March 31, 2003) and announced a statutory home confinement scheme (from April 10, 2003) (SARS Expert Committee 2003, p. 95). She also issued an unprecedented isolation order to those residents in Block E of Amoy Gardens *in situ* on March 31, 2003. However, when it transpired that the faulty sewerage and drainage system might have led to the vertical spread of the disease in Block E, the residents were evacuated to three government holiday camps to continue the ten-day period of quarantine (SARS Expert Committee 2003, p. 50). During this period, schools were closed and communication channels with central and provincial authorities were established to cooperate in the fighting of SARS.

At the height of fear and grief, many individuals and civil society organizations worked together to turn the crisis into opportunities for change, creativity, and innovation. The alumni of the Chinese University of Hong Kong, which runs the Prince of Wales Hospital, were among the first to set up the "We Care Foundation" in March 2003, to support frontline medical workers to fight against SARS (Loh and Welker 2004, p. 224). The University of Hong Kong started the WAY ("We Are with You") Movement, which redefined SARS as "Sacrifice, Appreciation, Reflection, and Support" (Chan 2003, pp. 138–9). SARS had actually made society's "invisible" social infrastructure visible: "NGOs set up hotlines and emergency services, and mobilis[ed] volunteers to … [help] underprivileged people to clean up their homes … senior government officials initiated an education trust for children who had lost their parents to SARS … [which] raised US$3 million in less than two weeks. A group of corporations and conscientious community leaders started another fund to help infected patients and their families. They raised more than US$2 million in one day for disbursement by the Social Welfare Department … The "Fear-buster" movement also pulled together a large group of expatriates to work together to promote Hong Kong locally and internationally … Individuals [contributed] time and expertise to help Hong Kong overcome this crisis" (ibid., pp. 139–40).

The number of new cases had continued to drop after April. Since early May, fewer than ten new cases were reported per day. The WHO removed its travel recommendations for Hong Kong in late May. After the last case of SARS was reported in Hong Kong on June 11, on June 23, 2003, the WHO removed Hong Kong from the areas with recent local transmission. In addition to Hong Kong, the SARS epidemic also died down in other areas, such as Toronto, Taiwan, Hebei, Guangdong and Tianjin provinces, and so on. The phase ended with the WHO's declaration, on July 5, 2003, that SARS had been contained worldwide.

Health Governance Issues Highlighted in the SARS Epidemic

The absence of regional health governance

According to the SARS Expert Committee (2003, p. 111), an expert investigation report on the outbreak of atypical pneumonia in the Guangdong province was produced on January 23, 2003, but it was not sent to the authorities in Hong Kong, nor to the WHO. In fact, the government of Hong Kong did not take any action until February. It was reported in *Apple Daily*, a popular newspaper in Hong Kong, on February 11, 2003 that SARS started in a place called Heyuan on January 3, 2003 and the patient died. On January 10, 2003 the epidemic spread to Zhongshan, infecting over 100 people, half of which were healthcare workers. In mid-January, infection was found in the cities of Shunde and Dongguan. According to the Legislative Council Select Committee on SARS (2004, p. 29), on February 10, 2003, the then Director of Health had instructed her colleague to follow up the news reports with health officials in Guangdong through telephone, fax, and letter on "the number of people affected, their age group, causative agent, signs and symptoms, treatment and fatality." However, there was no response to all these requests. Later, the Secretary of Health, Welfare and Food advised the Director of Health to contact the Ministry of Health in Beijing directly and then a channel of communication was established. This "circuitous" route of contact reflects the "One Country, Two Systems" mentality. As a SAR, Hong Kong should communicate directly with Beijing. Furthermore, since information on infectious diseases is classified as a state secret, this probably explains why the authorities in Guangdong had chosen to remain silent upon Hong Kong's request for information.

On February 12, 2003, it was confirmed by the Guangdong province that from November 16, 2002 to February 9, 2003, six out of the 21 cities in Guangdong had found 305 cases of atypical pneumonia, 105 of which involved healthcare workers. The epidemic had caused five deaths (*Hong Kong Business Journal* 2003). However, this announcement had little impact on establishing dialogue mechanisms between the health authorities on both sides of the border. As Hong Kong places an emphasis on Western medicine, whereas China blends Western and traditional Chinese medicine, the two systems are not compatible. Coupled with the "One Country, Two Systems" arrangement, few had thought about inviting medical experts from Guangdong to assist Hong Kong's battle against the epidemic when it started to unfold. Nor had the health sector dispatched any delegation to Guangdong to learn from their experience.

In fact, China's reforming medical system may not be ready for cooperation. For instance, the US-style Centre for Disease Control and Prevention on the mainland was only established in 2002, and also the Ministry of Health needs to head a national network of centers, so that the practice of reporting, tracking, and tackling new diseases can be further developed (Duckett 2003). In other words, the sudden spread of the epidemic had presented a huge challenge to the reforming and decentralizing healthcare system and might have exposed their lack of competence in the face of crisis. Luk (2003) argues that we can infer that the lack of pathology reports on the atypical pneumonia implies a lack of macro-control in the health sector by the central government. This speculation may contain some truth, as the central government had apologized formally for its belated reporting of the SARS outbreak, and it fired the Minister of Health and the mayor of Beijing after a retired Chinese military doctor claimed that there were more cases of SARS and resulting deaths than the official figures showed (Mingpao 2003). However, Fidler (2004, p. 107) argues that, "the saga of the SARS outbreak in China tells the story of the humbling of the sovereignty of a rising great power. The humbling of Chinese sovereignty occurred in both traditional public health areas, such as surveillance and response, and matters of political ideology. As a result of its response to SARS, China suffered extensive and withering scrutiny and criticism of its attitude toward public health, its health care system, and the political ideology underlying governance in that country." The episode points to the need of a mode of regional health governance to cope with borderless diseases.

Fragmented local health governance

According to the SARS Expert Committee (2003, p. 12), the HB, DH, and HA were responsible for the following during the SARS epidemic:

- The HB: mapping out a strategy for managing and controlling the epidemic, coordinating efforts in the health sector, and overseeing Hong Kong's emergency response.
- The DH: under the policy direction of HB, undertaking all the necessary public health functions, including disease surveillance, contact tracing, enforcement of public health legislation, liaison with HA and the health community, public education, and liaison with the mainland health authorities and the WHO and the international community.
- The HA: mobilizing and managing its resources in the public hospital system.

However, as commented by the Hospital Authority of Hong Kong Review Panel (2003, p. 19), the reality was that there was "an absence of a clear chain of command, contingency plan or formal mechanisms for bringing together the key decision makers in HA, DH and HB for the purpose of crisis management". In fact, the Secretary of the HB's repeated emphasis on the absence of a community outbreak in his communication with the lay public prior to March 24 (the day after the HA Chief Executive was admitted into hospital because of SARS infection) may have constrained a timely escalation of the government's position and action (ibid.).

HB: failed to conduct the "health orchestra"

The Secretary of the HB was looked upon to be the "commander" of the battle over SARS: preparing a strategy, and coordinating efforts within Hong Kong, and within the health sector in particular, to manage and control the epidemic. However, the HB does not have the necessary human resources support for policy formulation. According to the Legislative Council Select Committee's report, the Secretary of the HB first learnt about the outbreak at the Prince of Wales Hospital through media reports on March 11, 2003 (LegCo 2004, p. 69). Then he instructed the DH to inform the WHO (which triggered the global alert) to seek help. On March 13, 2003, he chaired a meeting with a senior expert from the Centers for Disease Control and Prevention in Atlanta, USA, a representative of the WHO, local experts in the field as well as health officials and executives, which led to the setting up of a HB Task Force on March 14, 2003 to monitor the outbreak of the disease, to oversee its control, to review the accumulated scientific knowledge of the causative agent, to develop a strategy to educate the public on personal hygiene, and to develop sector-specific guidelines (LegCo 2004, p. 235). However, no strategy was put forward to manage and control the epidemic.

The Secretary of the HB also lacked the capacity to coordinate the activities and responsibilities of the DH, the HA, and the private sector (SARS Expert Committee 2003, p. 88). In fact, a former legislator representing the constituencies of the health sector argued that "the private sector had been neglected in a compartmentalised health-care system. Private hospitals and doctors are looked at as problems, rather than as partners" (Benitez 2003). Although the line management relationship between the bureau and the department is clear, there is still a problem between the policy-making and the professional execution. For instance, the Secretary of HB has accountability for the health system as a whole, but the statutory public health powers are vested in the Director of Health (LegCo 2004, p. 88). If the Secretary of the HB has had problems coordinating the health sector, one can imagine how difficult it will be for him to be in charge of overseeing Hong Kong's emergency needs. After all, under the accountability system, his rank is the same as that of all the other Principal Officials.

Hence, at the height of the battle against SARS, the Chief Executive of the HKSAR set up and convened the first meeting of the CESC (Chief Executive's Steering Committee) on March 25, 2003 to take over the HB Task Force's role as the overall commanding body in steering the government's overall response (LegCo 2004, p. 238). The Inter-departmental Action Coordinating Committee was chaired by the Permanent Secretary of the HB and included members of over 25 bureaus, departments, and public bodies to coordinate the implementation of decisions made by the CESC and Secretary of the HB (ibid., p. 104). At that point, the Secretary of the HB's role was to personally coordinate the respective work of the HA and the DH and focus on the health sector (ibid., p. 238). The CESC had effectively directed a number of measures to contain the epidemic, reflecting to a large extent the power of a top-down, executive-led government.

DH: room for improvement in carrying out public health functions

The role of the DH is in the prevention, assessment, and control of the outbreak of infectious diseases in Hong Kong (LegCo 2004, p. 234). However, poor linkages with HA and private family doctors hampered surveillance work during SARS. Except for a sentinel surveillance scheme joined by selected family doctors, very little surveillance data were available from the private sector (SARS Expert Committee 2003, p. 115). There was an absence of comprehensive laboratory surveillance (ibid.). At the early stage of the SARS outbreak, the DH and the HA had two separate SARS databases for public health and clinical treatment purposes, which were not compatible (ibid., pp. 116–17). It was only on March 24, 2003 that the two systems were combined with the police database to form a commonly accessible database.

The DH's capability in contact tracing was also questioned. The DH was informed of Professor Liu's admission to the Kwong Wah Hospital on February 23, 2003 and investigation then started. According to the Legislative Council Select Committee's investigation, the medical officer in charge of investigation thought that for a respiratory tract infection, the place of residency was not significant and so the hotel was not investigated. On March 8, 2003, the same officer was informed by the Ministry of Health of Singapore that the three tourists who were hospitalized after traveling to Hong Kong had stayed at the Metropole Hotel. On March 13, 2003, the DH was notified of a severe community-acquired pneumonia case who had stayed in the Metropole Hotel, and still no action was taken to investigate the hotel. It was only after the DH learnt (from a fax sent by Health Canada on March 18, 2003) about an index patient in Canada for the SARS outbreak in Toronto, who had stayed at the Metropole Hotel, that investigations began at the hotel (LegCo 2004, pp. 38–9). Had the Metropole connection been identified earlier, the "global" infection might have been minimized.

The DH's exercising of legislative power through the Quarantine and Prevention of Disease Ordinance (Cap.141) was also heavily criticized. As early as March 19, 2003 (the day on which the Metropole Hotel link was recognized), a professor related to the Prince of Wales Hospital had written a letter to DH urging the Director "to consider all possible measures including quarantine to contain the outbreak before it was too late" (LegCo 2004, p. 60). In fact, as early as March 17, 2003, the deputy director had asked her whether SARS should be made a statutory notifiable disease, and around March 24 the Secretary of the HB asked her again whether Hong Kong should follow Singapore in enacting quarantine laws. However, the DH showed reluctance to do so (LegCo 2004, p. 63). When the DH finally decided to amend the legislation on March 27, 2003 and exercise her power to issue an isolation order to residents in Block E of Amoy Gardens, more than half of the residents had already left.

There are also clear deficiencies within the DH in terms of manpower and specialist expertise in "field epidemiology and infectious disease control, information systems support, and insufficient public health resources to cope with a large-scale community outbreak" (SARS Expert Committee 2003, p. 124). One reason, according to the SARS Expert Committee, is disproportionate funding for public health services *vis-à-vis* the public hospital system. In the 2003 financial year, recurrent public expenditure on healthcare services was HK$31.8 billion, HK$29.2 billion (91.8 percent) of which was allocated to the HA, compared to HK$2.6 billion (8.2 percent) to the DH.

The DH's interface with the HA and other academic institutions related to health matters also needs to be streamlined. During the SARS epidemic, there had been reports of the DH and academic units within hospital doing double contact tracing; and the HA and the DH issuing differing guidelines to elderly homes. Private-sector doctors had complained about the government's failure to provide private clinics with clear guidelines on how to identify patients with SARS, and so on (Moy 2003). According to the Legislative Council (LegCo 2004, p. 35), the DH should have taken proactive steps to obtain information through other channels, apart from approaching the Ministry of Health in Beijing and the WHO.

HA: unprepared and resource-strapped

In response to the atypical pneumonia rumors in China, a Working Group on Severe Community-Acquired Pneumonia (represented by the DH) was established in February 2003 by the HA head office. According to the Legislative council (LegCo 2004, p. 18), the HA head office had issued a memorandum on surveillance on Severe Community-Acquired Pneumonia (SCAP) on February 12, 2003 and a set of frequently asked questions on the management of SCAP on February 21, 2003, though frontline doctors did not seem to be aware of these documents. In response to the Prince of Wales Hospital outbreak, a "Cluster Meeting on Atypical Pneumonia" was established on March 13, 2003. Although HA had put in place an outbreak-control plan to deal with outbreaks of infectious diseases of public health significance, the plan did not specify: the command structure; an action plan; cross-cluster, inter-hospital, and other patient movement; manpower and expertise deployment; and guidelines for closing a major part of the facility and suspending certain hospital services (LegCo 2004, p. 255). It is no wonder that during the SARS outbreak there was a clear failure of communication and a lack of clarity about roles and responsibilities, such as frontline staff complaining about their being alienated in the decision-making process, and that HA Board members felt that they were not adequately involved in decisions being made by senior executives (SARS Expert Committee 2003, p. 90). Without a system for internal feedback, the management was perceived to be remote and busy in meetings (HA Review Panel 2003, p. 23).

The SARS epidemic shows that the HA has poor infection control knowledge, practice, and standards. According to the SARS Committee (2003, pp. 121–36), these include the absence of a predetermined outbreak control plan or communication strategy clarifying the respective roles and responsibilities of the HA, the DH, and the universities; poor infection control in terms of structure, staff training, and awareness of necessary practices; deficiencies in the hospital environment, such as ward design, spacing of beds, and ventilation; and problems with the availability, supply, and distribution of drugs and equipment, including personal protection equipment.

The situation was worsened with the admission of the Chief Executive of the HA to hospital on March 23, 2003, because the leadership role became fragmented. The key leadership roles during crisis had never been clearly established and became increasingly confusing, especially when the HA Chief Executive continued to be involved from his hospital bed after the first week of hospitalization (HA Review Panel 2003, p. 21). The designation of the Princess Margaret Hospital (PMH) as a SARS Hospital on March 6, 2003 turned out to be a mistake, because of the sudden surge of SARS patients associated with the Amoy Gardens outbreak (HA Review Panel 2003, p. 21).

An active civil society combating SARS:
under-utilized resources in the health territory

Over 1,000 civil society organizations, including community-based organizations, non-governmental organizations, labor unions, religious groups, professional organizations, universities, and foundations, had fostered partnerships, contributed knowledge and creative ideas, provided expertise, and shared social capital to fill the gaps that could not be plugged by an executive-led and top-down mode of governance (Thompson and Yow 2004, p. 218). For instance, in March 2003, a group of four young computer engineers started listing SARS-infected buildings in Hong Kong on the web, eventually forcing the government to publish its official list (Loh and Welker 2004, p. 225). SARS had revealed to the compartmentalized bureaucracy a strong and powerful message that it should not ignore: that civil society has a huge capacity in organizing itself, and should be duly treated as a strategic and significant partner in health governance.

Conclusion: Curbing the Global Epidemic at the Local Level

The Hong Kong experience has highlighted the intricate relationships of health governance at different geographical levels with varied and evolving histories, culture, and political economic practices. As reflected in the SARS battle, poor communication is probably the Achilles' heel of the local health sector: Hong Kong knew very little about the epidemic in China, not to mention about working together for disease surveillance; communication between the DH and the HA had left much room for improvement too, and the HB was not very effective in serving as the "commander in chief" during the crisis; there was almost communication breakdown during the early stage of the crisis between the HA management and the frontline healthcare workers; and communication between the government, the HA, and the general public had left a lot to be desired. All these can be blamed for a lack of foresight in formulating a strategy and a basket of measures to tackle the potential health impacts of an increasingly globalizing world. Such an oversight probably can be explained by the government's philosophy, which is that the protection and maintenance of health is a personal responsibility. Hong Kong needs to realize that "health" should be regarded as a fundamental human right and an important resource for development, especially in face of a "risk society," and should start asking itself questions such as: How can impact assessments be used to identify potential threats to our society? What must be done to ensure that "health" matters in all related policy areas? How can the private and public health sectors work together to promote a healthy society? How can a fairer, more objective, and transparent mode of health governance be instituted? How can intelligence of disease or related information between Hong Kong and its immediate hinterland be improved? How can forces be joined internationally to tackle the "risk society"?

The SARS drama in Hong Kong reminds us that global epidemics have to be curbed at the local level, within a well-connected multi-scalar network that is vigilant both in monitoring and internal communication. The virus that knows no political boundaries in a globalizing world has ironically unveiled the various levels and layers of invisible barriers to concerted efforts of tracking down and containing a deadly infectious disease. It is indeed a humbling exercise for *Homo sapiens* to realize that in order to survive and sustain on planet Earth, we have to network and co-learn together as a global community, and that such efforts have to start at home, with an open mind and a readiness to cooperate and work in partnership and navigate a way out of historical, cultural, environmental, social, political, and economic differences at various geographical scales.

5

Surveillance in a Globalizing City: Singapore's Battle against SARS

Peggy Teo, Brenda S.A. Yeoh, and Shir Nee Ong

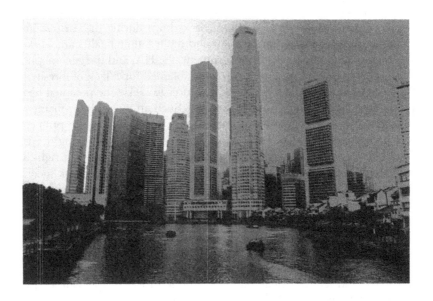

Introduction

With its rapid escalation between November 2002 and March 2003, SARS represented "globalisation's dark side" (*Streats* 2003, p. 3), hopping from Guangdong in China to other epicenters including Hong Kong, Taiwan, Vietnam, Singapore, and Canada. In response to what was undeniably a major challenge to urban governance based on a "hierarchical and hermetic system of nationally-based health policy" (Keil and Ali 2007, p. 848), Singapore, as with globalizing cities elsewhere, resorted to a slew of extraordinary measures to arrest the disease. In the absence of a coordinated global governance system to match the globality of SARS as a networked disease, governments tightened their grip on local containment strategies and in the process put to the test the reach of state surveillance and the degree of compliance among its citizens. In this chapter, we first explore the implications of surveillance strategies used during the outbreak in Singapore. For a city whose *raison d'être* depended on global connectedness, SARS resurfaced the dangers of overexposure, rekindled fears of security breaches, and renewed recognition of the city's material vulnerabilities. We show which specific groups of people were deemed as external threats and examine the emergent public discourse on the costs of keeping our borders open. Second, we investigate state and non-state, spatial and non-spatial strategies that had emerged to contain the disease. We unpack the broad public discourse on the contagion effects of SARS and the need to wage a "war" against the "epidemic" as well as how members of society recalibrate urban geographies through constructing "safe" and "unsafe" zones in reaction to contagious outbreaks.

By doing this, we are taking up Parr's (2002) call to understand the social lineaments around sickness and disease. Thus, we work through and understand SARS from a social perspective within the primary context of Singapore, taking into account the idea that specific locality issues are important to understanding outcomes (Moon 1990). Why was the island so successful (*Straits Times* 2003i,m) in its containment policies, disruptive as these were to economic and social institutions and to daily life? By examining the social responses to these measures, we hope to "relocate" public health research away from a purely medical focus. As Foucault (cited in Kearns 1994, p. 112) argued, illness may be biologically determined, but because it is observed and treated by others, we must address issues such as politics, discrimination, and civil rights (Swain et al. 1994; Gleeson 1996).

The Epidemiological Outbreak and Measures to Fence in SARS

Medical knowledge on SARS was very limited when it began its insidious spread in Singapore in early 2003. The disease was called "atypical pneumonia ... never before seen in humans" (WHO, cited in Chew 2003, p. 1). To separate the probable from suspected cases, temperature and other symptoms such as cough, breathing problems, laboratory test results, and X-rays were used. The index case patient, Patient A, was admitted into Tan Tock Seng Hospital on March 1, 2003 after returning from a trip to Hong Kong. While two others who accompanied this patient on the trip recovered, 24 of Patient A's primary contacts became infected. These included eight nurses, a health attendant, five patients in the same ward, and ten visitors. The first person to die, on March 25, 2003, was the father of Patient A. The second was the pastor of Patient A. SARS started off primarily as a nosocomial (hospital-acquired) infection. According to Gopalakrishna et al. (2004), the early stages were the most detrimental because lack of knowledge prevented quick action to isolate and contain, leading to the spread of SARS into the community. Infected individuals brought the infection from the hospital to another epicenter, Pasir Panjang Wholesale Market. Table 5.1 shows the profile of those infected. In total, there were 238 cases and a fatality

Table 5.1   Profiles of probable SARS cases

	Number	*%*
Gender		
Male	161	67.6
Female	77	32.4
Total	238	100.0
Median age in years (age range of infected persons in brackets)	35 (1–90)	–
Number of deaths	33	13.9
Date onset of first probable case	February 25, 2003	–
Date onset of last probable case	May 5, 2003[a]	
Profile of cases		
Healthcare workers	97	40.8
Family/household members	55	23.1
Inpatients	31	13.0
Visitors to hospital	20	8.4
Social contacts	15	6.3
Imported	8	3.4
Co-workers in Pasir Panjang Wholesale Market	3	1.3
Taxi drivers	2	0.8
Flight stewardess	1	0.4
Undefined	6	2.5
Total	238	100.0
Location of transmission		
Hospital/nursing home	178	74.8
Household	33	15.5
Overseas	8	3.4
Community	7	2.9
Pasir Panjang Wholesale Market	3	1.3
Taxi	2	0.8
Flight	1	0.4
Undefined	6	2.5
Total	238	100.0

[a] This does not include the single isolated case that occurred in September 2003, involving a researcher working on the virus in a research laboratory.
Source: WHO (2003c).

rate of 13.9 percent (WHO 2003c). It was not until May 30, 2003 that the WHO removed Singapore from the list of countries affected by SARS. On September 9, 2003, a new but isolated case occurred, as a laboratory researcher working on the virus became infected. No further cases have been reported since then.

The high fatality rate and the rapid spread caused much concern. To elicit the cooperation of the public to contain the disease, Singaporeans were warned about the methods of transmission; for example, close contact (droplets), and the length of time the virus was expected to stay alive on a surface (*Straits Times* 2003d). The incubation period was defined as ten days before the onset of symptoms. Singaporeans were also informed how the initial index case was imported from Hong Kong and the subsequent spread of SARS was traced over time and space, both locally and on a global basis.

Based mostly on biomedical information about the disease, the Singapore government designed isolation and containment strategies. In the first instance, Tan Tock Seng Hospital was designated the SARS hospital. Isolation wards were set up and arrangements made for special ambulances to transport SARS cases to the hospital. Doctors were not allowed to practice in more than one hospital during the SARS outbreak period and a certain number of healthcare workers were dedicated to provide care in the SARS wards. A "No Visitors" rule was imposed for all public hospitals except those treating children and obstetric cases. There was extensive use of N-95 masks, gloves, shoe and head covers, goggles, and gowns. Frequent hand washing, change of clothing, and disinfection of facilities and isolation rooms were carried out (Chew 2003; Leung and Ooi 2003). A ring of protection had thus been set up.

Outside the hospitals, contact tracing and home quarantine were put in place to further tighten the grip around the disease. Checks were constantly done to monitor people. In all public places, individuals had to have their temperature taken (later, thermal scanners were introduced) before they were allowed into public buildings, offices, and some residential locations. Common areas – for example, elevators, public toilets, and hawker centers – were disinfected more frequently. Schools, kindergartens and childcare centers were especially vigilant in an effort to protect the children. In fact, schools were closed for two weeks. In addition, a special television channel was set up to educate Singaporeans on preventive measures. Here, details were disseminated on what to do if one suspected oneself or family members to be infected. Doctors were instructed by the Ministry of Health (MOH) on diagnostics and containment/protection strategies such as the setting-up of fever stations away from the main human thoroughfare.

As a globalizing city-state, Singapore is extremely open to people coming for leisure, work, education, or other reasons. The airport, port, road, and rail openings into the country were equipped with thermal scanners, each costing SGD90,000 (*Straits Times* 2003h). Foreign workers who came to Singapore to work as construction workers, including those from the Peoples' Republic of China (PRC), were subject to a 14-day quarantine. Foreign professionals working in Singapore, as well as Singaporeans who had visited SARS-affected countries, were asked to voluntarily quarantine themselves for ten days. Students were likewise asked to do so and to declare their overseas visits to the school. Anyone who had a temperature above 37.5 °C was asked to stay away from school or work.

From the many recommendations and policies implemented in Singapore, it is clear that medical understanding of contagion guided policies on containment. These seriously affected the daily routines of many Singaporeans and disrupted people flows from outside the city-state. How did Singaporeans react to quarantine and confinement, especially if the former entailed the use of web cameras for policing? Should the names of those who were served such orders be made public? Would public naming infringe the privacy and rights of individuals? Did hospitals have a right to prevent Singaporeans from seeing their loved ones who were ill and who needed their moral support? Evidently, Singaporeans sensed unequal distributions of power (Dyck and Kearns 1995). Health, being basic to human endeavor, may be regarded as a foundational justification for government action. However, not everyone accepts the diminution of individual autonomy and privacy in exchange for collective benefits (Gostin 2001). Certainly there will be degrees of acceptance in such social contracts, even if they pertain to the "new global threat" (Koh et al. 2003). These form the grist for understanding the disease from a social point of view, with regard to which the next sections outline three broad areas of discussion: how security becomes redefined as global movements of people threaten to spread infectious diseases; social responsibility in maintaining surveillance and control for good public health; and fear in shaping perceptions of safe and unsafe places when infectious diseases threaten.

Global Linkages in a Time of Crisis

In conventional security terms, since statehood is tied to territory, movements of population can undermine security, as people have long been known to be responsible for the transmission of disease. As the flows of people increase in contemporary times, the rhetoric used in conventional discourse on security is now employed for disease; for example, we talk about the "fight against disease" or use the term "a time bomb" (Thomson 1997, cited in Graham and Poku 1998, p. 226). For nations that are well plugged into the global economy, such movements can only grow in the foreseeable future. Will the potential threats to health and security be put aside for more immediate benefits?

To understand Singapore's reaction to SARS, there is a need to understand Singapore's rationale for sustaining "exceptionalism" in the global context. Leifer (1998, p. 19), for example, wrote that Singapore's "circumstances and condition as a city state ... are *sui generis* in the modern world". Agreeing, Ow (1984) says that Singaporeans have a perennial "crisis mentality." They are constantly reminded by the government that Singapore's position in the global economy is a very vulnerable one. Singaporeans need to work hard to sustain the country's economic and social growth. This mindset has helped to direct Singaporeans' energies in the same direction. In 2003, Singapore recorded a GDP of SGD38,023 per capita, compared to SGD1,567 per capita in 1965 when the country first became independent (Statistics Singapore 2004a). Much of the growth has been attributed to the purposeful global engagement of the island's economy. While Foreign Direct Investments (FDI) into the country was SGD217 billion at the end of 2001, Singapore also invested SGD131 billion abroad (Statistics Singapore 2004b). As a business epicenter, Singaporeans have to act responsibly so that investors, entrepreneurs, and business executives will still continue to come. At all costs, investment confidence in the island should not be diminished by the SARS outbreak (*Business Week* 2003).

In addition, Singapore is a cultural marketplace in which "culture and the arts ... form important strands in ... our city life" (Ministry of Information and the Arts 1998/99, p. 1). The global linkages mean that fragments of people and cultures hailing from different parts of the globe are expected in Singapore. Many of these are sojourners, people circulating among different cities, or shuttling between the global city and the home nation. As national borders become more porous in keeping with the pace of globalization, transnationalism, describing the way people straddle "home" and "host," becomes more common. Thus, besides the 7.5 million visitors who passed through in 2002, Singapore's transnational profile also includes foreign talent who are highly skilled and highly paid professionals, the 650,000 low-waged unskilled migrant workers who come for two-year contracts to work on the construction sites or as domestic maids, and expressive specialists who are creative individuals and who participate in the cultural scene in areas such as art, fashion, design, photography, film-making, writing, music, and cuisine (Teo et al. 2004).

Openness of the economy and society has assisted the country in the past and this quality is fundamental to its global city aspirations. What happens, however, in a time of crisis such as the SARS threat? Will the fluid flows of people coming into the country for business, work, study, or leisure be deemed as "overexposing" Singaporeans to the SARS virus? Exactly who becomes labeled an "outsider" at this time, and how much will openness continue to be valued? It is to these issues and questions that the following sections will explore.

Social Responsibility, Surveillance, and Control

Social responsibility is a rhetoric that has often been used in Singapore to marshal the people toward the same goal. Chua (1995) suggests that the successes arising from this approach has given the People's Action Party (PAP) political legitimacy in Singapore and in part accounted for its re-election time and again. The ideological framework of "national survival," which sees threats emanating from outside of Singapore as well as from within (e.g., Singaporeans who broke quarantine orders), helps to discipline society. During the height of the outbreak, political leaders talked about the "war" against SARS and fighting at the "battlefront" (*Straits Times* 2003a) in an attempt to rally Singaporeans to work cooperatively with the state. What is the public reaction to this discourse?

In the neoliberal context of contemporary societies such as Singapore, Fischer and Poland (1998) assert that community policing in public health is no longer as coercive and interventionist. Instead, discipline and regulation is less punitive (Foucault 1979, 1991). Formal processes from the state recede in the governance of public health, while self-regulatory civil and individual mechanisms come forward. Using knowledge and raising issues related to risk and responsibility, individuals and communities are moved to act independently or as a group to manage and reduce harm in public health maintenance. Self-regulation by these "responsibilized" subjects (Fischer and Poland 1998, p. 188) is considered progressive, since it involves voluntary action from private, civil, and commercial institutions. However, in a country where state influence is as strong as it is in Singapore, how much confidence does the leadership place on self-regulation? Raising public consciousness is presumably insufficient, because the state continues to impose surveillance strategies and use legislation to enforce compliance.

Enforcement poses less of a problem when it is carried out in public spaces, as the state's jurisdiction in the policing of these spaces is seldom questioned in Singapore. However, when surveillance and control begins to intrude into private spaces, it becomes more problematic. Using the argument that medical privacy is not absolute in the case of infectious diseases (Bayer and Fairchild 2002), surveillance and control throws into relief many issues concerning human rights, freedom as well as equality. Since new technologies such as detection devices and cameras help to transcend space, we ask how much infringement can be tolerated.

Safe and Unsafe Spaces

For humans, spaces are not isotropic or homogeneous, but laden with meaning such that behavior becomes affected by perceptions of these spaces. For example, fear, especially of the unknown, can strongly influence behavior. In this study, we uncover the extent to which fear of SARS affected the spatial behavior of people as they constructed "safe" and "unsafe" locations in their minds.

Methodology

Ideally, in-depth qualitative interviews would be effective in teasing out the nuances in public opinion on SARS. However, there was the ethical issue of exposing interviewers to infection, in addition to time and money constraints. Hence, we opted for the telephone questionnaire survey method, as this would give us a good overview of public opinion. After an initial pilot study in early June 2003, the actual survey was conducted in mid-June to end July 2003 on Singaporeans and permanent residents. Snowballing was used to construct a sample that was close to the national profile. A team of 69 trained surveyors was asked to use its contacts to get the sample profile assigned to them.

The questionnaire survey comprised sections on the demographic characteristics of the respondents; the implications of SARS on Singapore's open economy and society; surveillance and control as preventive measures to curb SARS; and the spatial avoidance behavior of the public. Respondents were asked whether they agreed with the measures that were implemented and if they avoided certain places. As the study was conducted close to the height of the SARS outbreak, we did not find statistically significant variations across socio-demographic variables. This tallies with the findings of Quah and Lee (2004), who reported variations only for the preventive measure of washing hands. More women and people aged above 35 took this preventive measure.

A total of 650 surveys were completed, of which 634 were successful. The data was entered into SPSS for analysis and secondary sources of information were consulted, because newspaper reports and public inputs in the form of letters to the press provided valuable insights on public discourse.

Discussion

Global interconnections during SARS

As Singapore works toward global city status, global linkages figure prominently in the imagination of the average Singaporean. On the one hand, there was widespread support to curb the inflow of people who could carry the threat of SARS into Singapore. On the other, Singaporeans were practical enough to realize that total exclusion would have adverse effects on the economy and on jobs. This ambivalence over the "good" and "bad" aspects of globalization was revealed in the findings.

For instance, the high-traffic Malaysian border raised practical issues of surveillance because of its sheer volume and frequency. Open borders suddenly become problematic, as Singaporeans constructed visions of the "enemy" infiltrating into the country. Singapore was by no means the only country with such a perception. Thai airports turned back fliers who showed flu-like symptoms. Malaysia imposed a visa freeze on people from the PRC, Vietnam, Canada, Hong Kong, and Taiwan. The PRC hit back by banning tours to Malaysia, Thailand, and Singapore. At the height of SARS, many companies in Singapore imposed an informal non-essential travel ban. This measure is consistent with travel advisories about SARS-affected locations such as the PRC, Taiwan, Hong Kong, and Toronto. In our survey, 80 percent of the respondents were willing to stop travel to SARS-affected countries for business or leisure.

There were other nuanced imprints on globalization. While foreign talent and foreign workers are both necessary to the sustenance of a labor-short economy, the former is encouraged to take root in Singapore while the latter is subject to measures that ensure their transience in the city-state (Yeoh and Chang 2001). The cosmopolitanism in Singapore's vision of a global city is obviously not an all-inclusive one and when SARS presented a health problem, this discrimination became more apparent in the social landscape of Singapore. Although almost 78 percent of the respondents said that it was discriminatory to confine newly arrived foreign contract workers (the unskilled) compared to self-quarantine for employment pass holders (the skilled), the majority (83 percent) still agreed with the use of this measure as a way to combat SARS. In the end, one wonders if these exclusionary policies, which are for the most part supported by Singaporeans, relegate foreign contract workers to the equivalent of the "human flotsam and jetsam" mentioned by McNeill (1976, p. 120).

Besides the foreign workers, PRC students studying in Singapore also bore the brunt of SARS. Since there were over 23,000 PRC students at that time (Ministry of Finance, Singapore Government 2003), to prevent them from going on home visits or leaving the country during the outbreak, their existing student visas would be revoked if they tried to leave. In addition, they had to pay a $1,000 deposit before leaving the country. In spite of the general consensus that SARS was dangerous, 42.7 percent of Singaporeans felt that revoking the visas was harsh. Nonetheless, 50.6 percent still stood by the idea that the visas ought to be revoked for students who insisted on returning to the PRC.

Where SARS had negative economic impacts, Singaporeans were less stringent about protecting the borders. For instance, it was then Prime

Minister Goh Chok Tong who led the drive to get ASEAN (Association of Southeast Asian Nations) members to work out cross-border controls at a summit on SARS convened in April 2003. This included dialogue with the PRC, Japan, and South Korea (*Today* 2003). As tourism was badly hit, Singapore's national carrier, Singapore International Airlines (SIA) dropped airfares in an attempt to bring back the tourists, while at the same time cutting the number of flights by 20 percent to save on costs (*Straits Times* 2003g). Awareness of the volatility of Singapore's economy to external forces led 84.5 percent of our respondents to agree that the airlines were correct to lower their airfares to bring tourists back.

Besides the airlines industry, the Meeting, Incentive, Convention, and Exhibition (MICE) sector, retail, food, and entertainment were also severely affected (Lorne 2003). While the government tried to cushion the economic impacts of SARS, at ground level, the measures had limited impact. Compared to Vietnam, the PRC, and Hong Kong, where the loss to GDP by tourism was only 15 percent, 25 percent, and 41 percent respectively in 2003, Singapore's loss was 43 percent (World Travel and Tourism Council 2003).

Travel bans, monitoring inbound tourist traffic by the use of thermal scanners, limiting business travel and making foreigners working or studying in Singapore feel excluded represent an increasing wariness about external threats. Where inter-country movements were once embraced, SARS surfaced the issue of security threats coming from without. Spaces were once again carved by political boundaries governed by disciplinary regimes so as to articulate discourses of "safety" and "protection" within localized contexts. As is the case with many protocols to protect the world's environment, when SARS hit, countries acted "local" even if they thought "global."

Social responsibility in the Singapore context

The analysis of social responsibility in public health begins with an examination of the social construction of the disease. SARS is suggested above as contagious and dangerous. The term "super-spreader" was used in the Singapore context on index cases. Index case Patient A, who eventually recovered, had her encounter with the disease featured on television (Mediacorp Channel 5 2003a). Her name was mentioned in the newspapers, generating a great deal of debate. Her "wrongdoing" was to bring SARS into Singapore and to have caused the death of loved ones. The psychological trauma that she went through was also recounted in the program, but the damage was already evident. She had caused harm and she felt marginalized by Singapore society. She was not the only one to feel ostracized. A physician talked about feeling victimized: "When I go out, people point at me and give me funny looks," she said, because they wondered why she delayed her decision to send her SARS patients to the hospital (*Straits Times* 2003k).

The local newspapers also reported that healthcare workers, nurses in particular, were avoided by Singaporeans (Mediacorp Channel 5 2003b; *Straits Times* 2003l) when they boarded the Mass Rapid Transit System. They could be easily identified, as they wore their uniforms. Some hospitals attempted to overcome this problem by making the nurses change into street attire before they left the hospital. Indeed, how the body is represented and read has significant bearing on surveillance and the use of space in the context of SARS. Lim (2003) also showed that Singaporeans feared discrimination and were ambivalent about naming quarantined individuals to non-family members. As surmised by a newspaper correspondent, "SARS is SARS, single syllabled and sibilant. The name hisses with the clarity of a deadly snake" (*Straits Times* 2003f, p. 16).

Compared to other diseases such as AIDS, bird flu, mad cow disease, or other recent epidemiological outbreaks, SARS had a far higher level of exposure in this small island state. There was a mobilization of resources of a magnitude that is rare in the country's history. Government, health workers, NGOs and volunteers, the private sector, schoolchildren, the military, and the police all took part in the battle against SARS. The unknown created a landscape of fear and brought the problem to crisis proportions. There was less concern about bird flu and mad cow disease, as it was believed that the authorities could block the entry of animal carriers and that Singapore, being a non-rural society, would be immune. AIDS was conceived as a lifestyle threat, but SARS was different because the carriers were human and so little was known about the disease.

We found much support for negative social constructions in our survey. In the study, the majority (59.1 percent) worried about SARS. Of these 375 respondents, over 90 percent worried about fatality and contagion. Alarm was thus fairly extensive in Singapore. Many also agreed with the state's call to contain the disease by exercising social responsibility on a daily basis. This included washing their hands (of which 88.8 percent of the total sample of 634 agreed), and exercising and getting enough rest (85 percent of total sample). Only 59.1 percent felt they should wear a mask, although very few actually did (unlike Hong Kong and the PRC) because the weather conditions made it impractical. The cognitive dissonance tallies with the findings of Quah and Lee (2004), who found that only healthcare workers consistently wore masks because of their high exposure to infection.

The high proportion of "responsibilized" citizens willing to cooperate has a fairly long history in Singapore. In the past, Singaporeans were urged by the PAP to submit to state policies because they were for the common good of the people. Ethnic, religious, and class differences were put aside so that all could reap the benefits of economic progress in the nation-state. The "war" rhetoric used on SARS echoed a similar approach to galvanize

Singaporeans to work toward a common goal during this period of "crisis." No fewer than ten cabinet and junior ministers gathered together to meet 1,800 grassroots, business, and youth leaders in mid-2003. The leaders emphasized that, "there is no excuse for anyone in Singapore not to know the part he has to play ... All of us as ordinary citizens ... have a part to [play in] fight[ing] SARS" (*Straits Times* 2003b, p. 1). It therefore came as no surprise that 93 percent of the total sample was willing to self-quarantine if the need arose. In addition, 77.4 percent was willing to reduce movement within their workplace or school.

Tensions, however, did exist, especially if the policing impinged on peoples' private spaces or threatened to make private spaces public. For example, 60.9 percent protested against broadcasting the names of those who were under such orders. One-third (33.1 percent) of the total respondents were against the installation of web cameras and tag surveillance of those under home quarantine orders. While this is certainly not a majority, for those whose private spaces were actually infringed upon, the reactions were quite negative. In a letter to the forum page of the local newspaper, a complainant under quarantine asked "the relevant authorities [to] enlighten" why CISCO personnel had to call at his home at "the ungodly hours of 2.00am on the first day and 2.30am on the second" (*Straits Times* 2003c, p. 14).

Other complaints about over-surveillance included the inflexibility of some schools. Many parents complained that their children were turned away because their temperature was above the standard 37.5 °C. Some medical practitioners reasoned that children often had higher temperatures as they tended to be more active. Consequently, teachers became more flexible. Nevertheless, a problem had emerged as parents found it difficult to make alternative childcare arrangements. In our survey, almost a quarter (24.4 percent) felt that the closure of schools was unnecessary. This problem was quickly tackled when the Ministry of Manpower sent a circular to the civil service to be flexible about allowing one member of such households to stay away from work. Private enterprise followed suit. A last example of over-policing is the "No Visitors" rule in hospitals: 18 percent of the respondents said that this policy was excessive. They felt that their loved ones needed their emotional support. Ultimately, the state had to respond and video links were made available to disgruntled individuals.

The numbers discussed in the preceding two paragraphs are by no means large, but they help to reveal the cognitive dissonance regarding public health policies. So long as the measures did not infringe on personal spaces or inconvenience an individual too substantially, there was support. Where this was absent, the complaints were forthcoming, causing the state to fine-tune its measures.

SARS and spatial barriers

Some sense of territoriality has been alluded to in the previous paragraphs. This section discusses the practice of space differentiation by Singaporeans during the outbreak. Spatial boundaries can be very specific as a means of managing risk, as in the case of selecting Tan Tock Seng as the "SARS hospital." The Pasir Panjang Wholesale Market was the other location that was closed off by the police. Besides boundaries that distinguished the "inside" from the "outside," spaces were also sectionalized as a precaution. All tertiary institutions divided their campuses into zones that could be isolated in case of an outbreak. Many companies in the private sector that felt that they could not withstand or afford disruptions in their businesses (e.g., broking houses) implemented crisis plans that included putting their officers into two or more locations. Working from home and teleworking were also temporary strategies that were employed until normality returned.

In our survey, we asked respondents how the outbreak of SARS had affected their movement across space. We asked if they purposely avoided the SARS hospital and other hospitals where SARS cases were also reported. We also asked about the wholesale market and about Changi Airport, where SARS was likely to be "imported" into the island. A spatially proximate public location to the SARS hospital was also included in the survey; namely, Novena Square Shopping Center, opposite Tan Tock Seng Hospital. From Table 5.2, the majority of the respondents avoided hospitals as a whole (72.2 percent), with 15.5 percent singling out the SARS hospital. Pasir Panjang Wholesale Market is a popular place to make bulk purchases for wet groceries such as vegetables, meat, and fruit. Not only are hawkers and restaurateurs found there, but even housewives make their way to the center on a daily basis. Due to the high volume of human traffic, the location was closed for 15 days while disinfection was carried out. Two-thirds of the respondents (62.5 percent) said that they avoided this place. High-risk locations such as polyclinics, private clinics, the airport, and buildings in close spatial proximity to possible "epicenters" were also mapped onto respondents' avoidance zones. One-quarter of the respondents (24.9 percent) said that they avoided travel by taxi. This arose because a taxi driver was infected by a SARS patient who he had unsuspectingly ferried. This taxi driver eventually died, but it was only in the autopsy that the connection was made. As a consequence, taxi companies in Singapore had to disinfect their taxis twice daily and the drivers were asked to not use the air-conditioning in their vehicles. Taxi drivers took their temperatures twice a day and had labels pasted onto a prominent location to say that they were "OK." Perceptions of SARS did indeed affect the spatial behavior of respondents, creating an intricate geography of "safe" and "unsafe" areas.

Table 5.2 What was avoided during the SARS outbreak (%)

Locations where infections were reported	
Tan Tock Seng Hospital	15.5
Singapore General Hospital	4.3
National University Hospital	3.5
Kandang Kerbau Hospital	1.9
Pasir Panjang Wholesale Market	62.5
High-risk locations	
All hospitals[a]	72.2
Polyclinics	53.2
Private clinics	32.2
Changi Airport	30.6
Novena Square Shopping Center	36.3
Travel in airplanes	30.3
Dental clinics	40.4
Low-risk locations	
Public housing estates and town centers	12.9
Neighborhood markets and hawker centers	10.6
Restaurants	16.9
Orchard Road shopping belt	18.0
Government buildings	11.2
Public transportation	
Travel in MRT and public buses	12.0
Travel in taxis	24.9
Others	
Meeting friends and relatives	8.0

[a] If the respondent selected "All hospitals," he or she could not select the named hospitals.
Source: Survey data.

Conclusion

Biomedical understanding of SARS was limited when the outbreak begun. Until more knowledge could be gathered, the WHO recommended conservative actions in order to be safe. Singapore's vulnerability left its leaders no choice but to take this approach. Draconian measures described above were implemented with little hesitation as to their social implications. From travel bans to outright penalties against foreigners working or studying in Singapore, SARS erected physical as well as mental borders against the globalizing aspirations of this city-state. As the seemingly incalculable disease increased both the messiness of urban life (Keil and Ali 2007) and the urgency for public order, security concerns were accorded a much higher priority compared to civil rights and democratic processes. Military metaphors were evoked in calling for a "war on SARS," further legitimizing the more drastic curbs on civil liberties.

In addition, the high level of public consciousness raised led to general agreement and support for the many initiatives taken by the state, as well as endorsement of the speed with which the problem was tackled. Singaporeans put up with the spatial barriers erected and voluntarily avoided high-risk places, as these were conceived as potentially dangerous spaces. Nonetheless, the politics of containment revealed that discrimination, exclusion, and protection of privacy remain social issues of some contention. As much as Singaporeans worried about the SARS threat, they also expressed discontent with intrusions into their privacy.

There are several lessons to be learnt from the SARS outbreak. In the immediate term, steps can be taken to deal with future threats similar to SARS. In Singapore, the government has already ascertained that one hospital is not sufficient for control of infectious diseases. Containment as a strategy has worked and will continue to be employed. However, the old priority of cost efficiency is being reviewed, because many infections had been transmitted in eight-bedder wards (Tambyah 2003).

In the longer term, the social disruptions need to be properly considered. Singapore's specific local context in terms of its historical experience may not be suitable for other countries. Taiwan also implemented the ring fence concept, but the quarantine order failed miserably. It was the healthcare workers (nurses and doctors) who broke free from their confinement and fled (*Straits Times* 2003e). Similarly, China reported instances of rioting in quarantine centers in two provinces (*Straits Times* 2003j). The politics of containment must examine receptivity to legislative decisions in the light of the historic and cultural specificity of the location. Transparency is something of a recent phenomenon in mainland Chinese politics (White III 2003). The sluggish response of Hong Kong was blamed on the desire to maintain business as usual in this international hub (Ngok 2003), poor communication among government bodies and with the public, as well as the weaknesses of health governance under the concept of "One Country, Two Systems" (Ng, Chapter 4). In the case of Taiwan, Ho (2003) attributes excessive politicization – for example, laying the blame on China and on the opposition – as the main problems for ineffective management of the disease. While most would subscribe to greater transparency and better coordination between government bodies at a national level as well as with the WHO and the CDC (Centers for Disease Control and Prevention), ultimately the response to infectious diseases will depend on social values, social conditions, and political contingencies. In the case of Singapore, we have objectively shown that there was fairly widespread support for measures that other countries were unwilling to adopt. The SARS episode revealed that compliance is effective and necessary for the containment of infectious diseases. The limited amount of questioning, the rapid rate of adoption, and the smooth carry-through of many of the policies came down to two things in Singapore: strong social discipline and the crisis mentality of the people. Whether these are replicable in a different time and space is another matter.

ACKNOWLEDGMENTS

This chapter is an abridged and slightly modified version of a paper that first appeared in *Health Policy* 72: 279–91 (2005), an Elsevier journal.

Part III

The Cultural Construction of Disease in the Global City

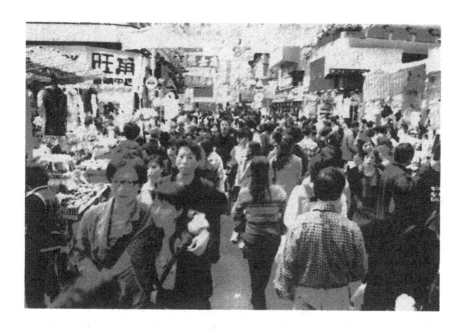

Introduction

S. Harris Ali and Roger Keil

Many facets of social relations and culture are taken for granted and therefore unquestioned during the course of everyday life. An extreme event may, however, shatter this taken-for-granted sense of reality to which we are accustomed under normal circumstances. In process, such events provide an opportunity to explicitly question and problematize those normally latent aspects of social and cultural life. By taking up this investigative opportunity, we may gain insights into how our culturally informed reality is constructed and constituted. Using the outbreak of SARS as an empirical referent, the chapters in this part implicitly adopt such an orientation. For example, in analyzing the North American newspaper coverage of the Toronto SARS outbreaks, in their chapter, Daniel Drache and David Clifton note that news coverage contributes to our social and cultural construction of reality by providing the public with important cues as to the scope, size, and importance of an outbreak. Furthermore, they point out that the cultural construction of an outbreak is critically influenced by the role played by media organizations as "gatekeepers" – that is, those in a position to decide where, when, and how the interests of various stakeholders, such as healthcare workers, governments, or members of the tourism/hospitality sector, are given voice in the public forum. In this light, the _framing_ of the outbreak by the media is one important factor in the cultural construction of disease. Thus, Drache and Clifton found that during the initial stages of the outbreak, the media coverage (particularly the international coverage) gave the *impression* that SARS was "out of control" in Toronto – a theme that is picked up by Claire Hooker's chapter on "SARS as a 'Health Scare.'"

Health scares are defined as those events that are perceived to endanger the lives of significant numbers in the population, thereby provoking strong societal reactions. Typically, health scares involve situations of large-scale fears, but with very low rates of actual mortality and morbidity – as Hooker argues was the case with SARS. For Hooker, the key dimension of SARS as a health scare was that it was a cultural construction that implicated economic systems, nationalist ideologies, and issues of border control; issues particularly relevant in our globalized age (for a more extended discussion of these matters, see the chapters in Part IV, "Re-Emerging Infectious Disease, Urban Public Health, and Global Biosecurity"). To analyze how these issues are implicated in health scares, as well as to address the more basic question of how health scares are promulgated or mitigated by social and cultural factors, Hooker focuses on the role of various actor-networks – professional or expert networks, communications networks, and staff or responder networks – which she analytically ties to existing research on the "social amplification of risk" framework.

The cultural dimensions of a disease outbreak may also vary in accordance with the political circumstances in which the outbreak occurs – a starting Peter Baehr adopts in his chapter, "City under Siege: Authoritarian Toleration, Mask Culture, and the SARS Crisis in Hong Kong." According to Baehr, the unique political circumstances of Hong Kong (i.e., the recent transition of political rule from the United Kingdom to China) fomented a unique reaction to SARS by the citizenry at both the political and cultural levels. To understand such reactions, Baehr develops the notion of "authoritarian toleration," in which the limited and circumscribed autonomy under the newly imposed Chinese rule had led to a political climate in which the Hong Kong citizenry distrusted and blamed the mainland Chinese officials for the problematic SARS response experienced during the early stages of the outbreaks. Baehr writes that although public wrath was directed toward upper-level mainland officials (and their Hong Kong representatives), public adulation was heaped upon local healthcare workers for their dedication, discipline, and sacrifice. In other words, "healthcare workers acquired prestige in direct proportion to the government's loss of it." At the same time, since much of the criticism of the government and praise for the healthcare workers came from non-mainland-dominated news outlets, their credibility increased. Interestingly, this was in contrast to the situation in Toronto, where Drache and Clifton found that the media coverage was problematic because their framing of the crisis was "drawing the spotlight away from healthcare workers and the more substantive health policy story."

Unique reactions to SARS were also found to have occurred at the cultural level. One notable example of this discussed by Baehr relates to the development of a "mask culture". It would be expected that in the chaotic times of an outbreak, a community might become socially fragmented as people searched for the parties responsible for the crisis. This was not the case in Hong Kong according to Baehr. Rather, a sense of social solidarity arose and the visible expression of this was seen in the donning of medical masks in public spaces. The wearing of such masks by citizens was taken as a gesture that socially acknowledged deference to the common good – that one was contributing to the public good by fulfilling one's obligation of taking action to protect the wider community. Baehr ends his piece by observing that an "epidemic is a menace to both the individual and the body politic" – a keen insight that especially resonates with the final selection of this part in terms of the cultural body politic.

In "'Racism is a Weapon of Mass Destruction': SARS and the Social Fabric of Urban Multiculturalism," Roger Keil and S. Harris Ali consider how racialized reactions to SARS in Toronto must be understood in terms of a broader conceptualization of how biopower is exercised in a post-9/11 era that is very much influenced in subtle and not-so-subtle ways by the master processes of globalized migration and neoliberalization. Since global cities are home to many different types of diaspora communities, the association of disease with race/ethnicity will have special significance for the lived experiences of such peoples. The cultural response to SARS in Toronto is illustrative of how disease outbreaks may touch the lives of such individuals on the micro level while also bringing to light the tenuous nature of urban multiculturalism at the more macro level – and it is the latter that is the primary focus of Keil and Ali's analysis. The racialization of SARS as a "Chinese disease" in Toronto could be traced to three broader, but inter-related, processes. The first is the historically based stigmatization of Chinese in North American cities, in which the space of "Chinatown" was symbolically associated with diseases such as smallpox, tuberculosis, and the bubonic plague, all of which were prejudicially attributed to the specific "habits and practices" of those living there. The second process involved in the linking of SARS with Chinese-Canadians was a function of more contemporary developments. Namely, the increasing public perception of modern China as a growing economic powerhouse has focused renewed Western attention to this part of the world. Accompanying this increased scrutiny is the reinforcement of particular Orientalist stereotypes, such as the allegedly unsanitary and unhealthy culinary habits of the Chinese. Thus, with SARS, an unusual amount of public and media attention seemed to focus upon the dietary choices of the Chinese, namely the consumption of civet cats, and the unhygienic conditions of the wet market where animals were slaughtered in preparation for consumption; both practices that were blamed for endangering the human population worldwide. Third, the popular press increasingly gave coverage to the idea that most, if not all, infectious diseases associated with the respiratory system have their origins in China. This notion in turn was linked to another prejudicial notion that served as the foundation for anti-Chinese racism, namely that Chinese should not be trusted because of their alleged authoritarian and secretive ways in covering up potential disease threats. The implications of these processes for the racialization of infectious disease, especially in the urban context, are only starting to be understood, but such issues will undoubtedly be of growing importance in the future as globalization intensifies the cultural and economic relationships between people from around the world (see Sarasin, Chapter 16, for a further theoretical discussion of this point).

6

The Troubled Public Sphere and Media Coverage of the 2003 Toronto SARS Outbreak

Daniel Drache and David Clifton

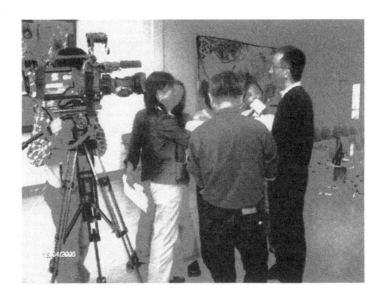

Introduction

As a center of the global SARS epidemic, Toronto was subjected to an extraordinary level of media scrutiny during the summer of 2003 (National Advisory Committee 2003). Nevertheless, most of the literature about the role of the media in the SARS crisis has focused on the Asian media or coverage of the Asian outbreak (Loh et al. 2004; Washer 2004; Wilson et al. 2004; Huang and Leung 2005; Ma 2005; Tian and Stewart 2005; Wallisa and Nerlich 2005; Wilkins 2005). While Bergeron and Sanchez (2004) examined the impact of the disease on Canadian students, and Bournes and

Ferguson-Paré (2005) examined the coverage of Toronto nurses, this is the first study to look holistically at the role of the news media in Toronto's SARS crisis.

Working in cooperation with the Canadian Media Research Consortium, Cormex Research, and the Robarts Center for Canadian Studies at York University in Toronto, we examined over 2,600 Canadian and American newspaper articles, and performed a detailed content analysis of slightly more than 1,600 SARS-related articles from the *Toronto Star*, the *Globe and Mail*, the *National Post*, *USA Today*, and the *New York Times*. The period researched was 91 days in length, running from March 16, 2003 to June 15, 2003. This chapter examines to what degree press coverage was balanced, fair, and adequate. It also carries out a content analysis of the coverage with respect to subject matter and tone; finally, it compares US and Canadian coverage of the SARS outbreak. The final section addresses the complex dynamics of the public sphere and information flows.

Framing the SARS Crisis

Fidler (2004) described SARS as the "first post-Westphalian pathogen," because it highlighted the extent to which globalization is impacting both the spread and containment of infectious diseases. Framing the SARS crisis in Toronto are what have become known as global cultural flows: the now ubiquitous and intense global exchanges of people, money, and information. These flows are asymmetrical, volatile, and disjunctive to markets and state authority (Featherstone 1990; Appadurai 1996, 2002; Drache 2004). Understanding the SARS crisis and communicating its nature requires an understanding of how global cultural flows have reshaped public events within far-reaching and complex chains of causality. While our analysis has covered the entire period of Toronto's SARS outbreak, four key moments were given particular scrutiny: the initial outbreak, the implementation of the World Health Organization (WHO) travel advisory, the end of the initial outbreak, and the second outbreak (see Table 6.1).

Table 6.1 Analysis periods

Period	Start date	End date
Initial outbreak	March 25, 2003	March 31,2003
WHO travel advisory	April 20, 2003	April 30, 2003
End of initial outbreak	May 14, 2003	May 18, 2003
Second outbreak	May 23, 2003	May 30, 2003

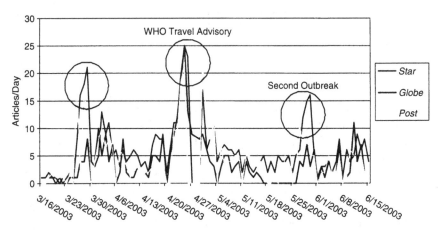

Figure 6.1   Saturation periods: *National Post, Globe and Mail,* and *Toronto Star*

During three of these periods, the initial outbreak, the WHO travel advisory, and the second outbreak, Torontonians were subjected to what we refer to as "saturation news coverage" of the SARS issue. On average, between March 25 and May 30, the *Toronto Star* ran 6.1 SARS articles per day, the *Globe and Mail* ran 3.6 articles per day, and the *National Post* ran 4.3 articles per day. As Figure 6.1 illustrates, during the three periods of saturation coverage, the number of articles per day jumped dramatically. For example, on April 25, at the height of the controversy over the WHO travel advisory, both the *Star* and the *Globe* ran 25 articles, and the *National Post* ran 22 articles. Importantly, these numbers include only those articles, op-eds, and editorials that were substantively about SARS, excluding letters to the editor and articles that made only a passing mention of the disease. If these latter groups were included, the numbers would be much higher.

With the exception of the coverage spike visible during the travel advisory, the *Globe and Mail* provided the most even volume of coverage, while the *Toronto Star* and the *National Post* appeared more prone to satura- tion spikes. While it is empirically difficult to measure the impact of media coverage on popular perception, agenda-setting research suggests that news coverage gives the public important cues as to the scope, size, and importance of an issue (McCombs and Shaw 1972; McCombs 1993). During periods of "saturation news coverage," the number of daily articles jumped to between 200 percent and 300 percent of average levels, with each paper printing as many as 25 articles per day about the crisis. Saturation news coverage in the local press reinforced the impression that SARS was out of control in Toronto.

Methodology

From the five newspapers, 1,600 articles were selected for detailed analysis. We examined issues of content, stakeholder representation, and tone (critical versus praising) as described below. Content coding was designed to assess three different types of coverage over the course of the outbreak:

- health coverage – medical information about illness and its management;
- economic coverage – stories principally concerned with the economic fallout of the illness; and
- political coverage – information about the role of public authority, regulatory preparedness, and the political reaction to the illness.

In any crisis, access to news organizations is critical, and different groups compete for voice and presence in the media. Using a list of 80 stakeholders, including patients, healthcare workers, local and national public health officials, the business community, citizens, the media, politicians, and foreign bodies such as the WHO, each article was coded to identify which stakeholders were given voice, when, where, and by whom.

A key variable in our study was the tone of the coverage in each paper. Tone is important in a crisis, because it contributes to the allocation of blame. We coded the criticism and praise directed at eight groups over the course of the outbreak. Specifically, these were the Government of Canada, the Government of Ontario, the public health authorities, healthcare workers, the World Health Organization, citizens, business, and foreign governments. For each group, it was noted whether the article was critical or congratulatory, and whether those comments related to the health, economic, or political aspects of the crisis.

The Competing Functions of the News Media

In a public crisis such as this, news organizations tend to serve four important and sometimes competing functions (Reynolds 2005):

- to channel local public health information by connecting public health officials to citizens, and, to a lesser extent, to serve as a channel for public health information between groups of professional stakeholders (e.g., medical officials, politicians, and businesses);
- to provide a national and international conduit for news reports and analysis;

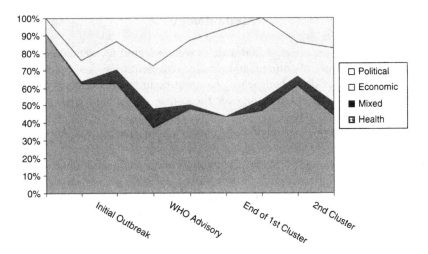

Figure 6.2   News content by type – Canadian: *National Post, Globe and Mail,* and *Toronto Star*

- to document the economic and other impacts of the crisis on businesses, frontline health workers, and the community as a whole;
- to offer a venue for public and political debate over the handling of the crisis.

Based on our data, the press coverage of the SARS outbreak did fulfill each of these roles to greater or lesser extents.

During the initial outbreak, coverage focused almost exclusively on health, with as much as 91 percent of Canadian coverage focusing on health issues. As the crisis progressed, the political and economic dimensions of the crises gathered momentum. A peak moment of intense media coverage occurred when the WHO issued a global travel advisory, warning international visitors of the risks of visiting Toronto. During the travel advisory, health coverage fell to its lowest point, accounting for only 37 percent of SARS-related news content in Canada. As Figure 6.2 illustrates, however, although economic coverage gained substantial ground, particularly after the travel advisory, it did not drown out the very real issues that the public believed were at the heart of the crisis, namely, the defense of public health, security, and well-being. Individually, the newspapers were quite similar to one another, with the *National Post,* conservative and right wing, devoting a slightly greater percentage of its coverage to health issues (65 percent), as compared to 55 percent and 53 percent in the *Toronto Star,* center-liberal, and the *Globe and Mail,* the national newspaper of record, respectively.

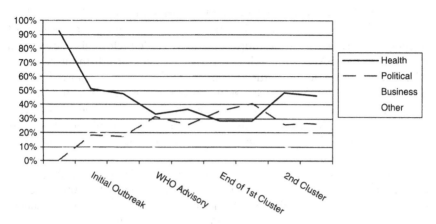

Figure 6.3   Stakeholder voices: *National Post, Globe and Mail,* and *Toronto Star*

The Canadian newspapers were also remarkably consistent in how they focused their attention on the competing claims of the various stakeholders as the crisis unfolded. As Figure 6.3 illustrates, during the emergence of the first and second clusters, the coverage gave special place to voices from the health sector, including local, provincial, federal, and international health officials. Later in the crisis, healthcare workers such as doctors, nurses, and Emergency Medical Service personnel received more attention, particularly as the Ontario Nurses' Association (ONA) became an important public advocate and critic of the government's lack of preparedness for the SARS crisis.

The tone and substance of the coverage changed as the economic costs of the outbreak mounted. After the WHO travel advisory, voice was increasingly given to politicians and business people, including those from the hospitality sector. One study conducted by the accounting firm KPMG at the behest of the Hotel Association of Canada estimated that the sector lost over a billion dollars of business during the crisis (KPMG 2003). There is no way of knowing if this figure was overstated, but it *was* part of the association's communication strategy to lobby the federal government. While successful in getting their issues onto the public agenda, the hospitality sector never succeeded in controlling the debate over the public dimension of the crisis.

Stakeholders, Political Spin, and Blame

Our analysis raises many questions about both voice and access to the media in times of crisis. Public interest advocates and healthcare officials such as Colin D'Cunha, Sheela Basrur, Donald Low, James Young, and other frontline healthcare workers dominated coverage of the SARS issue. This was because they represented the state and the not-for-private sector of society, and spoke with authority on the epidemiological causes and consequences of SARS. Still, while it is true that the health ministry under Clement, for example, had little credibility, D'Cunha (who reported to that ministry) Basrur, and Young were state officials who gained in stature during the crisis and had the same credibility as the local public health officials. While the allocation of voice is never a perfect predictor of the arguments made in the press, it is nonetheless useful in determining who held the press attention at key moments.

Inevitably, every major crisis takes on a political dimension. Writing in the midst of the crisis, a *Globe and Mail* editorial (April 26, 2003) drew a sharp contrast between the poise and professionalism shown by Lucien Bouchard, the iconic premier of the PQ government during the ice storms of 1998, and the leadership displayed by federal and provincial politicians during the SARS crisis. Significantly, Ontario Premier Ernie Eaves' low-key, feeble leadership was much criticized, and contributed to the fall of his government later that year. The handling of political crises makes and breaks modern political leaders – for example, US President George W. Bush's standing in the polls was boosted by his handling of the September 11 terrorist attacks, but undermined by his response to Hurricane Katrina and the flooding of New Orleans.

In retrospect, the press' framing of the SARS outbreak was problematic in that it politicized the crisis along partisan lines, drawing the spotlight away from healthcare workers and the more substantive health policy story. The Canadian press became an autonomous actor in the SARS crisis, in much the same way that the American media did after Hurricane Katrina flooded New Orleans (United States House of Representatives 2006a, pp. 163–82). Both of these examples illustrate just how powerful the press is in constructing reality in the public mind. Frequently, misinformation, rumor, and speculation compete for headlines with on-the-ground reporting and in-depth analysis. Truth is often a victim, and reporting in times of imperfect information can be speculative and highly personalized, focusing on individual triumph and tragedy.

As Figure 6.4 illustrates, after the WHO issued its travel advisory, healthcare workers, especially nurses, who had been so prominent in the news coverage were increasingly displaced by professional politicians. Healthcare professionals found themselves caught in the crossfire between the federal government in Ottawa and the Ontario provincial government at Toronto's Queen's Park.

One of the reasons why the role of the press is magnified in a national crisis is that the media strategies of the various actors combine to put news organizations at the center of the crisis, making print and electronic media

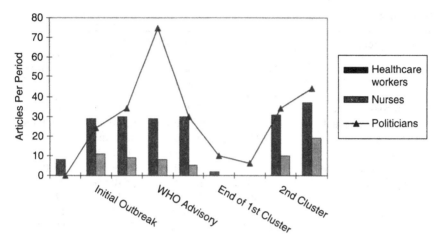

Figure 6.4 Stakeholder voices – healthcare workers and politicians: *National Post, Globe and Mail,* and *Toronto Star*

the primary sources of information for the public, and empowering the news media to become an actor in its own right. The *National Post* was formerly owned by Conrad Black, and is a mouthpiece for the far right in Canada. Its coverage, notably in its editorial section, tended to be highly critical of the federal government, which at that time was controlled by the centrist Liberal Party. In contrast, the *Toronto Star*, Canada's largest paper, which has historically aligned itself with the Liberal Party, was most critical of the provincial government, then controlled by the Conservative Party (see Table 6.2). The *Globe and Mail*, Canada's newspaper of record, has a "small-c" conservative orientation, and apportioned blame more or less equally between the provincial *and* federal governments.

The American Coverage of SARS

Among Torontonians at the time, it was widely held that US coverage of the Toronto outbreak was biased, alarmist, and inflammatory, blowing the story out of all reasonable proportion. On April 24, an article on the front page of the *New York Times* (April 24, 2003) read: "Travellers Urged to Avoid Toronto Because of SARS." Although the headline caught the interest of Canadians, less attention was paid to the editorial that ran in the *Times* the next day, which pointed out that the US Centers for Disease Control and Prevention did not agree with the WHO's travel advisory, and was advising Americans that travel to Toronto was safe, provided that they did not visit

Table 6.2 The apportionment of blame

Criticized group	Critical articles[a]			
	National Post	Globe and Mail	Toronto Star	Total
Federal government	34 (8.7%)	22 (6.7%)	37 (6.7%)	93 (7.3%)
Provincial government	24 (6.2%)	26 (8.0%)	60 (10.8%)	110 (8.6%)
Public health	14 (3.6%)	13 (4.0%)	13 (2.3%)	40 (3.1%)
Healthcare workers	3 (0.8%)	8 (2.4%)	6 (1.1%)	17 (1.3%)
World Health Organization	24 (6.2%)	16 (4.9%)	24 (4.3%)	64 (5.0%)
Citizens	3 (0.8%)	10 (3.1%)	5 (0.9%)	18 (1.4%)
Business	2 (0.5%)	1 (0.3%)	5 (0.9%)	8 (0.6%)
Foreign governments	13 (3.3%)	17 (5.2%)	23 (4.1%)	53 (4.2%)
Total number of critical articles	117 (30.1%)	113 (34.6%)	173 (31.1%)	403 (31.7%)
Total number of articles	389	327	556	1,272

[a] The number of critical articles as a percentage of the total number of stories run by each newspaper.

Table 6.3 Coverage types

Area	Content types (%)			
	Health	Economic	Political	Mixed
Toronto	52	24	17	7
National	51	24	19	6
Foreign	59	23	12	6

healthcare facilities (*New York Times*, April 25, 2003). In this respect, US reporting was remarkably more balanced than initially expected.

The greatest difference between the American and Canadian newspapers was the volume of their coverage. Using standard criteria, our study examined 556 articles from the *Toronto Star* as compared to 273 from the *New York Times*. While the American papers treated SARS as a big story, the disease nonetheless shared the news agenda with the war in Iraq, a story of far greater interest to American readers. In fact, when local (*Toronto Star*), national (*Globe and Mail* and *National Post*), and foreign (*New York Times* and *USA Today*) coverage is compared, what is most striking is how similar the coverage patterns were. As Table 6.3 outlines, in each area about half of the coverage was devoted to health issues, a quarter to economic coverage, an eighth to political coverage, and the rest to mixed coverage.

Table 6.4   Health sub-topics

Health sub-topics	American sources (%)	Canadian sources (%)
Cites current list of probable/ active cases	2	4
WHO travel advisory	5	5
Reports of new clusters, cases	7	10
Deaths/fatalities from SARS, profiles of victims	4	5
Changes in social practices/customs	9	8
Quarantine and infection control measures	40	40
Research on disease (spread)	27	14
Impact on healthcare system	1	13
Other	3	3

A further illustration of common cross-border journalistic standards can be seen in Table 6.4. The SARS articles that focused on health issues were broken down into nine subcategories, based on their emphasis. In seven of those categories, the distribution of the Canadian and US stories was almost identical. The only significant differences were between the categories of *health research* and *healthcare delivery*. The Canadian papers focused a great deal of attention on Canada's healthcare system and its inability to deal with the outbreak, while the American papers gave more attention to the need for research.

Finally, we were interested in whether Toronto was differentiated from other SARS-affected areas where, *unlike* Canada, the disease was active in the general population. Canada received some form of mention in 45 percent of the *New York Times'* SARS-related articles, and 61 percent of those in *USA Today*. As Figure 6.5 illustrates, these references were of two types. In the *New York Times* and *USA Today*, respectively, only 17 percent and 20 percent of the SARS-related stories were actually about Canada, whereas a much larger percentage (28 percent and 41 percent) simply listed Canada as a SARS-affected area, along with Hong Kong and China's Guangdong province. The inclusion of Toronto on this list reinforced the impression that the risks in Toronto were higher than they really were.

Media Strategies in a Public Crisis

It is significant that all of the major players in the SARS crisis had media strategies with specific goals and objectives. Public health officials used the media to communicate the severity of SARS, and the need for citizens to

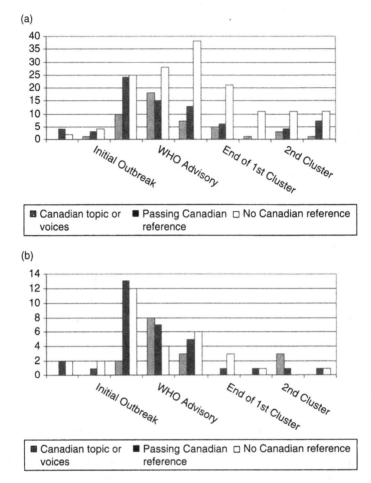

Figure 6.5 Canadian references in American newspapers: (a) *The New York Times*; (b) *USA Today*

respect the quarantine measures (National Advisory Committee 2003). Not surprisingly, the business community used the media to communicate the severity of their economic plight. Private-sector organizations were highly visible in demanding compensation and special government programs for the hotel, convention, and restaurant and travel-related industries that were most affected by the outbreak. The Ontario government had a media strategy to pressure the federal government to help offset some of the costs of containing the outbreak (Taber 2003). In turn, the federal and city governments used the media, most notably during its dispute with the World

Health Organization, to show that they were actively working to have the travel advisory lifted (Lewington and Rusk 2003). As a letter submitted to the National Advisory Committee on SARS and Public Health, signed by the heads of nine major health associations, pointed out, this lack of unity in official communication was detrimental to the public interest:[1]

> How the crisis or emergency is reported is just as important as how it is actually handled. It is also crucial that the public, and the media have a clear understanding of the language of the crisis so that clear, consistent messages are communicated and received. Governments across jurisdictions must develop an emergency plan to which all parties are committed regarding leadership in communications. (cited in National Advisory Committee 2003, p. 32)

Significantly, competing stakeholder groups worked to capture the sympathy and attention of the media in order to advance their own agendas. Sometimes they operated at cross-purposes to one another. The provincial Campbell Commission noted that: "Poor public health communication can also have a negative economic impact, if messages intended for a local audience resonate negatively on the international scene" (Campbell 2004, p. 58). In order to contain the outbreak, public health officials had to communicate the message that SARS was a serious threat. The message that SARS was a serious threat impacted the travel industry in all of the affected countries (Arguin et al. 2004; Mason et al. 2005). In Toronto, hotels, restaurants, tourist sites, and Asian businesses were hit particularly hard, and many in the private sector use the growing sense of economic uncertainty in their media strategies (Canadian Federation of Independent Business 2003; KPMG 2003; PKF Consulting 2004). On balance, the public interest was not served by the fact that the public health message and the economic recovery message were working at cross-purposes, competing with and undermining each other at key moments. In a crisis situation where every major stakeholder has a media strategy, it is naive to argue that the press simply reports the news as it unfolds. Media organizations function as "gatekeepers," consciously choosing where, when, and how to divide their attention among the various stakeholders (White 1950; Snider 1967).

SARS, the Media, and Global Cultural Flows

Understanding the SARS crisis requires an understanding of how global cultural flows behave in complex chains of causality. A global cultural flow is an intense movement of people, capital, ideas, and information that has unanticipated consequences for institutions, social values, and public expectations. It is critical to make a distinction between the global effect of

SARS on national institutions, and the capacity of the international community to form a public response (Marginson and Sawir 2005). This enables us to understand just how complex the chains of causality can be. In this case, an infected woman gets on a plane in Hong Kong and flies back to Canada, bringing the virus with her. As the virus spreads through the city, local media and public health officials generate a constant flow of public health information that is transmitted around the world. The news that Toronto is under a WHO advisory disrupts the flow of tourists and travelers. As economic losses mount, all three levels of government adopt aggressive media strategies aimed at countering the image of Toronto as a SARS-affected area. Social scientists have described this phenomenon of novelty and surprise as "unintended consequences"; all flows have such consequences for people, states, and businesses, and governments are not easily equipped to react to multi-level public health crises. Much of the blame game that was greatly in evidence stems from the lack of effective emergency planning and coordination between different levels of government.

By Way of a Conclusion

The SARS crisis reveals that governments face three discrete and interrelated challenges in managing public crises in an era of global cultural flows:

- First, the media coverage of SARS in Toronto demonstrates the need to think more systematically about the growing importance of the public domain as the sphere of communicative interaction. Our understanding of the modern public sphere owes much to Habermas' (1989) original theorization. In the SARS crisis, as this study reveals, the public domain remains pluralistic and diverse, because it is the privileged site of critical debate, informed discussion, and opinion mobilization. When the public inhabits this privileged sphere of interaction, it grows more robust and democratic norms are strengthened. When elite frames and filters dominate discourse, the public domain shrinks as a place of open debate and discussion (Herman and Chomsky 2002). In the SARS crisis, coverage vacillated between these two sharply contrasting poles as modern theorists have predicted.
- Second, fascination with new and emerging diseases such as SARS, West Nile, and Ebola leads to media coverage that far outweighs their actual mortality, while diseases such as influenza, hepatitis, malaria, and diarrhoea each claim more than half a million victims a year and go largely unreported (Glass 2004). Toronto is a site of intense competition for

audience share, a commercial imperative that contributes to what some critics have called "pack journalism" (Crouse 1972; Sigal 1973). Large 16pt headlines, disturbing photos, and persistent focus on the number of deaths are interpreted by the public as a situation spinning out of control. An unintended consequence of such coverage is public fear and mis-understanding. The public was to an extent manipulated by misinformation and speculation, even though public health officials and health professionals, such as nurses, demanded accountability and transparency. These tensions cannot be papered over or underestimated.

- Finally, new technologies such as the Internet and the cellular phone were also critical sources of information during the SARS crisis. Alternative sources of information, paradoxically, served to enhance and reinforce the importance of print media. While it is fashionable in many circles to hype the technology of the information age, in times of national crisis, print journalism, radio, and television remain as important as ever. In the SARS crisis, the public authorities needed to tell Torontonians that SARS was deadly serious, while at the same time trying to tell potential tourists that the city was safe. In an age of ubiquitous information flows, there was no way to insulate each audience from the message meant for the other. The result was confusion and contradictory messages.

If there is a simple lesson to be gleaned from media coverage of the 2003 Toronto SARS outbreak, it is that people remain dependent on their local news providers to understand, react, and take preventive measures when faced with a health crisis. Public authorities have immense regulatory power that has not been diminished in an interdependent world. With respect to health needs, the state is the instrument of first response and last resort. Certainly there is no evidence that public authority has been hollowed out. Intensive public health crises inevitably raise fundamental questions about legally entrenched rights and freedoms, and how each level of government intends to balance concerns about individual rights and community con-cerns about infectious disease (Jacobs 2005).

Still, the principal finding of this study is that news remains socially con-structed, and that in pluralist democracies, where "news shapers" from across the political spectrum actively work to manage the news, journalistic neutrality and objectivity are frames that need to be interrogated (Manheim 1998). The modern public sphere has become more complex and multi-leveled. An optimal response to a post-Westphalian pathogen requires focused com-munication strategies, proactive public health systems, and a realistic under-standing of the global reach of local communication. The public was never a "phantom," as Lippmann (1925) falsely characterized it; instead, it was active, engaged, and informed. The question that is not addressed, and that needs to be, is whether the frontline health workers, the key health and political officials, and the public as a whole believe that media coverage of SARS was fair, balanced, and responsible. The press itself, in a public forum, may also find it salutary to review its own role in dialogue with all stakeholders. It is only with this further research in hand that definitive recommendations can be made as to the management of future crises.

ACKNOWLEDGMENTS

This research was undertaken as part of the Global Cultural Flows Initiative, and the authors would like to thank and acknowledge the contributions and support of Professors Seth Feldman and Fred Fletcher of York University, and Andrew Laing, President of Cormex Media Research in Toronto.

NOTE

1   The letter was signed by the heads of the Canadian Medical Association, the Canadian Public Health Association, the Canadian Nurses Association, the Canadian Healthcare Association, the Canadian Dental Association, the Association of Canadian Academic Healthcare Organizations, the Canadian Pharmacists Association, the Canadian Association of Emergency Physicians, and the Canadian Council on Health Services Accreditation.

7

SARS as a "Health Scare"

Claire Hooker

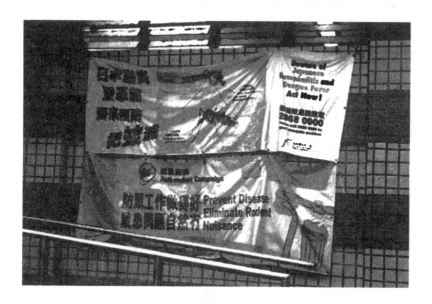

Introduction

How, moreover, might epidemics of fear if not disease be sociologically explained and understood?

Stephen Williams (2001)

Epidemics of fear, perhaps also of disease: these are two most prominent anxieties. Health professionals genuinely fear the possibility of a vast out-break of a new or re-emerging infectious disease. But they don't just worry about these events – they (we) also worry about fear-mongering as well. Many health professionals worry about the enormous impacts that public fears may have on economies and societies: "the problem with SARS," I have heard several in Canada say, "was not SARS itself, but fear" (Skinner 2003). By this they mean that the disruptions of SARS were vastly disproportionate to its body count of 44 deaths, a very small number in comparison with the mortality rate commanded by, *inter alia*, smoking, drinking, driving, and not getting a flu vaccine.

In this chapter, I will join these conversations to reflect on current concerns about, and responses to, the threats of infectious disease, specifically in an urban context. First, I will situate these concerns and reactions in a more general conceptual framework, concerns about "health scares" – events in which there is a strong social reaction to a specific hazard that appears to threaten the health of a significant portion of the population. This is, if you will, the problem of not-disease-but-"fear itself" that was mentioned above. I briefly discuss concerns with epidemics of new and re-emerging infectious diseases as a particular category of health scare. In asking how we can analyze, predict, and, perhaps, prevent or resolve health scares, I then turn to the "social amplification of risk" framework and to the role that networks – actor-networks that link humans and non-humans in specific responsive alliances, and social networks, including intra-urban networks, professional networks, and global cities networks – may play in the amplification or attenuation of risk issue signals, and so to the resolution or otherwise of health scare situations. In the remainder of the chapter, I show how networked social amplification and attenuation effects played out in the outbreaks of SARS in Toronto in the spring of 2003. I conclude with comments on the central importance of social and professional informational networks and connectivity in the ecology of the urban landscape for successfully managing health scares in the future.

Health Scares

Like a haunted house the morning after Halloween, many a bloodcurdling health hazard looks less frightening in the daylight of follow-up studies than it did in the first shriek of publicity.
Avery Comoraw, Less than 'Scary Health Scares: Killer Cranberries?, *2000*

In U.S., Fear Is Spreading Faster Than SARS
New York Times *banner headline, April 17, 2003*

Since the subject of "health scares" has not yet attracted scholarly analysis (but see Leiss 2001; Gwyn 2002), in this section I offer some evidence about what kind of social phenomenon health scares are.

First, health scares are a new social phenomenon. They are hybrid representational–physical entities. They are real not as epidemics or earthquakes are real, but real in a social sense: products of recent politico-cultural concerns, they are events marked by sudden mass insecurities about the consequences of an increasingly globalized, fluid, late-capitalist world. I will demonstrate: A search using the term "health scare" on electronic indexes – those for news sources, such as CBCA Direct, or for health and medicine, such as PubMed or Medline, and those for the social sciences, such as sociofile – shows that colloquially at least, there is a widely accepted concept of "health scares" as bounded events in which a group of people hold significant fears for their health. This search collected 56 news articles, many of which contained the term "health scare" in their titles, and 160 publications in scholarly and professional literatures. The overwhelming majority of articles in both categories were published in the mid- to late 1990s. As the earliest studies in the scholarly/professional collection were published in the early 1970s, this indicates that our preoccupation with "health scares" is a relatively recent phenomenon. Moreover, although one news article contained references to health controversies from the 1950s and 1960s (Rosner and Markowitz 2002), all the health scares discussed in the scholarly/professional literature occurred in the period after 1970. This period has also seen the growth of scholarly and professional attention to emergency preparedness and planning, and of preoccupations with concepts of "risk" in the health sciences in particular.

So what kind of events do we think "health scares" are? It turns out that health scares occur in a wide variety of domains. The scholarly/professional literature contained 178 individual discussions of 49 health scares topics, including BSE/prion diseases, HIV/AIDS, SARS, fluoride in water, X-rays, genetically modified foods, hormone replacement therapy (HRT), vaccine side effects, channel blocker side effects, radiation from mobile phones and powerlines, Tylenol tampering, dioxins, radon gas, *Cryptosporidium* in water supplies, flesh eating disease, hazardous wastes, food irradiation, acrylamide in foods, West Nile virus, breast implants, Ebola, phthalates, polluted apple juice, lead, vinyl chloride (PVCs), swine flu, bioterrorism, alar, and hormones in the milk supply. These health scares came from six domains: disease, especially communicable disease; toxins and contaminants of air, food or water; environmental pollution; side effects of medical products or procedures; intentional harm; and the unanticipated consequences of products or industrial operations (e.g., genetically modified foods (GM foods) and silicone breast implants). Several health scares fitted more than one domain: BSE, for example, was represented as both a disease and as an outcome of late industrial agribusiness practices (Ratzan 1998; Miller 1999). The news literature added new local examples from the same domains.

All health scare events discussed in the sample could be classified according to three fears/outcomes profiles, as depicted in Table 7.1. The overwhelming majority fell into square G: fears of large-scale destruction, but with low to non-existent actual mortality (so far): examples include BSE, inhalation anthrax, SARS, GMOs, radiation from powerlines and mobile

Table 7.1 Fears/outcomes as described in articles

	Fears of catastrophe	Fears of severe outcomes	Fears of tiny increase in risk
Large-scale devastation	A	B	C
Significant mortality	D HIV/AIDS (developing world)	E Cholera, water-borne disease outbreaks, lead poisoning, meningitis	F
Low or non-existent mortality to date	G BSE, anthrax, SARS, Tylenol tampering, dioxin, GM foods, flesh-eating disease, radiation from cell phones, terrorism, acrylamide, Ebola, alar, PCBs, swine or avian influenza	H Radon gas, West Nile virus	I Oral contra-ceptives, HRT, vaccines, fluoride in water, X-rays, channel blockers, cancer mortality, phthalates, interferon

phones masts, dioxins, and radon in homes. A small group, largely composed of events involving new hazard notifications warning of small rises in the risks attached to specific medical products or procedures, fell in square I: low fears and low outcomes. Examples include scares around brands of oral contraceptives, vaccines, and channel blockers. (It should be noted for this profile that: (1) whilst the reported rise in risk was majoratively very small, the numbers of people using these products or procedures and thus affected by the hazard notification was often very large; and (2) in several cases later reviews of scientific data found no rise in risk at all (e.g., Spitzer 1999). Largely, therefore, I is a subset of G.) Finally, a few "health scares" really did become crisis events, falling into square E: severe fears and severe anticipated outcomes. Examples include food and water-borne outbreaks such as the epidemic of *E. coli* related disease in Walkerton, Ontario, and tuberculosis among the homeless. These cases, except HIV, were localized. I conclude from this spread that "health scares" are not so much events in which there is a strong fear response from the public but no "real" threat – which is how health professionals often describe them – but events in which fears of possible but unlikely catastrophe are entertained in conditions of scientific uncertainty and cultural insecurity, which is a corollary of my conclusions in the previous paragraph.

Finally, although they seem unreal because of their low mortality rates, virtually all health scares have commanded attention and concern from journalists and health professionals because of the all-too-real economic cost and social disruption that they have caused. The two are intertwined, of course: often, the "problem" was not so much that people ceased eating cranberries or beef, or even that they ceased using the contraceptive pill mid-cycle or pulled their child out of a school built near powerlines – in any case many of these behavior changes were fairly short lived – but the enormous, sometimes devastating, impact that these actions had on industries and the communities they sustained. And, while local consumer behavior has been significant in generating many of these impacts, it was often trade embargoes and drops in tourism that did most of the damage (Powell and Leiss 1997). Consider BSE: it was the context of international trade that made this the costliest health scare the world has ever seen (Ratzan 1998). The trade embargoes first put in place by France as a kind of quarantine, and then strategically implemented elsewhere (as Canada found to its cost in 2003) bound notions of health to national identity and economic power. Trade barriers have to a large extent become the lines of hygiene (Bashford 2004) of the market-driven, deregulated new world order of the early twenty-first century, lines that mark nations as pure or as contaminated. Amid an effectively global, interconnected, and highly networked economy, health scares reassert the validity of borders: prosperity is equated with *security*, which decodes to border control for health.

I note here that urbanicity is an important, though relatively unexplored, dimension of health scares, for three reasons. First, health scares can be a product of a particular urban setting, as for example when a system breakdown (such as a power failure at a local supermarket) causes a sudden mass or concentrated health impact (unsuspected cases of food poisoning). Second, apart from specific agricultural sectors, it is urban areas, particularly global cities, that are likely to directly experience the economic impact of health scares, as industries dependent on prosperity (tourism, entertainment) reduce. And, third, the social inequalities of urban geographies can exacerbate a health scare. Cities are resource machines producing and distributing resources according to location (Fitzpatrick and LaGory 2000). Social inequalities expressed through hazard exposure – the less privileged, the more vulnerable – and through expectations of response, such that those areas within cities with the fewest response resources also experience lack of trust, shaping landscapes of fear and despair (Fitzpatrick and LaGory 2000, Slovic 2000; see also Rodwin, Chapter 2).

In sum: health scares are events typically characterized by large-scale fears but very low actual mortality and morbidity. As a recent feature of early twenty-first century "Western" societies, their existence supports the contention of "risk society" theorists that we have become very anxious about the intrusion of those catastrophes to which we – as opposed to those "Others" in the "third world" – have hitherto felt immune (Adam et al. 2002). This is the context in which responses to infectious disease are created. Health scares are "problems" (as in my opening quotation, "the problem with SARS ...") because of their devastating economic (which means, social) consequences. This means that health and economic concerns must be regarded as interdependent and as shaping one another: one cannot understand responses to, and reflections on, SARS, for example, without understanding these connections. Finally, the economic context clearly demonstrates the tensions between the globalizing, border-crossing tendencies/realities in economic systems, and the reification of nation-hood, of national economies held and patrolled within national borders. This tension operated in responses to contemporary concerns with infectious disease also.

Disease Scares: Pandemics

In a world where diseases respect no borders, it is important that we cooperate across borders internationally as well.
                Canadian Health Minister Ujjal Dosanjh to the United Nations,
                                                        November 17, 2004

[Pandemic preparation] has been done through programs ... focused more generally on increasing preparedness for bioterrorism and other emerging infectious disease health threats.
                US Department of Health and Human Services (HHS 2004)

Among the panoply of health scares, there is a special place reserved in our cultural imagination for fears of a mass outbreak of disease. This is attested to by movies such as *Virus* and *Outbreak* and novels like Robin Cook's *Contagion*. When I asked Canadian health professionals and policy-makers for examples of health scares, they typically thought first of Ebola, West Nile virus, Norwalk, meningococcal disease, *Clostridium difficile*, SARS, avian influenza, and monkeypox.

Above all, right now we're all supposed to be worried about a global pandemic of influenza. Health professionals on television repeat that the question is not *whether* this will happen, but *when*. "During the last few years, the world has faced several threats with pandemic potential, making the occurrence of the next pandemic just a matter of time," says the World Health Organization (WHO)'s website (WHO 2005). Accompanied by well-publicized exhortations from the WHO, Western nations such as Canada, the US, and Australia have drawn up pandemic influenza preparedness plans, publicly stating strategies on everything from vaccine manufacture and stockpiling to data collection and management systems.

One key reason for our current anxiety about pandemic influenza is encapsulated in the reiterated phrase "because we are living in a world where diseases respect no borders." On the face of it, this phrase is a little puzzling: What other kind of world have we ever lived in? It indicates a new preoccupation among health professionals – and let us not forget, also among (Western) security and economic policy-makers as well – about the health consequences of the dissolution of formerly strong social boundaries, between peoples, communities, professions, and nations. In particular, the physical movement of people through increasingly globalized socio-economic networks, especially, as discussed elsewhere in this volume, the global cities networks, has created fears of contagion, both literal and ideological. Diseases of travel – of which SARS was considered the precedent-setting example – represent the discomfiting reality of the connectivity of the developed and developing worlds in late capitalism (Wilson 1995; de Hart 2003). The phrase also evokes modernist anxieties about *transgressions* – the theme, common in stories of health scares, that danger results from either nature's capacity to elude the artificial boundaries that humans construct, or from human violation of "natural" boundaries. Pandemics are frightening because they are represented as the consequences of particular mobility regimes – the rapid movement of peoples and organisms, agricultural and industrial practices that constantly cross boundaries between species – that are regarded as unsettling in themselves by many westerners, and which are uncomfortably linked by multiple networks to ourselves. The notion of a "pandemic" itself is defined by the traveling of a disease: the WHO's stages of pandemic alert are built around a disease's geographical movement (Public Health Agency of Canada 2005).

Borders may be meaningless to a microbe, but in pandemic preparedness planning our security is perceived to rely on our requiring microbes to respect them anyway. (Hence the conceptual and practical entanglement of bioterror – which attacks a state – and influenza preparedness, as shown in the quotation above.) Our first move in combating new and re-emerging infectious diseases has been to double the guard: to put in place more extensive and rigorous quarantine and border screening regimens, to examine travelers and prospective immigrants and exclude those believed to harbor illness, to identify, cordon off, and patrol dangerous places in the world (Hooker 2006). Yet at the same time, the successful *resolution* of a pandemic is believed to be vested in global networks of another sort: informational networks, managed virtually through technology, directed by an international body, the WHO, and rooted in formal and informal social networks between scientists and health professionals (Fidler 2004).

In sum, network society (Castells 2000) and contemporary global mobility regimes have facilitated expansions of actual microbial traffic along with the transgressive, or at least threatening, movements of people and goods. When novel diseases enter the urban ecologies of Western cities, especially global cities (Sassen 1991), place and the health burdens shaped by inequitable urban geographies can facilitate their spread. As discussed above, this is the primary socio-political-economic context in which health scares occur. How the "lifecycle" of a health scare plays out can be tracked by examining what social mechanisms contrive to amplify or attenuate collective responses to the health risk as the event progresses.

Network Amplifiers: The Social Amplification of Risk

Understanding how the numerous factors of geographies, media reporting, expert decision-making, and so on fit together and influence each other in real time to produce a health scare is challenging by reason of the complexity of these interactions. In my view, the model that can best capture this complexity is the social amplification of risk framework (Pidgeon et al. 2003). Developed to understand, predict, and manage public response to industry-related hazards (nuclear power, the "Love Canal," chemical contamination), the model may be easily adapted for use in understanding the causes and effects of major types of health scares, side effects of existing therapies, and outbreaks of disease.

The social amplification of risk framework begins with the assumption that hazards and risk events are only given meaning by being observed and communicated by human beings. In the communication process, hazards and risk events are portrayed through *risk signals* (images, signs, symbols), which change as they are decoded and transmitted by different "receivers"; that is, stakeholders and social groups. These signals are subject to (somewhat predictable) transformations as they pass through different information channels and various *social stations*, such as government bodies, expert or professional groups, the news media, community organizations, and individual people. These transformations will *amplify* or *attenuate* the signals by such means as increasing or decreasing the volume of information about an event, heightening the salience or availability of certain aspects of it, or reinterpreting, elaborating, discarding, or adding symbols or images (Kasperson et al. 1988). The system is dynamic: transformations in one station will feed back into the system to affect others. This is how a health scare is socially produced.

The social amplification of risk framework also explains the impacts of health scares. Signal amplification or attenuation will lead to particular responses by social actors. These responses produce "ripple effects," secondary and tertiary consequences that spread far beyond the impact of the hazard itself, and include mental perceptions, economic, political and social pressure, social disorder, liability, loss of credibility or trust, and stigmatization. Some ripple effects may be positive, including revised hazard response planning or a reduction in the risk posed by the hazard itself.

The advantages of using the social amplification of risk framework to analyze health scares can be summarized as follows. (1) It helps identify and focus attention on the different social actors involved in a health scare, and demonstrates how the health scare is the outcome of interactions within and between these actors – including scientists and health experts. This is important because health scares are not uncommonly seen as the result of "irrational" behavior choices or "misinformed" action, usually on the part of the public or the media. (2) It demonstrates why responses to, and the impacts of, risk events are so often incommensurate with expert risk assessments. Risks are no longer "real" or "false": they are both empirically demonstrated (with real consequences) *and* socially constructed by amplification processes. (3) It demonstrates the temporal aspect to health scares: how perceptions and relationships alter with changes in hazard notification sequences (Pidgeon et al. 2003) or communications by specific bodies. (4) It shows how factors such as loss of trust between actors can lead to perceptions and responses that serve to amplify risk signals and spread ripple effects. As discussed above, this may be crucial in local urban ecologies. (5) It can be used to show how and why amplification processes cause ripple effects such as the Othering and stigmatic-marking of particular social groups, an issue that was of particular importance during the SARS outbreak, as discussed by Keil and Ali in Chapter 9 of this volume.

The social amplification of risk framework as it is currently used and understood also has certain disadvantages, of which two are particularly important. The first is that the framework, which was conceived from the same circles that produced the foundational psychometric studies of risk perception, offers no mechanism for analyzing how power operates within or around the system – of whose interests are involved in the definition of an event in particular terms ("outbreak" versus "pandemic," for example), of what kinds of knowledges are developed and legitimized throughout the process, or of the political context in which the event took place. Of course the framework may include discussion of power relations where the perceptions or interactions of the various stakeholders reveal this, but in general the framework treats amplification/attenuation as occurring in a politically neutral context. Consequently, the social amplification of risk framework would not automatically reveal what the commissions of inquiry into the

SARS outbreaks so stunningly revealed; namely, that the 20 years of neoliberal policy-making that dismantled so much public health infrastructure in Ontario enabled the outbreak to occur in the first place (Keil and Ali, Chapter 3). The second major disadvantage of the framework is that it is descriptive rather than explanatory: it does not offer a causal model of how signals are amplified at particular stations nor of how different social stations affect each other – only *that* they do. However, combining the framework with other social theories may help rectify this second defect and perhaps even mitigate the first. I suggest that one fruitful combination lies in joining the insights of network society theory to the framework.

So far, the importance and functioning of network society (Castells 2000) to the social amplification of risk framework has remained unexplored. And yet clearly social networks are immensely powerful amplification or attenuation devices in a health scare situation. The global cities network and other social networks among different diaspora have already been identified as a strong amplifier of infectious disease risk (Ali and Keil 2006). In natural disaster situations, social networks are crucial management and survival devices, often altering their character and constituency in ways that attenuate fear (especially by building trust) more efficiently than the provision of external resources. Informational networks – from the informal to those entirely dependent on technology – can act as very strong risk signal amplifiers (as in the case of SARS) if their structure causes their content to bear characteristics such as novelty, mass impact, or dread (Pidgeon et al. 2003), or as equally strong risk signal attenuators (as in the very beginning and the aftermath of SARS). Indeed, given the centrality of the network enterprise in the contemporary world and its reliance on the information flows made possible by new technologies (Castells 2000), the social amplification of risk framework might be more usefully constructed around risk signal transformations in *kinds of networks* than in categories of social station. In fact, I suggest that this approach may thus solve some of the problems so far encountered in rendering the framework analytical and predictive rather than merely descriptive, as it allows for the factors that relate amplification effects in different social domains – the media, policy-makers, and the public for instance – to be studied (Breakwell and Barnett 2003).

In the concluding section, I examine SARS as a health scare using the social amplification of risk framework. For this case study, I conducted an extensive documentary analysis of published reminiscences, reports, talks, discussions, and research reports produced during and after the outbreaks in Toronto in addition to the materials, including the Commissions of Inquiry, made available through the websites of local, provincial, and federal health authorities. In addition, I conducted interviews with 18 medical and communications experts who were professionally involved in responding to the outbreak and five focus groups composed of eight people randomly drawn from the Greater Toronto Area. Analysis proceeded thematically and was interpretively guided by the social amplification of risk framework used as a mapping device to identify stakeholders, social stations, and the risk signals that became associated with the disease. In what follows below, I concentrate on which networks acted to amplify or attenuate signals about the risk of SARS, and what ripple effects these signal transformations produced.

SARS as a Health Scare

I genuinely thought that we were going to see a different world by the next month. I thought we were going to be remembered as the people who failed to stop SARS.
Paraphrased comments from the Toronto SARS scientific advisory committee

Risk signals about SARS amplified hugely and rapidly in Toronto during the first days and month of the outbreak. There is a basic psychometric explanation for this. The qualities associated with SARS were those that are typically associated with amplified risk perception: the disease was *novel*; knowledge about it was very limited and its behavior was *uncertain*; it spread through momentary coincidences, such as sharing an elevator with an infected person, and so appeared extremely *uncontrolled*; it threatened to cause *mass* mortality; there was a certain amount of *dread* associated with its onset and mortality rate; and having crossed from the developing to the developed world, it was highly *salient* (Slovic 2000). But such cognitive biases do not explain how social context influenced the construction of this "scare." I argue that SARS risk signals were amplified and sometimes surprisingly attenuated through three major kinds of networks: professional or expert networks; communications networks; and staff or responder networks. It is important to note that in so doing I intend no criticism of the actions or decisions of any responder to SARS.

Expert networks

Experts are not immune from psycho-social amplification effects, though their knowledge and training may to some degree may to some degree substitute the rules of rational decision-making (Slovic 2000). If "fear" was a problem during SARS, creating "irrational" decision-making with consequent negative social and economic effects, as some have suggested (Skinner 2003), then it was a significant problem within the SARS scientific advisory committee (SSAC), a close network of scientists and public health professionals which, though constituted *ad hoc* from semi-formal professional/personal networks, had formal responsibility for responding to the outbreak. The risk signals attached to SARS, including images and symbols of the 1918 "Spanish" influenza pandemic – a model that has been used as the standard for measuring possibilities and fears about contemporary infectious respiratory illnesses, and that has generated at least one very infamous health scare before SARS, the 1976 "swine flu" affair (Neustadt and Fineberg 1983) – generated significant amplification effects in the SSAC. In the committee process members were guided by two important and related decision values. First, they were attentive to all cases of completely contingent, unpredicted spread, which might indicate a threat to the community. They were particularly alarmed by the reports that arrive at the end of March of the outbreak of SARS amongst the residents of a large apartment building (the Amoy Gardens) in Hong Kong. Second, they therefore made decisions based on worst-case scenarios, preferring the costs of over- to under-reacting (interview data). These values were also held by the community (focus group data).

The result was recommendations for disruptive containment measures that, since *actions* are powerful communications in themselves, greatly amplified risk signals. These "social distance" measures targeted particular public mobilities within the networked social space in the city (Sheller 2004). The extensive quarantines – 30,000 people were examined for quarantine in Toronto alone (Hawryluck et al. 2004) – the closure of one hospital and cancellations of visitor access and non-essential services in many others across the province, school closures, and event cancellations (Campbell 2004, 2005; Naylor et al. 2004) were very strong signals about the magnitude of the risk. The consequent impacts, such as those unable to visit mortally ill loved ones or those who suffered or died as a result of inability to access medical services during SARS (Svoboda et al. 2004), generated their own amplification effects through local social networks.

The composition of the responding professional network, especially the lack of connectivity with a particular node (see Urry 2004a), a person of significant professional standing but who had previously had troubled relations with other health experts, led to a block in information flow and a consequent loss of ability to generate internal critique of committee decisions. A prominent former Chief Medical Officer of Health, now the CEO of a major hospital affected by SARS during the outbreak, very early queried the extent of the outbreaks within healthcare settings on the basis of incidence data that showed the rate of infection had peaked and as declining before the end of March – about the time the Amoy Gardens outbreak was reported – and hence called into question the extent of the containment measures. However, he was unable to access the SSAC, as some of its members felt that they had previously had unproductive professional relationships with him. Severing this node from the network led to risk signal amplification, as he then made his objections publicly (Dwosh et al. 2003;

Schabas 2003). I remind the reader once more that the purpose of mentioning this story is not to suggest wrongdoing or misjudgment on either side, but because the exclusion of dissent through network constitution is a structural bias that has also existed in other health scares (e.g., Neustadt and Fineberg 1983) and tends to contribute to amplification.

Having demonstrated how network composition and structural connectivity can generate amplification effects, I should now draw attention to its potential for attenuation. Professional networks strongly attenuated SARS risk signals in two ways. First, clinical learning through local professional networks meant that responders could soon make decisions based on technical information rather than on values. In Canada, this new security augmented outrage at the travel advisory issued by the WHO at the time of the second outbreak (interview data), which local experts felt to have been unwarranted. Second, the international network of scientists and health professionals that raced to gain knowledge about SARS functioned as a brilliant example of the successful "network enterprise" (Castells 2000), circulating both the virus (for experimental work) and scientific information at record speed around the globe, coordinated by the WHO. The rapid genetic sequencing of the virus and the accumulation of clinical information generated containment and treatment actions that brought the epidemic under control much faster (see Ali, Chapter 14).

Communication networks

Two communications networks were explicitly subject to extensive criticism for amplifying risk during and after the outbreaks (Campbell 2004, 2005; Naylor et al. 2004). The first were intra- and intergovernmental. The failures in communication between local, provincial, and national government levels were legion: epidemiological tracking done painstakingly by Post-It™ notes in the "war room"; cross-country daily briefing conference calls for communications officers involving literally thousands of people; the absence of contact details for the province's family physicians (a common feature of health scares – Skouby 1998). Issues about data ownership and access between the three levels of government generated risk issue signal amplification at the WHO in relation to Canadian government capacity that led to the travel advisory (Naylor et al. 2004). Again, lack of connectivity and limits on the (literal) space of flows generated by poor communications resources (Castells 2000) amplified risk signals during SARS.

Unsurprisingly, the mass media, especially newspaper and television coverage, was also commonly identified as a risk signal amplifier during the outbreaks. For example, images of people wearing masks were criticized as atypical and were perceived as crucial risk amplification symbols (focus group data). However, criticism was not uniform. Local media, at least in

Toronto, was in general praised for reporting timely and accurate information and, despite constraints in their professional position, for intelligent engagement in the story as it unfolded (interview data; see also Drache and Clifton, Chapter 6). It was international media networks that were blamed, along with the travel advisory, as major contributors to the severe economic impact of SARS on Toronto, because they simplified, decontextualized, and hence sensationalized the story.

Employee networks

As has been discussed by Keil and Ali in Chapter 3 of this volume, the physical extent of the outbreak in Toronto directly resulted from neoliberal policies that saw the underfunding of healthcare systems and the casualization of the healthcare workforce, particularly in nursing. Semi-formal social networks among healthcare workers therefore acted as SARS risk signal amplifiers in two ways. First, because these responders were working for very long hours in stressful conditions but were reliant on each other for support, informal communication through the networks acted to validate experience but also to deepen the sense of crisis (Schull and Redermeier 2003). Second, outrage about exposure to the risk and inadequate safe-guarding, backed by longstanding anger over the gendered inequities of their position within the healthcare system, immensely amplified risk signals among nurses (Naylor et al. 2004). Many felt stigmatized in the general community, in part as a result of selective media reporting (Campbell 2004). Because some of them threatened to walk off the job, this amplification had the potential to greatly magnify the extent and impact of the epidemic itself.

Conclusion and Implications

We can understand SARS as a health scare by an analysis of the kind of network dynamics proposed by Castells (2000) as central to modern social organization in a globalizing, interconnected, and information technology dependent world. This analysis fits the conceptual structure provided by the social amplification of risk framework (Pidgeon et al. 2003).

Risk signal amplification during SARS was productive of the kind of severe social and economic impacts that are characteristic of health scare situations. SARS carried strong risk signals – it was a novel disease arising in part from the environmental pressures of the late-capitalist, globalizing era, and appeared to threaten the security of developed nations. As in other health scares, information and symbols flowing through local and international professional networks raised great fears about its possible mortality toll, but in fact the number of deaths was miniscule compared with many forms of preventable death in the nations that it affected. The fearful and precautionary response from experts and governments at various levels was, as in many other health scares, greatly exacerbated by lack of connectivity, node exclusion, and other network disruptions that impaired the enterprise and blocked feedback processes. The huge negative impacts suffered as a result of the outbreaks of SARS were, as in other health scares, both economic and social.

It should not be forgotten that risk signal amplification also generated positive actions, some of which in turn generated attenuation effects. Among these can be included the swift response of the highly networked international scientific community, coordinated through the WHO, which greatly strengthened the organization's role as the central node for disease control networks in a globalized world (Fidler 2004). The advent of SARS has also strengthened pandemic preparedness planning in many nations, in which the explicit creation of response networks through different sectors of government has been made central.

Health scares are largely testimonies to western anxieties and have been productive of global and local inequalities and "Othered" identities, reinscribing the boundaries between the "first" and the "third" worlds despite the fact that increasing connectivity has generated an increased likelihood of a primary health scare category, a new infectious disease (King 2002). But the reality of the potential threats remains, and so does the uncertainty. Whether or not to react to a particular constellation of raindrops as if it were the hundred-year flood is a question that worries most of those to whom the responsibility of intervention falls. In these scenarios, the network enterprise is a crucial provider of speedy and effective answers, leaving us the luxury of debating the values that we wish to guide our choices in health scare situations in the future.

8

City under Siege: Authoritarian Toleration, Mask Culture, and the SARS Crisis in Hong Kong

Peter Baehr

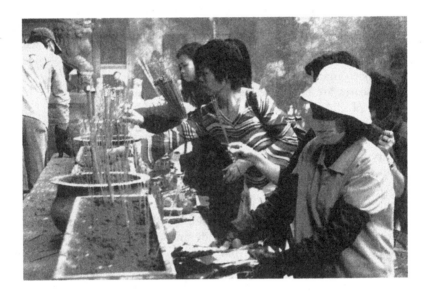

Introduction

The SARS outbreak of 2003 is an occasion not only to detail the impact of a mysterious disease on an unprepared city. It is also an opportunity to reflect on the political and social dynamics of crisis. Already, much has been written about SARS. Yet to understand what happened in Hong Kong (and elsewhere) during the SARS crisis, we need concepts and theories to guide us. Up to this point, we have had all too few; discussion of SARS remains limited to an overwhelmingly descriptive register. In this chapter, I propose to introduce two concepts – "authoritarian toleration" and "efface work" – that enable us to discern why and how SARS took the shape it did in Hong

Kong. I begin with some background information before moving on to discuss the political debility that SARS revealed, its consequences on the mainland, and its implications for a post-Westphalian health order. A final section examines the ritual aspects of mask culture in a diseased city; I contend that the mask symbolized a complex form of solidarity.

Life and Death in a Time of SARS

The SARS outbreak of spring 2003 was a major blow to the people of Hong Kong. Between the end of March and June 23, when the World Health Organization (WHO) removed the territory from its list of SARS-affected areas, the very face of Hong Kong changed. The mask became ubiquitous. Crowded shopping malls and restaurants emptied as people retreated to their tiny apartments. Schools and universities closed. The property market sagged still further, swelling the number of owners in negative equity. Expatriates and others flew home, often to be met by friends and relatives less than delighted to see them. Tourism plummeted and with it hotel occupancy, which in April and May fell to 20 percent. Cathay Pacific – Hong Kong's flagship airline – flies on average 33,000 people a day; in April, that decreased to 4,000. Workers were laid off in droves as over 3,800 businesses folded between March and the beginning of June: by May, unemployment at around 9 percent was the highest since 1975. Fewer tourists exacerbated deflation as retailers cut prices to promote sales.[1] And from abroad a series of interdictions revealed Hong Kong's emerging pariah status. The Swiss government told Hong Kong exhibitors planning to show their wares at the Basel World Watch and Jewellery Show to stay away. In May, a number of American universities – Berkeley, the University of Rochester in New York, and Washington University in St Louis, Missouri – imposed a series of restraints on Hong Kong students: summer school programs were postponed or cancelled; students were advised to miss their graduating ceremony. Hong Kong athletes were debarred from participating in the 2003 Special Olympics World Summer Games.[2]

Compared with other diseases, the death toll of SARS patients was tiny at 299, and even that number is likely to be inflated because few post mortems, the gold standard of death attribution, were conducted.[3] (A person might suffer from SARS but expire because of some other condition.) In 2002, 370 people died of atypical pneumonia in Hong Kong. Each year, influenza kills 20,000 people in the United States alone. By the turn of the new millennium, HIV/AIDS had taken 20 million people globally and infected 36 million more (Kiple 2003, p. 5). According to the 2004 Report on the Global Aids Epidemic, 7.4 million Asians have AIDS. It was the mystery of the SARS coronavirus, and the suddenness of its appearance, that created most anxiety. And no one knew at the height of the outbreak what the final death tally would be. Making matters worse was the correct perception that health workers – the people who are supposed to be the protectors of others – were themselves a disproportionately high victim group. Of 1,755 people classified as having SARS in Hong Kong, 386 were medical staff. To help them, civil society and media organizations launched a series of campaigns. "Fighting SARS. It's Everyone's Business" proclaimed the *South China Morning Post* (SCMP) in a May 1 report that described how transport operators, hotels, banks, arts and recreation venues, supermarkets, restaurants, and other businesses were all playing their part in a city-wide alliance. So, too, was the SCMP itself, which organized "Project Shield" – a mass fund raising campaign to provide medical supplies (superior goggles, face masks, protective hoods with respirators, DuPont Barrierman protection suits, etc.) for the embattled public health sector workers. Within a week of being launched in late April, it collected over $HK10 million.

Paradoxes of Authoritarian Toleration

And what of the Hong Kong government's response to the SARS outbreak? It is simplistic to argue that the government's tardy and confused response was the result of a few ineffectual individuals. Overall, individual ministers acted in good faith and with integrity. So did the much-maligned Chief Executive Tung Chee-hua. To explain how the authorities mishandled SARS, we need to go deeper and examine the peculiar political order that constitutes Hong Kong.

A "political order," in this usage, refers to something more elemental than either a particular administration or the stream of policy decisions that every administration must expedite to run a modern state. It denotes, instead, the structural framework of governance, the political rules of the game, within which policy decisions are grounded and executed. This suggests another distinction: between a policy blunder on the one hand, and a political defect on the other; that is, a deficiency, tension, or contradiction that shapes the broader policy arena. Much recent critical commentary on Hong Kong has focused on a series of ministerial scandals, chaotic equivocations, and disastrous political decisions that show the incompetence of a particular administration. Though these incidents are, as unhappy mishaps, comparable in principle to the misjudgments that governments commit everywhere, they are also connected to a predicament that goes to the fundaments of Hong Kong's political arrangements. The SARS crisis of 2003 exposed a government not simply unprepared for the disease itself – no government was prepared – but one whose *system* of governance was chronically fragile, commanding very little confidence among most Hong Kong people. The source of this fragility goes beyond the widespread disenchantment that most citizens feel today for the vocation of politics, or ideological antipathy to particular party programs or policies. The problem lies in the very nature of the Hong Kong Special Administrative Region as a legal or corporate "person," the rival principles of legitimacy – liberalism and Leninism – to which that person is subject, and the tensile field of opportunities and restraints it affords Hong Kong people.

To understand the structural weaknesses of this political order, it is instructive to examine some key features of Hong Kong's Basic Law, adopted on April 4, 1990 at the third session of the Seventh National People's Congress of the People's Republic of China (PRC). The Basic Law, a tortuous by-product of the Sino-British Joint Declaration (1984), is often described as Hong Kong's "mini-constitution," a label that is simultaneously true and misleading. It is true in the sense that the Basic Law formally allocates various powers to the executive, legislative, and judicial branches of the Hong Kong Special Administrated Region (HKSAR), and sets up a *modus vivendi* among them. In such wise, the Basic Law enshrines the "constitution" of Hong Kong.

Yet the label "mini-constitution" is misleading to the point of being absurd if one imagines the Basic Law to be a constitution in, for instance, the American republican sense. First, and most obviously, Hong Kong is not itself a state, the Basic Law is not a product of Hong Kong people, and the territory over which it distributes its powers has no sovereignty of its own. Unlike republican constitutions that stand on their own feet, the Basic Law is subordinate to, and an appendage of, Article 31 of the Constitution of the PRC. It is thus a derivative document, rather than a founding charter *sui generis*. Article 1 of the Basic Law defines the HKSAR as "an inalienable part" of the PRC. Article 2 stipulates that it is the "National People's Congress [that] authorizes" the HKSAR "to exercise a high degree of autonomy and enjoy executive, legislative and independent judicial power." Article 2 continues by granting Hong Kong's courts "final adjudication," but this is not as final as it first appears. Though the power of "final adjudication" of the HKSAR is vested in the Court of Final Appeal (Art. 82), the "power of *interpretation*" of the Basic Law itself belongs to the Standing Committee of the National People's Congress (Art. 158), as is the power of amendment of the Basic Law (Art. 159). It transpires that it is the National People's Congress in Beijing – and behind it the Politburo – rather than any Hong Kong court that is empowered to settle definitively a controversial legal issue that has been referred to it by the HKSAR government. The appointment of the Chief Executive (currently Tung Chee-hwa) by an 800-member, Beijing-dominated, nominating committee, and the bifurcation of Hong Kong's legislature into functional (corporate) and geographical constituencies, also militates against democratic representation.

A second feature follows. Despite the impressive panoply or rights of mobility, association, communication, conscience, welfare, and domestic security that Hong Kong residents enjoy under Chapter III of the Basic Law, these liberties have no independent status. They ultimately depend for their existence and exercise upon the *authoritarian toleration* of the Sovereign. Hong Kong's freedoms are, in other words, the result of permission. And their basic precariousness became obvious in the autumn of 2002, when the Hong Kong government belatedly commenced its consultations over Article 23 of the Basic Law. Article 23 requires the local government to "enact laws on its own to prohibit any act of treason, secession, sedition, subversion against the Central People's Government, or theft of state secrets." Article 23 also instructs the HKSAR to "prohibit foreign political organizations or bodies from conducting activities in the Region, and to prohibit political organizations or bodies of the Region from establishing ties with foreign political organizations or bodies." The coincidence of Article 23's introduction and SARS could not have been worse for the government. Hong Kong people knew of the SARS cover-up on the mainland. They knew, also, that disease information is strictly controlled by the CCP. If Article 23 had been up and running in Hong Kong, what would have happened to its media? Would it have been able to monitor and criticize the government's performance? And here we come to a paradox of authoritarian toleration. Simplifying a more complex picture, one can say that while SARS in pluralist Hong Kong served to weaken the local government still further, SARS on the mainland probably contributed to the strengthening of the Communist state. The Hong Kong government suffered a blow to its prestige for at least two reasons.

To begin with, the Basic Law simply does not allow the government to be truly representative, legitimated by popular consent and participation. This is the authoritarian face of the system. In consequence, the travails that Hong Kong people endured since the handover of 1997 – the financial crash, persistent deflation, falling property prices – were blamed not on a ruling *party* that could have been ejected at the next election, but on an immobile system that had become hopelessly out of touch with public opinion. SARS deepened the sense of malaise because bureaucratic guardianship, couched in juridical and scientific language, came to be experienced as remote and patronizing by those subject to it. Politicians graced with the popular touch, skilled in political electoral battles, and able to speak a discernibly visceral language were nowhere to be found at the upper echelon of decision-making. Hong Kong people looked for the vibrant leadership associated with Rudy Giuliani; they found instead the avuncular and ineffective Tung Chee-hwa, an erstwhile shipping magnate, unable to steer the ship of state.

Moreover, as Ma Ngok (2003, pp. 113–4) perceptively observes, "the relevant policy decisions on SARS were mostly made by medical professionals.

Secretary [for Health, Welfare and Food] Yeoh, Head of Health Department Margaret Chan, and top executives of the Hospital Authority are all medical doctors by training." So, too, was Arthur Li Kwok-cheung, the Secretary for Education and Manpower. The result of their scientific mindset was a pronounced tendency to consider public fears as irrational, exaggerated, and unenlightened. Health Secretary Yeoh Eng-kiong originally downplayed the seriousness of SARS; throughout the crisis he refused to don a mask in public, believing that the virus was transmissible only through intimate contact. On March 15, Arthur Li insisted that school closures were unnecessary because schools were the safest place to be. That may or may have not been true. But the corollary of such an Olympian attitude was to make him appear dilatory or indifferent to the urgent desire of parents to protect their children. To make matters worse for Mr Tung's administration, while the medical leaders of the government and Health Authority took the brunt of public anger, health workers on the front lines assumed the aura of public heroes facing not only the hazards of a mystery pathogen but also the ill-coordinated efforts of those who should have been their champions. Admired for their dedication, discipline, and sacrifice, healthcare workers acquired prestige in direct proportion to the government's loss of it. *It was they who came to represent the people of Hong Kong* in the spring of 2003. The most basic justification of any state to exist is that it can protect its own citizens or subjects. By failing to be, or to look, effective in the "war" against SARS – the ubiquitous military language revealed the stakes involved – the administration forfeited public trust.

A second reason SARS weakened the Hong Kong government has to do with the pluralism of the wider society it manages. Because genuine liberties do exist permissively in Hong Kong, under authoritarian toleration, people were able to take advantage of them, initiating courses of action independent of the government and, in the process, making it look even more feeble. As Michael DeGolyer (Loh and Civic Exchange 2004, p. 124) recalls:

> Members of the public ... pulled students by the thousands out of schools and made the decision to close scores of schools voluntarily, even over Government threats, weeks before the Government closed all educational facilities until preventative measures could be put in place. The media led a campaign to raise money for and purchase and distribute protective clothing to front line hospital staff – after the Government was patently failing to do so. Businesses launched informational campaigns to inform themselves and their overseas colleagues of the situation in Hong Kong, weeks before the Government could organize its own version.

In short, SARS weakened the Hong Kong government because it played on the frailties and opportunities afforded by authoritarian toleration. If Hong

Kong's political order had been open to greater participation, selecting politicians who enjoyed popular confidence and who spoke a "language" that ordinary people understood, it would still have faced major obstacles. But the chances of surmounting them without major political damage would have been higher. Conversely, if the regime had been based on a less open and more repressive system – if, in short, there had been less toleration and more authoritarianism than on the mainland – it would never have allowed residents to organize themselves independently, to monitor relentlessly government activity (and inactivity), and on July 1 to hold a protest demonstration consisting of half a million people. The protest was aimed ostensibly at the government's activation of Article 23, the Basic Law provision discussed above. But it was the administration's mishandling of SARS, above all, that galvanized the streets.

Mainland China and the Emergence of a Post-Westphalian System

A contrast with mainland China is instructive. It is very difficult to judge the extent to which SARS increased or weakened the Communist Party's mandate. Many who visited China in April 2003, and some of my own students who returned there during the university's Easter vacation, paint a picture of anger and bitterness at a party that thought more of its own reputation than its citizens' lives. Maochun Yu (in Congress of the United States 2003, pp. 83–4), a professor at the United States Naval Academy, remarks that the SARS crisis "discredited" the government's image in many quarters, and ruptured the "banality of deception" in China – the uncritical acceptance by many ordinary Chinese of government positions on Taiwan, Tibet, and US foreign policy. In contrast, the credibility of non-Chinese news outlets – excoriated since the days of Mao for being the "mouthpiece of international anti-China elements" – gained credence from the government's about face in April, a belated admission that the foreign media had been right all along. More than that, SARS provoked muckraking attacks on Chinese Communist Party (CCP) ineptitude and corruption by cyber mavericks such as Ren Bumei, Zheng Yichun, and Donghai Yixiao. It also gave vent to a stream of anti-CCP vitriol that appeared as satirical rhyming couplets or puns, a veritable "bonanza of materials ridiculing the surreal dimensions of the situation" (ibid., p. 84). If parody is to respect what acid is to metal, it would appear that CCP authority was badly corroded by recent events. The government is now determined to improve its internal reporting system. But far from this being a Chinese *anno mirabilis*, presaging greater openness and reform – or even "China's Chernobyl," as *The Economist* speculated in its April 26, 2003 edition – neither the Party nor the government it dominates have yet admitted that it told lies or deceived the Chinese people. The reason given on May 30 by Gao Qiang, the Vice Health Minister, for the leadership's decision to fire the Minister of Health and the Mayor of Beijing was not that they had concealed the scale of SARS. It was that they had been lamentably remiss in locating and transmitting factual ground-level data from their respective jurisdictions to the Central Committee. Slipshod working practices were at fault (ibid., p. 83). The lesson learned was that a modern country requires enhanced Party efficiency and regulatory consistency, something quite different to social transparency or accountability. Yet again we see in China not the oft-predicted fluorescence of civil society, let alone democracy, but the forward march of a Party determined to manage better.

And the Party may well succeed. Besides, the domestic verdict on President Hu Jintao's handling of the crisis was by no means uniformly bad. Publicly exposed by the international media, facing mounting fury at home, and belatedly aware of the potential consequences of SARS for public health, public authority, and international investor confidence, the CCP machine went into full gear. The "old" Maoist institutions – neighborhood and campus committees, the *danwei* (work units) – were mobilized to coral carriers of the epidemic (though thousands fled the cities or were ordered to return to their villages). Ministers and their secretaries, seeking to restore confidence, gave live press conferences charting SARS' course and solemnly reiterating their commitment to abide by WHO diagnostic standards. Since April 2003, more than a billion dollars has been "allocated to build China's national and regional centers for disease control and prevention."(Congress of the United States 2003, p. 103). In Beijing and the coastal cities, at least, the result of the scare was to persuade many Chinese citizens that, whatever the initial bungling, only a strong party, equipped with draconian powers, could have bested SARS or now be able to restructure on a national scale its ramshackle, decentralized health system. And among a rural populace that numbers 700 million, it may be hard to visualize any other organization of national scope that can deal with a public emergency.

On the other hand, never before has the Communist Party been subject to such effective outside pressure. David Fidler (2004), a professor of law, with a keen eye on the interaction between disease and international relations, argues that SARS marked the culmination of a new approach to public health governance in which state sovereignty was trumped by global actors, foremost among them the World Health Organization (WHO). Unofficial sources of information, Fidler shows, were instrumental in tracking the disease. SARS, David Fidler maintains, delivered the *coup de grace* to the "Westphalian" system of public health governance; the term is an allusion to the Peace of Westphalia (1648), which marked the end of three decades of brutal strife in Europe. Attempting to limit the ruinous effects of religious fervor and dynastic ambition, the Westphalian peace sought to stabilize Europe on the basis of three principles: state sovereignty, non-intervention, and international legal agreement among independent states. Henceforth, domestic governments alone would decide what was best for their subjects. Concert among nations would take place on the basis of enlightened self-interest. No recourse would be made to a putative common and supreme authority. From the middle of the nineteenth century until the last decade of the twentieth, Westphalian governance typified the international health regime too. Article 2.7 of the United Nations Charter (1945) endorses the non-intervention principle. The WHO's International Health Regulations (IHR), now in the process of radical reformulation, enshrine it. Adopted under Articles 21 and 22 of the WHO constitution, the IHR (an outgrowth of the 1951 International Sanitary Regulations) were unabashedly minimalist. Only three diseases – plague, cholera, and yellow fever – were subject to IHR rules of reporting. In turn, relevant epidemiological information had to issue from a government body, as distinct from a non-governmental outlet. The IHR architecture was designed principally to avoid undue interference with trade and travel. By the 1980s, the IHR were plainly antiquated. HIV/AIDS fell outside the IHR purview, yet few health threats were greater. Emerging and re-emerging diseases testified to an urgent need to supplement horizontal (inter-state) rules by vertical (intra-state) ones that would eradicate disease at source. Yet the Westphalian governance system had never accepted that it was the job of "outside" bodies to interfere with a nation's "internal" disease-control measures. Accordingly, "WHO member states routinely violated their IHR obligations to report outbreaks of diseases subject to the Regulations" (Fidler 2004, p. 35).

So it was neither surprising nor against the letter of the IHR for China to balk at international pressure for full disclosure. The WHO's Global Outbreak Alert and Response Network (established in 1997) had no pan-national "right" to demand information from recalcitrant states. It still has no right. But, and this is the key to Fidler's analysis, SARS gave it the legitimacy to intervene. Never before on such a scale, and with such vigor, had the WHO so brazenly employed information from non-state actors (individual citizens, lobby and political interest groups, Internet reporting systems such as the Program for Monitoring Emerging Diseases [ProMed]), to evaluate government statements. Never before had it become the virtual arbiter of travel, through its advisories and alerts. The WHO's Global Network had no formal legal authority to do any of this, or even to advise individual travelers to reconsider their plans; the "correct" procedure would have been a recommendation to governments that *they* advise their nationals to postpone travel. But the WHO did not wait for permission. Instead, it minted its own authority during the SARS crisis, despite being angrily denounced for exceeding its remit by agencies such as Health Canada.

In May 2003, the World Health Assembly put the official, retrospective, seal of approval on the WHO's actions. True, prior to 2003, the WHO was already inching toward a more activist role, spurred particularly by HIV/AIDS and re-emerging diseases. Further back, its own constitution was "the first international legal instrument to state that the right to the highest attainable health standard of physical and mental health was a fundamental human right (WHO 1948, Preamble). The human right to health is radically counter-Westphalian because it makes the individual rather than the state the central governance focus" (Fidler 2004, p. 38). The WHO's response to SARS dramatized this seditious idea by acting as if it were consequential. Meanwhile, in mainland China, the WHO's pressure prodded the government to recognize the seriousness of the threat that it faced. Eventually, Beijing sought the world's help until the early summer, when SARS appeared to be defeated.

The Masked City

SARS can be understood epidemiologically as a virus that tested Hong Kong's healthcare system and governance to the maximum. Sociologically, it can be seen as a test of Hong Kong's moral existence: how the city and its environs coped with fear. The ancient notion that plague is a sign of evil is no primitive superstition. It grasps the reality that any threat to the group as a whole is simultaneously a "sacred" violatory event of the most extreme kind (Gordon 1999, p. 7). The specter of plague or any other pandemic summons up the possibility of a collective death: the extirpation of the social itself. How did Hong Kong deal with such an eventuality? Let me focus on one salient response.

Durkheim claimed to find the index of forms of solidarity in law and attitudes toward punishment and compensation. Another vital index, I suggest, is to be found in the "social language" (Goffman 1974 [1959], p. 159), symbols and "codes of representation" that people use to describe their predicament. More precisely, solidarity can be located by investigating *what* people saliently speak about, *how* they speak about it – that is, with what terms and metaphors – and with *what sensibility*.

Elsewhere, I examine this language, particularly its Chinese articulation, in some detail (Baehr 2006). Here I will only sketch its main dimensions. What Hong Kong people spoke about was the disease itself. Was it abating or spreading? What could be done to stop it? How safe were one's children and relatives? Should domestic helpers be permitted to leave their employers' apartments for the usual Sunday gatherings in Central (the financial and government district) and elsewhere? By definition, this is not the usual language of everyday life, but when it momentarily becomes so it articulates by repetition the new reality. How did Hong Kong residents speak about SARS? Short of a genuine ethnography, we cannot be certain. But in both Chinese and English language media, metaphors of war were pervasive. Tung Chee-hwa, Hong Kong's Chief Executive, announced early on that "we [government ministers] are confident that we [Hong Kong people] will win the war."[4] Nurses and doctors were described ubiquitously, by government officials, media and citizens as "frontline" workers (*qianxian*) and, albeit with militaristic hyperbole, as "troops" (*jundui*) that are "marching through the fog."[5] Hong Kong's premier English-language newspaper, the *South China Morning Post*, organized "Operation Shield" to raise funds for the "embattled" medics. Medals were dispensed to the dead; their bodies buried in Gallant Garden.

Much of this disease-as-war language was government and media "frame." Its plausibility in the popular imagination can only be conjectured. More evident is Hong Kong's response to its "heroes," a term widely used during the outbreak to describe medical staff who died trying to protect others. And here we approach the issue of moral sensibility. For at the same time that Hong Kong people were bitterly criticizing their own government for what they deemed to be its general incompetence, their hearts went out to those in the front line. Georg Simmel (1950 [1908], pp. 387–8) reminds us that gratitude is an emotionally charged form of giving, supplementing the legal order; unlike monetary exchange, it is "practical and impulsive." He adds that although gratitude "may remain, of course something internal, it may yet engender new actions." It forms part of "the moral memory of mankind." That memory is today discernible in the bronze busts, titular scholarships, and commemorations through which Hong Kong people now recall the dead health workers.

If language was one key medium through which people communicated a danger to their own existence as individuals and to the mortality of the society of which they were part, social ritual was another. Here I am less concerned with the persistence of established rituals than I am with the emergence of new ones, peculiar to the situation itself. Durkheim argued, in *The Elementary Forms of Religious Life* ([1912] 1995), that social solidarity requires the existence of bodies in close and regular interaction, face-to-face encounters, to charge up a sense of a common reality. In a powerful recent adaptation of this argument, Randall Collins (2004, p. 41) glosses:

> Society is held together more intensely at some moments than at others. And the "society" that is held together is no abstract unity of a social system, but is just those groups of people assembled in particular places who feel solidarity with each other through the effects of ritual participation and ritually charged symbolism.

Of particular importance, in Collins' theory, is what he calls "emotional energy": the variable confidence, élan, initiative, and purposefulness that people derive from ritual interactions and that by social disposition they seek to maximize. Emotional energy is localized and situation specific; it is most intense at the moment of the ritual itself, tending to drain away thereafter unless and until it is periodically renewed. It both belongs to and, in feedback loops, constitutes a ritual encounter. In a figure that schematizes the ritual process, Collins (ibid., p. 48) itemizes its four necessary ingredients: group assembly (bodily co-presence), barrier to outsiders, mutual focus of attention, and shared mood. Let us apply these ingredients to the Hong Kong case.

What kind of society was Hong Kong during the SARS crisis? I am not thinking here of intensive units of interaction such as health workers – or New York firefighters in the aftermath of 9/11 – who handled the crisis around the clock, lived together for weeks on end so as to avoid infecting their own families and who, by so doing, intensified the bonds of their own solidarity pocket. My interest is in the wider society, the ostensible spectators on events, as it were. What, if anything, distinguished it symbolically from its previous social character? A shared mood of trepidation was one feature, aggravated by the fact that SARS was a new virus for which there was no known cure and that mutated in unpredictable ways. A mutual focus of attention was another factor, centered on daily (sometimes hourly) updates of SARS casualty statistics, and information about where the disease was spreading. And there was a double barrier to outsiders: one elected by foreigners who stopped coming to Hong Kong; the other generated, under pressure, among Hong Kongers themselves for whom domestic strangers – and even intimates – became a source of jeopardy as unwitting carriers of the pestilence. Where, then, was the group-assembly, the close interaction that gives people a sense of belonging? Had it momentarily disappeared? Or was there still some means by which it made an appearance? Disease repels people from contact. It puts a premium on co-absence. By minimizing bodily contact it must also attenuate solidarity and moral density, and thereby the presence of society itself. The reality is more complex.

In a seminal essay, Erving Goffman coined the term "face work" to exemplify the many ways in which individuals publicly challenge, apologize, cooperate, and forgive one another in situations of co-presence. "A person's performance of face work, extended by his tacit agreement to help others perform theirs, represents his willingness to abide by the ground rules of social interaction" (Goffman 1967a [1955], p. 31). For Goffman, the self consists not just as an assemblage of "expressive implications" but also as "a kind of player in a ritual game who copes honourably or dishonourably, diplomatically or undiplomatically, with the judgmental contingencies of the situation" (ibid., p. 31). "By repeatedly and automatically asking himself the question: 'If I do or do not act in this way, will I or others lose face?,' he decides at each moment, consciously or unconsciously, how to behave" (ibid., p. 36). As is well known, Chinese culture attributes an especial importance to "face" and its requirements.[6] The paradox of *efface* work begins, however, with the face out of sight. Disease, too, is faceless, invisible, unlike a marauding army, a volcanic lava flow, a tsunami wave, or the violently swaying trees that announce the arrival of a hurricane. And the more mysterious it is, the more a disease is likely to induce generalized hypochondria. All kinds of sundry illnesses are read as its symptoms: diarrhea, coughing, fever.

Disease in Hong Kong is a remarkable laboratory to examine how even in situations of social repulsion a collective existence is affirmed. Isolation has its social patterns and consequences. Granted, where possible, people in Hong Kong vacated the usual packed public spaces: shopping malls, restaurants, churches, and cinemas. But for the most part flight was impossible. People still went to work and, for at least half of the period in which SARS was active, to school and to university. Those without their own vehicles (the majority) were compelled to employ public transport. Thus bodies remained co-present for much of the time. Families still met, even if there was reluctance to keep up contact with elder members – the key target group of SARS deaths.

In a masked city it was difficult to recognize the identity even of one's friends and colleagues as they passed. Yet mask-wearing became the quickly improvised, if obligatory, social ritual; failing to don one was met with righteous indignation, a clear sign of ritual violation. The mask symbolized a rule of conduct – namely, an *obligation* to protect the wider community – and an *expectation* regarding how one was to be treated by others (Goffman 1967b [1956], p. 49). More simply, the mask was the emblematic means by which people communicated their responsibilities to the social group of which they were members. Through mimicry and synchronization – key mechanisms of emotional contagion (Hatfield et al. 1994, pp. 156–8) – mask-wearing amounted to a joint action, normatively embodied, the entrainment and attunement of the society as a whole. By disguising an individual's face, it gave greater salience to collective identity. By blurring social distinctions, it produced social resemblance. Mask-wearing activated and reactivated a sense of a common fate; it was a mode of reciprocity under conditions that supremely tested it. Accordingly, mask demeanor was much more than a prophylactic against disease. It showed deference to public emotions and the decision to respect them. That throughout the crisis Health Secretary Yeoh refused to wear a mask, saying that the virus was only transmissible through intimate contact, was a social gaffe of the first order. Note too that efface work – precisely because it is a performance – requires effort. Though this is not the emotional energy of attraction and enthusiasm, and the antithesis of collective celebration, mask-wearing demands activity: donning the mask, changing it every couple of hours, feeling it become fetid with spittle, speaking through it in frustratingly muffled tones, buying new masks, ripping them off in relief when backstage. As a contribution to general sociological theory, I suggest that SARS showed that social ritual (as mask-wearing) can function even where *there is resistance to bodily contact*, even where *emotional energy is very low*, and even where a group *uses an emblem that appears to symbolize the opposite of integration.*

Conclusions

Societies, like individuals, forget easily. They crave normality, a reflex that has advantages. Existence cannot be lived as if it were a perpetual crisis. Forgetfulness and distraction allow us to let go of past injury; inconsistency is a welcome impediment to fanaticism. Yet understanding and memory are vital too. Epidemic is a menace to both the individual body and the body politic. In this chapter, I have sought to locate theoretically the political and social responses to SARS. Other chapters in this volume do more, urging vigilance and action. As we brace ourselves for an avian flu outbreak, their message could not be more timely.

NOTES

1   For economic data, see Sung and Cheung (2003). See also Brown (2004b). The first book on SARS, entitled *SARS War. Combating the Disease,* was by P.C. Leung and E.E. Ooi (2003). It was published in late April 2003 [sic].
2   All these prohibitions were quite quickly lifted, but by then the emotional damage had been done.
3   The WHO's gross total worldwide, as of July 11, 2003, was 8,437. Of these, 7452 recovered, while 813 perished, a case fatality rate of 9.6 percent.
4   *Ta Kung Po*, March 28, 2003, A01 (no reporter's name cited). Chinese has various terms for war and battle, notably *zhang* and *zhan.*
5   *Apple Daily*, March 17, 2003, A02 (reporters Leung Shun-yu, Chui Doi-ling, Chui Wan-ting, and Lai Ka-kui).
6   Significantly, the first footnote of Goffman's "Face-Work" essay is devoted to Chinese conceptions of face. For a more recent analysis, see Bond (1991, pp. 58–71).

9

"Racism is a Weapon of Mass Destruction": SARS and the Social Fabric of Urban Multiculturalism

Roger Keil and S. Harris Ali

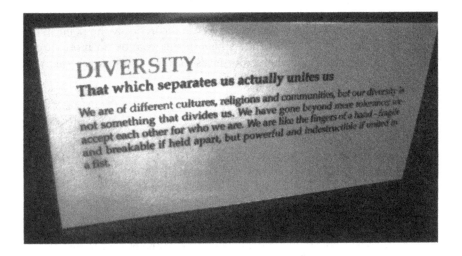

DIVERSITY
That which separates us actually unites us

We are of different cultures, religions and communities, but our diversity is not something that divides us. We have gone beyond mere tolerance; we accept each other for who we are. We are like the fingers of a hand - fragile and breakable if held apart, but powerful and indestructible if united in a fist.

Introduction

Dis-information is a weapon of mass destruction
You could a Caucasian or a poor Asian
Racism is a weapon of mass destruction
Whether inflation or globalisation
Fear is a weapon of mass destruction

Faithless, "Mass Destruction," 2004

In early June 2006, Canadian security forces arrested 17 individuals for the alleged plotting of terrorist acts. All 17 were Muslims from various immigrant communities in the larger Toronto area. In the days after the arrests, which were based on a series of Internet-communicated schemes hedged by the young men and a shipment of ammonium nitrate (the main ingredient in the 1995 Oklahoma City bombing), discussions about diversity, tolerance, and rac(e)ism flared up in Toronto. The windows of a mosque were shattered in acts of vandalism. The police chief, Bill Blair, vowed to protect the innocent and to avoid a hunt on Toronto's Islamic population. A few weeks earlier, Toronto police had staged a similar raid. This time, the suspects (of whom there were more than 100), were nabbed in an early morning, through the military-style action of 600 officers. These were not suspected terrorists but allegedly common drug dealers, consisting of the "Jamestown Crew" gang members and weapon-wielding neighborhood crooks. Furthermore, the majority of the suspects belonged to the Caribbean-Canadian community, mostly black youth. In the aftermath of these arrests, too, a discussion ensued about the racial aspects of the police action (and subsequent court proceedings). As the American paper *Christian Science Monitor* reported, "while police and the public applauded the hard-line approach, social pundits and criminology professors are sceptical that the approach is getting at the roots of the problem: poverty, illiteracy, dysfunctional families, and racism in a diverse ethnic population" (Newman 2006). Although most would agree that terrorism is a bad thing and drugs and guns are a seriously dangerous combination, there may be reason to reflect on the prospective fallout of such pervasive police action against a clearly identifiable group in a city that prides itself on its diversity. In such moments of violent clashes between the state and some of its citizens in the diverse globalizing city, the ripple effects of the fight against certain kinds of crime and terror can backfire. These conflictual situations, which pit certain groups in society against others and against the state, reveal the fundamental volatility of the arrangements that govern diversity in globalizing urban regions such as Toronto. Recalling a line from the British band Faithless' 2004 hit song "Mass Destruction," we note that "racism is a weapon of mass destruction." We argue that the vulnerability of complex multicultural or diverse cities such as Toronto to violent racist incidents has been pervasive in a post-9/11 environment. We maintain further that the threat of terrorism and violence is similar to the possible effects of the threats posed by pandemic infectious disease. As became clear in the case of the 2003 Toronto SARS outbreak, racism against the perceived carriers of the virus, mostly Chinese-Canadians, developed into a potential "weapon of mass destruction" capable of the unhinging of the carefully crafted, albeit profoundly fragile, community relationships of the multicultural Canadian city.

The potentially explosive effect of SARS on Canadian society is that it (or the "Asian" flu, the avian flu or some other pandemic like it – Davis 2005; Dyer 2006) fundamentally endangers the precarious compromise between the settler society and postmodern multiculturalism. If Canada/Toronto is billed as the postmodern model of lived diversity, will it be able to withstand the new biopolitical and disciplinary onslaught of the crisis an emerging infectious disease pandemic? And to what degree can a more emphatic concept of biopower emerge from the incipient crisis of multiculturalism as witnessed during the SARS outbreak of 2003? We are asking now: What happens when biopolitics meets the multicultural society? The important issue here is the transition from a unilateral (usually state-based) biopolitical intervention to a contested terrain, in which biopower is produced in a process of competing forces. In this sense, biopower is enmeshed in a larger context of societal relations (actor-networks, if you will), where racism is one, multiculturalism another mode of regulation. This means that there are competing options here for the structuration of relationships of racialization and disease through biopolitical regulation (e.g., state measures against certain migrant groups suspected of being carriers of disease), and the biopower assertions of various social groups (e.g., community organization against the articulation of medical practices with processes of racialization) (see also Allahwala 2006).

SARS and Racialization in Toronto[1]

While the human and economic losses associated with SARS were central to most reports and academic analyses of the outbreak, there was also reason to be concerned about the less-publicized aspects of racialization of the disease and subsequent incidents and tendencies of racism in affected societies, especially large multicultural cities such as Toronto, Hong Kong, or Singapore (*Asian Pacific Post* 2003; Leung and Guan 2004). All this occurred in a situation where race and disease are linked already. The racialization of poverty and disease is not an epiphenomenon but a structural condition of the global city. In relation to the health field in particular, Galabuzi has found, for example, that "the racialization of poverty" has also led to inequalities in the health and well-being of visible minority populations: "Such documented characteristics of racialized poverty as labour market segregation and low occupation status, high and frequent unemployment status, substandard housing combined with violent or distressed neighbourhoods, homelessness, poor working conditions, extended hours of work or multiple jobs, experience with everyday forms of racism and sexism, lead to unequal health service utilization, and differential health status" (Galabuzi 2004, p. 235).

The main consequence of a disease like SARS might ultimately not be its impact as a killer of infected individuals, but its impact as a destroyer of the tenuous multicultural fabric of Toronto. Implying that the disease might be linked to China (its place of origin) or to the Chinese (as carriers of the virus) has had severe implications for the relationship of East Asian immigrants to other people in the Greater Toronto Area (GTA). Canadian citizens of Chinese origin comprised about 7.5 percent (348,010) of the 4,647,955 people living in the Toronto metropolitan area in 2001 (Statistics Canada 2005a). The city is the preferred destination of most immigrants from Asian countries to Canada.

Toronto is often referred to as the most multicultural city in the world. About 50 percent of its population of 2.5 million are people of color ("visible minorities" in the official Canadian parlance); about 50 percent are immigrants to Canada. Most Canadian immigrants come to the GTA, a global city region of 5 million people and the economic engine of the country. By the middle of the next decade, more than half of the population in the region will be non-white. This diversity is governed by an official federal policy of multiculturalism as well as various time-honored institutions of multiculturalism at other governance scales, most prominently in the City of Toronto. Still not all is well as far as the inter-ethnic and inter-"racial" relations in Toronto are concerned, and as such, the policy of multiculturalism is often criticized as acting as a smokescreen that masks various institutional forms of racism in the housing and labor markets, in the education system, in law enforcement, and so on (Goonewardena and Kipfer 2005). While the topic of racialization of social relations is painstakingly avoided in public discourse, on the radio, in schools, and so on, the Canadian settler society, with its own history of secondary imperialism, continues to have huge unresolved issues of racism related to Aboriginal communities, Black Canadians, as well as, increasingly, Asian immigrants. The question we are asking here is: Will multiculturalism be challenged by the phantasmagoric articulation of virus and race (Sarasin 2006)? Is there a collusion in the public perception of seeing alien viruses in alien bodies?

Our chapter will provide a narrative of the racialization of infectious disease in the context of Toronto's multiculturalism and the region's formation as a major global city. We will advance the hypothesis that the SARS outbreak strained the usually happy appearance of this particular multicultural urban fabric of diversity. The chapter is not a systematic empirical discussion of racism in connection with SARS. There is overwhelming structural and anecdotal evidence of racialization in public discourse, everyday practices, and institutional policies, as documented in the comprehensive study by Carrianne Leung and Jian Guan (and as witnessed by several important submissions to the expert panels of the three SARS commissions; see Chapter 11). Rather, this chapter presents a conceptual argument on the relationship of globalized urbanization, emerging infectious disease, and racism. The history of cities and the history of migration are intertwined. This is an old story. It has recently been punctuated by the emergence of a specific type of urbanization that arrived with the latest phase of globalization of capitalism: global or world city formation (for an overview, see Brenner and Keil 2006). This process is fundamentally connected to the migration of labor, both at the high and low ends of labor markets, to global cities. Flows of capital draw flows of labor (Sassen 1991; Samers 2002). For some, the diasporic movement of people to the burgeoning global cities is the hallmark of the current period.

Urbanization, Racism, and Disease

Keeping cities safe from disease has long meant keeping certain racialized groups either outside or controlled. The individual body that is infected with the virus is seen as a threat to the "popular body," which is always racialized (Sarasin 2003, 2006). The conundrum of racism as a decision "between what shall live and what shall die" (Foucault 2003; Sarasin 2003, 2006) is hence inscribed in a multitude of regulations of urban migration and settlement, daily conduct, and emergency behavior. Racism appears as both a central element of societal/urban normalcy and as the source of many forms of social death (Lemke 2003). The structural racism of the urban morphology (expressed in historical processes of ghettoization and segregation) is compounded with a set of more or less opportunistic rules that govern how bodies move in these morphologies. Fighting infectious disease is always tied up closely with spatial strategies of control, particularly linked to the use of urban spaces. Historically, attempts have been made to confine disease through ghettoization of infected populations, along with their often racialized or otherwise marked segmentation from mainstream societies. There are basically two kinds of segmentation possible: expulsion or ghettoization. Although not well examined (Craddock 1995, p. 957), most of the ways in which we view infectious disease have a clear geographical dimension. How are connections made between the control of populations who are real or perceived carriers of disease, their residence, and their economic utility for the system? The interaction of local/global economic interests, domestic/foreign health concerns, and race/residence concocted a brew of victimization that proved positively uncomfortable and potentially dangerous to the Asian community in particular and the entire fabric of Toronto multiculturalism in general. SARS endangered the social fabric in a physical and political way. The virus represented a corporeal threat to the body politic. Canadian urban multiculturalism was the result of the specific processes of societalization of a white settler society, which is now transformed into a society strongly shaped by non-European immigrants.

SARS, Biopolitics, and the Crisis of Multiculturalism

The story of SARS in the global city is a new narrative. In the process of global city formation, it has been argued that place becomes race (Razack 2002a,b).

The usual story on Toronto's history of diversity goes like this: "The city has transformed, in less than a generation, from an overwhelmingly white Christian society to a multicultural, multi-faith society. While commonly referred to earlier in the century as 'the Belfast of the North,' following the 1998 municipal amalgamation, the newly established mega-city of Toronto adopted the phrase 'Diversity is our Strength" as its official motto" (Isin and Siemiatycki 2002, p. 189). During the 1990s, the Toronto story was rewritten accordingly and became a big chunk of the national mythology itself:

> The land, once empty and later populated by hardy settlers, is now besieged and crowded by Third World refugees and migrants who are drawn to Canada by the legendary niceness of European Canadians, their well-known commitment to democracy, and the bounty of their land. The "crowds" at the border threaten the calm, ordered spaces of the original inhabitants. A special geographical imagination is clearly traceable in the story of origins told in anti-immigration rhetoric, operating as metaphor but also enabling material practices such as the increased policing of the border and of bodies of color. (Razack 2002a, p. 4)

Official multiculturalism is meant to regulate the demographic diversity on the basis of the traditional "diversity management" between Aboriginals and French and English colonists (Wood and Gilbert 2005). But multiculturalism as a state policy, together with the commodified, market-regulated everyday life of neoliberal capitalism, also represents a new form of "differentialist" racism, which differentiates between people less on the basis of (constructed) biological difference and more on the basis of (assumed and reified) cultural characteristics (Goonewardena and Kipfer 2005). Viewed in such a way as a form of racism, multiculturalism displaces racialized social conflicts (over jobs, residence, police behavior, etc.) onto a placated cultural terrain. It needs to be added that the official multiculturalism in Canada entered the historical stage when Canadian politics changed from its post-World War II doctrine of social equity to the current programs based on neoliberal competition politics (Rao 2002; Wood and Gilbert 2005). Since arriving in the 1970s, the new, mostly visible minority immigrants, the majority of whom settle in Toronto, have been predominantly employed in the low-paid and precarious occupations of the neoliberal, post-Fordist model. Non-white migrants who came to Canada between 1976 and 1995 earned between 17.1 and 27.7 percent less than white immigrants in the same period. The rate of poverty among visible minorities is twice as high as among white Canadians (Galabuzi, cited in Rao 2002, pp. 18, 23). The official policy and ideology of multiculturalism perpetuates the myth of the classless immigrant society, while in reality ethnic communities are being disorganized. Professionals and other members of the ethnic intelligentsia are separated physically and in their everyday lives from their communities, and must be content with jobs in manual labor or in low-wage services (Rao 2002). With the changing composition of the immigrant population, the spatial pattern of settlement has changed as well. The settlement of new migrants, especially of non-white, non-European people in the suburbs, altered the social geography of center and periphery in Toronto. Visible minorities can now also be found in spatially peripheral areas of the urban region. Instead of moving to the classical immigrant quarters in the central city (Little Italy, Little Portugal, Chinatown, etc.), newcomers now move directly into suburban (single-family home or condominium) or exurban enclaves of ethnic and religious minorities. So-called "ethnoburbs" (Li 1998) evolve now in the old and new suburbs of Toronto. Scarborough, Markham, Brampton, or Mississauga are examples of this type of suburban immigration. There are, of course, tremendous differences in class and origin that give nuance to this settlement pattern. Wealthy Chinese families often settle in areas where their preference for big suburban single-family homes and the colonization of the existing business community has sometimes led to friction with the existing Anglo population. The traditional suburban population has great difficulty reconciling the visual and cultural "intrusion" of Chinese Theme Malls with their traditional idea of suburban life. In the past, this has led to racist statements on street signs and construction plans (Isin and Siemyaticki 2002). Other migrants, such as Africans or Afro-Caribbeans, find their first home in Toronto mostly in the high-rise towers of the old, inner suburbs, where the supply of affordable housing in public or private apartment buildings affords them a "port of entry." In these older suburbs, in addition to affordable housing, there are also emerging ethno-national service networks and jobs in the increasingly peripheralized manufacturing industry (Murdie and Teixeira 2000, p. 217).

Making Chinatown: Histories of Racialization and Disease in Canada

The new diaspora culture is grafted onto an existing system of segregation and discrimination, which has historically linked space, race, and place in Canada.

The history of immigrant settlement in Canada still has an impact on today's racialization of communities. Following Kay Anderson (1992; cited in Craddock 2000, p. 69), settlement of non-European immigrants to Canada tended to produce a separated urban geography, a "landscape type" distinctive to groups that were considered different from the European norm. Craddock notes: "The Chinese were the furthest away from the European ideal; they were, more than any other immigrant group, the 'Other' as distinct from the 'us,' a separate category requiring ascription to a particular space within the urban landscape" (Craddock 2000, p. 69; see also Anderson 1992). Craddock continues: "More than just spaces encompassing the Chinese population of a city, though, these landscapes were social constructions with ascribed images and practices that in particular ways served the ideological needs of the larger urban arena" (Craddock 2000, p. 69). The notion that Chinatowns were constructed as "headquarters of disease" was the most powerful guarantor of the enshrined difference experienced in these places (ibid.).

When assessing the spatial strategies with which the local state encountered the SARS epidemic in Toronto, the historical example of the original settlement of Chinatown is a useful guidepost. Susan Craddock has looked at smallpox infection in relation to the Chinese population in nineteenth-century San Francisco. She writes: "Chinatown was considered an extension of the Asian 'threat' into the boundaries of the city, and these shifting perspectives on smallpox were inextricably intertwined with increasingly negative perceptions of this city within the city" (1995, p. 962). This important observation lays down a certain pattern, which is both universal and specific in time and space. Toronto, for example, has three Chinatowns (both residential and commercial) and a smattering of Chinese populations in the rest of the city. Toronto's Chinatowns are a far cry from the immigrant ghettos of the nineteenth century. Yet the pattern remains: the perception of vulnerability of the entire urban region to problems such as infectious disease is refracted through specific social and spatial communities of "the other." In the case of SARS, it was the Chinese and other South East Asian communities' neighborhoods that were stigmatized and publicly associated with the spread of disease. Individuals of East Asian ancestry or origin were subject to racism on a daily basis, and Chinese restaurants and shops suffered immediate and long-lasting economic consequences as customers shunned neighborhoods, which were considered to be frequented by people from Asia who could be possible carriers of the virus (Leung and Guan 2004).

Since the suburban Chinese enclaves of Toronto are not as easily defined and its populations are not as easily contained as historical ghettos and their residents, a potential state biopolitical strategy to contain disease associated with these places and their people could not possibly be easy (let alone desirable and advisable). Similarly, the movement of people into and out of these places and communities was unmappable after they left the prescribed pathways of international air travel and disappeared into the capillary system of the urban region. To return briefly to Susan Craddock: "The coded meanings – and spatialization – inherent in responses to diseases must be uncovered in the 'density of the social fabric', not just the surface" (1995, p. 967). In Toronto, any "symbolic mapping" (Craddock 1995) of the spread of infectious disease in and through urban communities will have to take into account the wild unpredictability of the topology of the global city (see Ali, Chapter 14).

Making Racism: The Complexity of Anti-Chinese Racialization in Toronto

From the perspective of SARS in Toronto in 2003, we can identify three interrelated processes through which identification of Chinese population with disease took place. These processes are all discursive-cultural and ascriptive. There are, of course, other factors at work, which we exclude for the moment: for example, the class- and gender-related material oppressions that Chinese workers and citizens have had to endure in a global city; that is, those resulting from the integration of new East Asian immigrants into the pre-structured registers of class, race and gender, immigrant labor, and so on. The three actor-network processes below combine the physical, natural, cultural, and symbolic flows through which the realities of Chinese-Canadians are constituted. They thread together numerous material and ideological factors of the diaspora experience, including diasporic connections with mainland China, Hong Kong, and other Chinese communities worldwide, microbial traffic, images of China as a global superpower, consumptive practices – old and new, food, and even insects.

1   The first area can perhaps be considered classical. It follows the historical patterns of stigmatization Chinese populations in North American cities have experienced since their first arrival in the nineteenth century. The association of Chinese urban population with disease in San Francisco had its origin in the nineteenth century, when smallpox, tuberculosis, and the bubonic plague were considered consequences of specific "habits" and forms of settlement in Chinese enclaves. In this way, the construction of an association of Chinatowns with disease reveals an important aspect of socio-spatial urban patterns in white settler societies: places are products of complex processes of the production of space. There is of course the myth that "[u]rban space seems to evolve naturally. We think, for example, that Chinatowns simply emerged when Chinese people migrated in sufficient numbers to North America and decided to live together" (Razack 2002a, p. 7). The reality of legal, economic, social, political, and other processes that produce the space of difference is more complicated than just "massing" of likeminded or ethnically similar individuals in the settlement process. In fact, the specific history of recent Chinese settlement patterns in Toronto adds to the puzzle: while the SARS outbreak in the Chinese community was really a suburban phenomenon, centered around Scarborough Grace Hospital in the city's east end, it was the inner-city Chinatown at Spadina – the most visible and symbolically laden settlement location of the Chinese diaspora in Toronto – that bore the displaced brunt of the anti-Chinese

reaction in the population as customers stayed away from restaurants and shops in the area. The space of these Chinatowns were not, as they were in the past, made into the physically controlled and constricted prisons of Chinese people, they became rather symbolically charged globalized stages in which the dynamics of related actor-networks are spurred into action.

2   The second identification builds on a largely ignorance-fuelled imaginary of realities in today's China. When the SARS outbreak occurred, the larger public of North America and Europe was just beginning to grasp the enormous emerging presence of China as an economic, political, and cultural power. Largely overlooked as an exotic and mysterious land considered to be caught between classical Confucian ways and brutal communist modernization (Tiananmen Square), China has entered the world stage with massive investments in technology and industry, with industrialization at an unprecedented scale, and with military power. At some point between the end of British colonialism in Hong Kong and Beijing's successful Olympic bid in 2002, the Chinese enigma had entered the Western consciousness in a new way. This new transparence of China, fueled incessantly by exquisitely illustrated press reports on the country's magnificent story of progress – be it critical (as in the case of the Three Gorges Dam) or admiring (as in the case of China's surprising entrance into the space age) – opened the door to a closer scrutiny of the country's ways and habits. This increased Western interest was also at the heart of the racialization of the disease in the SARS outbreak. While previous associations of Chinese populations with disease focused on deviant social habits in North American Chinatowns (Anderson 1992; Craddock 2000), the new wave of such racialization had at its center the allegedly unhealthy ways of living that are understood as dominant in China. In a replay of similar dynamics in the 1980s, when bushmeat-eating Africans were blamed for the spread of HIV (and subsequently other diseases such as Ebola or Marburg viruses), the Chinese habit of consuming wild animals such as civet cats was blamed for endangering human populations worldwide. This connection became even stronger as the avian flu threat grew and not just exotic but rather mundane forms of meat production and consumption came under scrutiny in the West. After the term "wet market" entered the vocabulary of Western discourse, the realization of less than sanitary practices of raising chickens and other fowl in and around people's living quarters in East Asia (and Turkey and else where) did not follow far behind (Spiess 2003; Davis 2005; Jacmenovic 2005; Sooksom 2006). In fact, the closer economic integration of Hong Kong (the Western lens on China) with the Pearl River Delta industrial developments in the Guangdong province of

China was the very precondition for this kind of ascription of disease proneness to regionalized (and racialized) cultural habits reflecting on Chinese populations globally. The implication here is, as Zhan has shown, "an exoticized bodily continuity between the wild animal and the Chinese people who readily consume it" (2005, p. 33). And Zhan adds: "The proliferation of these 'you-eat-(animals)'s in everyday discourses of Chineseness (and even Asianness) underscores the viscerality of racialized Orientalist tropes that produce various exotic Others through their excessive pleasures and enjoyments. In the case of scientific and popular discourses of SARS, we see the recurrence of a familiar narrative strategy that visceralizes the traditional and the uncanny as the origin of a culturally specific disease that – if not contained – threatens to destroy the global" (Zhan 2005, p. 38; and we might add: "the global city network"). In contrast to the racist and developmentalist ascriptions of the origins of HIV to the eating or sexual habits of central Africans, the association of disease to wild animal markets in China was placed mostly in a discourse of "development-out-of-control." Rather than pointing to the pre-modernity of such habits, commentators insisted on inscribing the SARS-origin story into the lore of rapid (and threatening) Chinese modernization: it is exactly the luxury character of the civet cat as a culinary delicacy devoured in the boom-fueled specialty restaurants in China's exploding cities that is focused on again and again. This combination of boom, luxury, and exoticness resonated with the images that had been produced and popularized of the settlement of Chinese immigrants in North American cities. Instead of the crowded, filthy immigrant slum of the traditional Chinatown, the new image of Chinese settlement was now built on a caricature of bustling and economically successful exurban enclaves with two-car garages in front of monster homes, with adolescent children in gold-plated Acuras and ravenous appetites for consumption of electronic gadgets and strange foods. The images that the West began to receive during the SARS crisis, of lifestyles in giant Chinese cities that nobody previously even knew existed, fell nicely into place in places such as Toronto, where the new Chinese immigrant landscape had produced very similar stories of high-tech based development and success, most visibly in the region's eastern suburbs of Scarborough, Markham, and Pickering. The symbol of this development was Pacific Mall, just north of Steeles Avenue, which appears as an awe-inspiring, dazzling branch of that distant economic miracle in Asia.

3　The third discourse of origin for the new association of disease with China (or East Asia in general) is related to the second one, but is different in perspective and language. The basis for this association is the scientifically grounded yet rapidly popularized idea that most infectious diseases, and more directly all such illnesses that affect the respiratory system (influenza, bird flu, SARS, etc.) have their origins in China. An entire industry of infectious disease specialists has emerged over the past 15 years to study (and possibly prevent from spreading) the emergence of killer viruses in China (Reynolds 2004). In addition to the suspicion that all evil in the shape of disease comes from China, there is a second dimension to this foundation for anti-Chinese racism: the fundamental mistrust in China, its authoritarian and secretive ways, and its allegedly less than trustworthy public health system (Abraham 2004; Fidler 2004). *New York Times Magazine* writer Gretchen Reynolds reports, in what can be considered a typical China-critical section of her otherwise excellent article on the threat of a flu pandemic: "China did not cooperate in a useful way with the international investigators, as its own health ministers have since acknowledged. Chinese officials released little information about cases among its citizens and declined to have outsiders visit the affected areas. One frustration for modern epidemiologists is that although viruses don't respect borders, doctors must" (Reynolds 2004, p. 43). This is not to say that Chinese officials did not, in fact, hinder or even sabotage global efforts to fight the disease. They did (Abraham 2004; Fidler 2004). But the identification of China's ways with SARS increased the readiness on side of the world's public to exhibit racist inhibitions and animosities toward all things (considered) Chinese. Further, the scientifically based narrative of the origin story of most infectious diseases in general and SARS in particular provided, unintentionally and by implication, a scientific basis for the development of expressions of racism (Foucault 2003; Sarasin 2004). The question we may ask in the context of our work is: How could Toronto health officials continue to insinuate that the virus had come from "outside" (China), while Toronto became the "outside" for the rest of the world when the virus threatened to spread from here?

Ultimately, the combination of these three strands with other events make anti-Chinese racism a highly specific localized affair. This process is composed of cultural events and markers as well as judgments on certain behaviors that add up to orientalization and racialization by implication. Mei Zhan has observed: "At stake in the production and representation of Chinese bodies of both human and nonhuman sorts are not just imaginaries of China's past but also visions of cosmopolitan futures – futures that depend not so much on the transition to a new stage of consumption, globalism, or neoliberal governmentality as on situated, contestatory projects and processes out of which unruly subjectivities and identities emerge" (2005, p. 32).

Racism without Race

Racism is not fixated on phenotype and skull shapes but also defines – in eugenicist terms – what has to be considered "healthy" and "sick," "strong" and "degenerated," and so on (Foucault 2003; Sarasin 2006). "In the age of biopolitics, racism is the function, which separates the healthy from the diseased, to the degree that 'the healthy' is sought on the level of the body of the people; racism is a selection, which expels those parts of the population that are presented as 'sick', 'impure' or 'racially different'" (Sarasin 2003, p. 62). As a product of the emergence of modern nation states in a colonial world in which race and nation became determinants of difference, racism as we know it today has had a specific historically determined biopolitical function (Foucault 1999, pp. 282–319). It is possible to argue that today, under the conditions of neoliberalization and globalization, this changes quite significantly indeed. As borders are perforated for some people and some business, they become closed to others. The nation state as a hermetic "race-container" shifts shape. Not just multicultural settler societies experience a redefinition of "race" as a concept of ordering power relations, but also those (Germany, Spain, Japan, for example) that have been rather impervious to immigration (in a formal sense) and settlement. It is possible, therefore, to think of racism today as a biopolitical regulator of a post-national kind to a certain degree. Clear distinctions into white and black, for example, don't work as well as "creolized" societies become the norm in many cities and countries (Goonewardena and Kipfer 2005). Emerging infectious diseases are both reactive to and productive of the new, globalized, creolized, and de-nationalized forms of racism and racialization that we encounter everywhere. This development is very much captured by Philipp Sarasin's provocative yet precise phrase of "infection as the metaphorical core of globalization" (Sarasin 2006, p. 160). This development leads to a new urban "biopolitics" that focuses on border control and internal control of infected bodies or those that could be suspect. Infection and migration are considered intertwined as cities are reaching an unprecedented multinational character. Infection and bioterror are likewise interconnected. Urban decision-makers, local public health officials, and others are actively reliving the political dream of discipline that allows them to potentially force the anarchic dynamics of the neoliberal city back into the harness of public (if not democratic) control. Sarasin correctly asks, then, whether we might need the phantasmagorical construction of the pandemic as part of the biopolitical regime of our time. Are the dreams of globalization and the nightmares of the pandemic the hallmarks of our post-9/11 societies (Sarasin 2004)?

Conclusions

We have suggested that the relationships of urbanization, disease, and racism have had a longstanding relationship on a colonially set stage in a settler society, in which visible minorities have in fact been largely invisible as active participants in Canada's national history (despite their significant and real actual contributions). More specifically, there has been a continuity in the linking of disease occurrence to racialized bodies – often, in fact, Chinese bodies. In the past, disease and urban built environments were linked, as was the case with smallpox and other epidemics in Chinatowns in the nineteenth and twentieth centuries in Canadian and American cities (Craddock 2000). In contrast to the traditional ghettoization of disease in space, the quarantine of individuals was the only spatial measure employed to regulate bodies in the SARS crisis. No incidence of racialization was linked to quarantine itself. Instead, as we demonstrated through the three steps we presented above, racism was present through association and articulation with discourses of racialization that were largely external to Chinatown as a specific place. Although Chinatown became a symbolic and economic site for the SARS theater by virtue of the fact that it was abandoned by clients and was patronized by politicians and community leaders, who wanted to show their solidarity with Chinese Torontonians, it did not become a site of disease *per se*. It was therefore also not subject to direct biopolitical regulation as had happened in previous decades. Chinatown, in fact, became part of the story of victimization rather than part of the story of accusation. Racialization through association occurred through the association of the disease with things Chinese, exotic and familiar, that were extraneous to the existing Chinatowns in downtown Toronto and to the formation of new Chinatowns in Toronto's suburbs, but central to the constitution of a globalized story of tying SARS to its origin in Chinese bodies and communities worldwide. The chain of association is maintained through the network of diaspora and immigration, which connects cities differently than in previous centuries: globalization has created a network of global cities, which are not joined through unilateral and unidirectional hierarchical links but through topological, multi-relational, and constitutive relationships that are performed through the bodies of migrants as much as through the socio-technical networks that sustain them. All stages of these topographies are racialized in a thoroughly globalized world where the incidence of disease and the construction of bodies are intertwined at all scales (Zhan 2005). Racialization and SARS are sutured through the discursive and material networks that sustain the global economy.

In the words of Foucault, racism is about the decision what will live and what will die. There is no reason to assume that Chinese Torontonians were treated differently than others as patients. There is evidence that they were treated different as citizens. A lesson was learned for all, though. Multiculturalism is not just something for sunny days and "red-boot" dance performances. It is also articulated with processes of disease governance in which it needs to safeguard its carefully crafted institutions, which are under fire in the best of times, against collapse brought about by the biopolitical pressures of globalization of disease and urbanization. These pressures are articulated through global actor-networks that engage microbes, humans, cities, and transportation networks in previously unknown ways. Literal and metaphoric "camps" and "labs" are littered along these networks and they are the structural nodes through which racialization takes place. As the "ghetto" metaphor of old loses explanatory power in today's global city spatialization processes, racialization becomes linked to the network's globalized reality. Accordingly, racialization today occurs through the symbolic interactions that take place through the globalized topographies of global city formation (Smith 2003).

NOTE

1   A longer version of this argument can be found in Keil and Ali (2006).

Part IV

Re-Emerging Infectious Disease, Urban Public Health, and Global Biosecurity

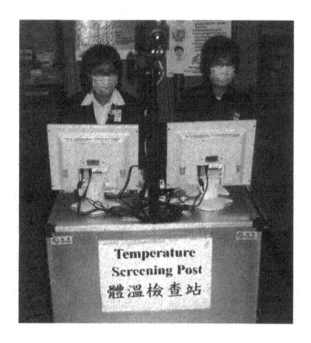

Introduction

S. Harris Ali and Roger Keil

A focus on the global politics of public health brings to light the fallacy of viewing infectious diseases as being exclusively limited to specific regions of the world or to only specific social groups within a city. Today, under the conditions of globalization, diseases are interrelated and networked together in complex and non-discriminatory ways. The chapters in this part explore some of the implications of how such networked interconnections, especially in relation to such phenomena as the macro forces of economic globalization and neoliberalism; global inequalities based on characteristics such as race/ethnicity and gender (both *between* the cities and regions of the world and *within* each of these); and the political economy of the pharmaco-industrial complex, all of which interact with each other to dramatically influence the distribution of networked diseases and the ability to respond to such diseases. Most notably, these processes have great significance for evolving issues related to biopolitics – or more specifically, in the post-9/11 era, to biosecurity. In this light, all four chapters in this part, in various ways, discuss some of the issues that arise as a networked global society is forced to deal to with the biopolitical machinations associated with such contemporary phenomena as border control and population mobility, the politics of inclusion/exclusion, and the ethnical implications of new and increasingly intrusive technologies of surveillance.

As documented persuasively by Laurie Garrett (2000), the foundation of today's crisis in global public health is a lack of resource allotment, distribution, and funding predicated by neoliberal reforms. Such circumstances, as Matthew Gandy notes in his piece, serve to reinforce and amplify existing forms of inequality, which in turn, have implications for the global spread of infectious disease. For example, with reference to HIV/AIDS in Africa, gender inequality in disease distribution is starkly revealed by the fact that women (and children) are by far the most severely affected subpopulation – an outcome that reflects a general societal neglect of this group within patriarchal societies. To combat this disease, therefore, a greater and more equitable distribution of resources to those in need will be required. Reflecting the dependency bias of structural adjustment plans, health resource distribution is based on tied aid. Consequently, resource distribution tends to follow patriarchal patterns whereby resources are preferentially directed toward males, while ignoring the plight of women and children. A second example is seen in the case of tuberculosis, where cuts in primary health, along with increasing poverty and homelessness, have resulted in a resurgence of tuberculosis in the 1980s in the global city of New York.

In her chapter, Susan Craddock observes that in a mobile society, not all groups are equally perceived as threats. Furthermore, these differential perceptions of threat reflect the social inequalities noted by Gandy. It is worth remembering here that the intersection of inequality with differential perceptions of infectious disease threats is a very important issue in studying the relationship between global cities and disease, because such cities, in particular, host different subpopulations. For example, there are those economic, cultural, and political elites who frequently travel from global city to global city; those marginalized diaspora communities who are often involved in occupations that support the activities of such elites (for example, domestics, nannies, migrant workers in various sectors), and those experiencing the highest level of disenfranchisement, such as the homeless and destitute. The association of disease with certain groups, but not others, based on social class factors is one important association that leads to differential perceptions of threat. Craddock focuses on the vulnerability of such groups to disease. Specifically, using the analysis of tuberculosis as an entry point, Craddock discusses the relevant discourses related to disease vulnerability in terms of such concepts as mobile populations, urbanization, and globalization. For example, she notes that race-based genetic research on susceptibility to tuberculosis tends to divert attention away from a broader social analysis of why those in a certain racial/ethnic category are more vulnerable to tuberculosis in the first place. This impedes progress in developing effective interventions by enabling conflating public health issues with other issues, such as immigration. Craddock's analysis of tuberculosis substantiates Gandy's arguments about how the contemporary politics of public health is marked by the politics of inclusion/exclusion, but she takes the argument further by developing in more detail the biopolitical implications involved, especially those related to current anxieties over the permeability of international, national, and urban borders.

Building on the theme of permeable borders, Nicholas King argues that the framing of highly mobile populations as infectious disease threats has led to a new and historically unparalleled emphasis on the technologies of surveillance, and in particular, the development of networks of syndromic surveillance. With syndromic surveillance, different data (types of drugs sold, physician diagnoses, hospital admissions, etc.) are analyzed together to monitor and detect changes in the distribution of signs or symptoms of disease in a population, in order to identify patterns that may indicate the early stages of a disease outbreak. The biopolitical implications of this are discussed in terms of how the emergence of syndromic surveillance can be understood in terms of the unprecedented convergence of the ideologies and practices of public health and national security under the rubric of biosecurity – or, more specifically, on the basis of the idea that the response to bioterrorism and emerging diseases require identical technological resources. Such an emphasis, as King explicates in his contribution, has implications for the study of networks in different ways, not the least of which is that at the level of contemporary discourse, the term "network" itself may serve as a powerful metaphor for interpreting the causes and significance of problems related to disease distribution. For example, today, the use of the term "network" may tacitly connote the reconfiguration of the spaces of global networks as the significance of territoriality wanes in our increasingly globalized and "borderless" world, which in turn, has implications for the way in which increasingly intrusive biosecurity measures are accepted and/or tolerated by society at large.

Biosecurity, as a set of procedures and infrastructures that police and control movement, is not limited to people; they are, as Steve Hinchliffe and Nick Bingham note in their chapter, applicable to other living things such as birds. Focusing on the practices rather than the ideas of biosecurity, these authors consider the case of avian influenza (bird flu) preparation in the city of Cairo. Similar to King, Hinchliffe and Bingham are interested in the question of convergence, this time, not in the convergence of surveillance technologies and techniques *per se*, but the issue of how various practices, places, and things interacted with one another to "produce" the city's response to the threat of bird flu. For example, in attempting to deal with this threat, Cairo officials banned the common practice of residents in city households to raise ducks and chickens on their properties. It was argued that in contrast to poultry raised on factory farms, those grown in the urban setting could not be closely monitored for avian flu, nor could their interaction with migratory birds carrying the virus be prevented as effectively. This had major repercussions for certain subpopulations within the city. First, the small-scale raising of poultry was a way of life for lower-income families and represented a cheap way of adding expensive animal protein to the family diet. As such, the ban disproportionately affected an especially marginalized group within society. Second, the ban reinforced a government initiative to eliminate the "backward" ways of Cairo citizens and to move toward the making of Cairo into a modern global city. Such an initiative included an emphasis on the pursuit of private corporate interests such as the expansion of the factory farming industry. The case of Cairo and avian flu clearly illustrates how the political economics of globalized urbanization may inform the biopolitics of a city in unexpected ways.

10

Deadly Alliances: Death, Disease, and the Global Politics of Public Health

Matthew Gandy

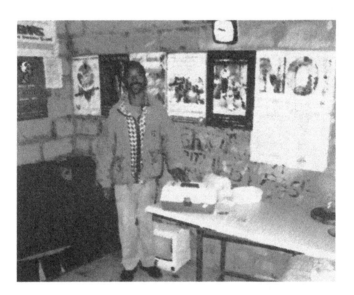

Introduction

The rancor surrounding the Bangkok AIDS summit of July 2004 and the more recent New York AIDS summit of June 2006 has exposed a series of fundamental disagreements surrounding the global politics of public health. These tensions range from access to cheaper life-saving drugs to disputes over the role of poverty and gender equality in the promotion of sexual health. The world is now experiencing the most profound public health challenge of the past 40 years: we have witnessed the appearance of new diseases such as Ebola, SARS, and in particular AIDS, combined with the alarming spread of diseases previously thought to have been under control, such as malaria and tuberculosis.[1] The AIDS pandemic in particular threatens to devastate entire regions and has already fundamentally altered the life expectancy and demographic profile of many countries in sub-Saharan Africa: in the past decade, life expectancies have fallen by 20 years in Lesotho, 19 years in Botswana, and 18 years in Zimbabwe.[2] Billions of people lack access to adequate sanitation and safe drinking water, and the UN predicts that slums will become the dominant urban form within the next 15 years.[3] With the recent emergence of the deadly H5N1 strand of avian flu, there is now urgent research into how viral mutations led to the 1918 influenza, in which over 40 million people lost their lives. Yet the very idea of "public health" sits uncomfortably alongside the current emphasis of biomedical science on the molecular realm of DNA coding and the development of lucrative Western markets for new pharmaceutical products such as sildenafil (Viagra). The needs of the majority – the global poor – scarcely feature within this tactical alliance between the biomedical sciences and corporate power: since most people threatened by AIDS, tuberculosis, unsafe drinking water, and other health threats are poor, they have little or no influence over the global politics of public health.

The contemporary city finds itself in the maelstrom of this escalating global crisis in public health. When we compare the nineteenth-century "epidemiological transition" with the contemporary dynamics of urban change, we find a mix of similarities and differences that caution against any teleological reading of current developments. There is now widespread acceptance that levels of morbidity and mortality in the nineteenth century were lowered through the rapid expansion of new technological networks, improvements in nutrition, widening access to health care, and other integral dimensions to urban modernity, even though the relative role of these different developments has been subject to extensive scholarly debate. Whilst epidemiological dimensions to the contemporary public health crisis share important parallels with the past – most notably the impact of poverty and inadequate sanitation – there are a number of aspects that warrant further reflection and analysis. The impact of enhanced global mobility on the spread of pathogens raises immediate questions about the biosecurity dimensions to globalization that have thus far been dominated by reactionary responses to immigration in the popular imagination. Similarly, the effects of neoliberalism, especially within the global South, have profound implications for public health policy where a more fractured and individualized response can be observed. And cities themselves are producing new political ecologies of disease as pathogens spread and mutate in the face of new opportunities precipitated by factors such as war, economic instability, or the rapid growth of informal settlements on the urban fringe. The day-flying *Aedes* mosquitoes that carry dengue fever, for example, have been able to expand their range in Southeast Asia through the use of breeding sites offered by construction sites or in puddles of water located in half-finished or abandoned buildings.[4]

The earlier connections between public health and political reform associated with the growth of the industrial metropolis appear far more attenuated in the contemporary city, where the generalized threat of disease can be extensively contained or obviated through the use of individualized medical interventions. What is especially significant about some of the newly emerging public health threats such as avian flu, SARS, or XDR-TB, however, is the degree to which these pathogens may reveal latent weaknesses in ostensibly effective public health systems that expose global interconnections in disease epidemiology. If we are to make sense of the current public health crisis, we need to explore connections between political, economic, and social developments that are ignored by the fragmentary emphasis of the biomedical sciences. The improvements in public health since the nineteenth century have paradoxically deflected attention away from the underlying causes of disease that the public health advocates of the past sought to highlight. The emergence of the "bacteriological city" during the second half of the nineteenth century rested in large part on the biopolitical reframing of the urban arena as a focus for modern forms of governmental intervention and public administration, if only to safeguard the role of cities as pivotal nodes for trade and commerce. Yet the political ambiguities of scientific urbanism in the field of public health – most sharply captured by the technical focus of the Chadwickian drive to rationalize urban form – laid the foundations for a growing tension in the twentieth century between the technical mastery of urban space and the persistence of political demands to transform modes of urban governance.

The success of antibiotics, vaccines, and other modern medicines had, by the middle decades of the twentieth century, led to a situation in which public health was increasingly viewed as a somewhat anachronistic and declining field of interest. Public health was increasingly characterized as an unglamorous field of study, or simply a specialized branch of "tropical medicine," with few prestigious research programs or career opportunities. The earlier emphasis on issues such as poor nutrition and the affordability of medical care had become progressively displaced by a biomedical preoccupation with the efficacy of new prophylactics and specialized medical interventions. Primary health care in particular began to lose its critical role within a holistic conception of social welfare for society as a whole, and state-funded primary healthcare programs became extremely vulnerable to macro-economic developments since the 1970s associated with the fiscal crisis of the state. In subsequent decades these trends have become intensified, with new inequalities in health care emerging at a global scale: wealthy people with private health insurance enjoy access to an unparalleled array of advanced medical care, including the most frivolous of cosmetic procedures, whereas in the poorest African states one in four children die by the age of four. In much of sub-Saharan Africa, healthcare systems are in a state of near collapse, with inadequate facilities, an exodus of trained staff, and shortages of essential medicines, and even where medical facilities are available these are often no longer free at the point of use, so that the onset of chronic illness spells economic ruin for poorer households (see De Cock et al. 2002; Eastwood et al. 2005).

The current impetus toward economic globalization is causing widespread social and economic disruption, ranging from wild currency fluctuations to the systematic collapse of viable agricultural systems (see Glyn 2005; Harvey 2005). Periods of rapid social and economic change both now and in the past have had profound implications for public health and pose immense risks for human welfare (Szreter 1997). The imposition of austerity packages – widely referred to as structural adjustment programs – in combination with the forcible extension of global markets for Western products is plunging millions of people into poverty and economic dependence. Whilst debates about globalization frequently focus on issues such as migration and terrorism, there has been a relative neglect of the public health consequences of neoliberalism. It is not only the fall in real incomes that has increased vulnerability to disease and ill health, but also the externally imposed pressures to reduce expenditure on primary health care. Existing primary healthcare services in much of the developing world and the former states of the Soviet Union have been drastically cut back, and services that were once freely available are now increasingly beyond the reach of the poor. The disruption of primary health care for diseases such as malaria and tuberculosis has other even more ominous consequences: incomplete or intermittent treatment fosters the development of drug resistance that renders many existing treatments ineffective, and necessitates a reliance on much more expensive alternatives that may only be available to a tiny minority of people in the worst-affected countries.

These deleterious public health trends also extend to the wealthiest global cities, such as London and New York, where a combination of poverty, homelessness, and cutbacks in primary health care during the 1980s has contributed to the resurgence of diseases such as tuberculosis. The spread of tuberculosis and other preventable diseases in the so-called "de-developing" enclaves of urban America and the poverty-stricken cities of the former Soviet Union can only be fully understood with reference to the dynamics of global political and economic change over the past 30 years.[5] Changing patterns of economic and social investment have contributed to a new geography of wealth and poverty, with significant implications for the epidemiology of disease. With the advent of more diffuse patterns of urbanization and the greater mobility of capital investment, it has become far easier for public health crises to be effectively ignored where they appear to present no generalized threat to the overall well-being of an increasingly globalized economic system.

Gender, Poverty, and the Global Public Health Crisis

An examination of the social impact of the global public health crisis shows that it is women and children who have been most badly affected: in the case of AIDS, for example, almost half of those infected are women. One of the least addressed dimensions to the structural adjustment programs externally imposed on developing countries is the deleterious impact on the sexual health of women caused by their increased economic dependence on men. Sexual health programs based on abstinence, for example, ignore the difficulties women face in negotiating safer or non-penetrative forms of sex: it is married women in sub-Saharan Africa and South Asia who make up the largest and most vulnerable group of women, since they are at risk of being infected by their husbands (see, for example, Akeroyd 2004; Susser and Stein 2004). In a common pattern, truckers, migrant workers, and other men who must travel in order to earn enough to support their families frequent brothels and then infect their wives, yet social mores and popular prejudice inhibit open discussion of sexual behavior. In India, for example, there are emerging disparities in rates of HIV infection linked to the prevalence of effective sex education: in more socially liberal states such as Maharashtra and Tamil Nadu, the promotion of condom use and extensive public health campaigns appear to have brought about a fall in rates of infection among women (Ramesh 2006b). Despite these localized successes, however, India may yet become the new epicenter of the global HIV pandemic. With 5.7 million people infected with HIV, India has now edged ahead of South Africa as the country with the greatest number of people carrying the virus. There is growing evidence that HIV is now spreading rapidly from at-risk groups such as sex workers and drug users into the general population: rates of HIV infection are already estimated to exceed 2 percent in Mumbai and are also rising in Hyderabad, Chennai, Bangalore, and many other major cities (Boseley 2006a; Fredriksson-Bass and Kanabus 2006; UNAIDS 2006). As in sub-Saharan Africa, it is women who remain at greatest risk from HIV infection, but social ignorance, the stigmatization of illness in women, and patriarchal power structures threaten to stymie national efforts to control the disease.

At the 2006 New York AIDS summit, the UN Secretary General, Kofi Annan, pleaded with delegates to take the threat of AIDS to women more seriously and lambasted the international community for its "unconscionably slow" response to gender inequalities and vulnerability to HIV infection. Yet the need for a new gender politics to underpin the development of a more effective response to the global public health crisis is being undermined by a coalition of religious conservatives extending from the Christian Right in the United States to some governments in Latin America and many Muslim countries, including more moderate states such as Egypt. The United States, under pressure from the Christian Right, refuses to emphasize the use of condoms unless it is specifically tied to the promotion of sexual abstinence or the restriction of sexual activity to marriage (MacAskill 2006). Hitherto successful AIDS prevention strategies in Uganda, for example, have been placed under threat by the increasing influence of US evangelical groups on public health policy, and the forging of alliances with Pentecostal churches and other religious groups in Africa who oppose the promotion of condom use or the support of sex workers (Vasager and Borger 2005; Berkowitz 2006). In a parallel development at the 2006 New York AIDS summit, the Organization of the Islamic Conference (which represents 56 predominantly Muslim states) refused to allow the conference declaration to make any reference to at-risk groups such as sex workers, drug users, or men who have sex with men. What we are now witnessing is an ideological convergence between religious fundamentalists – both Muslim and Christian – who wish to subvert public health policy into a discourse over sexual morality. Ranged against these conservative voices, however, are a new generation of HIV-positive women activists such as Rolake Odetoyinbo Nwagwu in Nigeria and Beatrice Were in Uganda, who are engaged in a vital struggle to challenge the social attitudes and economic inequalities that have driven the devastating impact of AIDS on women and children in developing countries (see SARPN 2006). The spread of AIDS in more traditional societies is closely linked with patriarchal power structures, whose sustenance is assured by the rise of poverty-fuelled ethnic and religious chauvinism that undermines the prospects for developing more progressive approaches to social policy. And in regions where war or civil strife prevail, the vulnerability of women and children to sexual violence, economic exploitation, and disease is even greater, so that we cannot consider public health questions separately from issues surrounding political stability and social justice.

Urbanization and the Biopolitics of Modernity

In order to understand better the political dynamics behind public health, we need to recognize how the development of the modern state emerged in tandem with new approaches to the administration of human populations. Biopolitical interpretations of history, following their lead from the work of Michel Foucault, emphasize how the emergence of modern systems of government rested in part on the recognition of distinct categories of people. The collection of information through the use of census data and surveys gradually enabled modern states to bring complex problems into the public domain. The public health crisis afflicting the industrial cities of Europe and North America became the focus of professional discourses in fields such as medicine, civil engineering, and urban planning. The emergence of modern methods of government was, however, a contested process, so that the scope and purpose of state activity was frequently the focus of intense political conflict between different interests (see Kearns 1991). A fragile consensus over public health policy really only emerged toward the end of the nineteenth century, when new advances in the bacteriological sciences could begin to dispel rival interpretations of disease epidemiology. In the pre-bacteriological era, the politics of public health were complicated by the persistence of traditional beliefs surrounding morality and ill health and the role of vested interests in the restriction of reformist political discourse. And even in the bacteriological era, the environmental claims of the German biologist Max von Pettenkofer and his allies continued to play an influential role in deflecting attention away from the systematic need for technological and governmental modernization: in the place of a city-wide approach, they insisted on tackling localized phenomena such as variations in groundwater levels. Yet outbreaks of cholera, typhoid, and other infectious diseases caused massive disruption and necessitated the introduction of better scientific knowledge into the management of cities. Most critically, the threat of disease and declining standards of living in the nineteenth century challenged those social and political institutions that appeared unable or unwilling to provide an adequate response.[6]

There are clearly lessons to be learned from the nineteenth-century politics of public health for current debates over the global public health crisis, but we should be careful not to overstate the historical parallels. Arguments for new forms of governmental intervention in the nineteenth century rested on perceived instances of market failure, so that private interests could be overridden without ideological contradiction to enable complex and expensive improvements to urban infrastructure. Over time, intense conflicts over the funding of better housing, water supply, and other elements within the fabric of the modern city became conjoined with wider reformist agendas facilitated by the extension of the political franchise to the urban poor. Yet the nineteenth-century industrial city, with its burgeoning working-class movements, presents a very different political arena to many contemporary cities in the global South, where we find a medley of different social forms ranging from humanitarian self-help organizations to sectarian militias and gang fiefdoms. In such situations, community-based forms of political mobilization are placed under severe strain by the extensive breakdown in social relations to produce a highly volatile and unpredictable context for the emergence of urban social movements. The politics of slums is very different from that of the nineteenth-century industrial city, and is increasingly a seedbed for new forms of religiosity and ethnic chauvinism rather than the wellspring for new visions of social justice (Davis 2004). The contemporary emphasis on "governance" in the wake of various forms of "state failure" raises profound questions about the capacities of civil society to provide basic services such as primary health care, sanitation, and transport. Although some scholars have tended to see the decline of the state as an opportunity for new forms of grassroots globalization (see, for example, Appadurai 2002), there remain real questions about what these small-scale networks and initiatives can actually achieve in practice in comparison with the historic transformation of cities in Europe, North America, and elsewhere.

The demands for improvement in the living conditions of the nineteenth-century industrial city necessitated sophisticated forms of governmental intervention in order to tackle the threat of epidemic disease. But these new spaces of public health control, deploying the latest advances in civil engineering and public administration, had a shadowy "other" represented in the increasingly squalid conditions endured by the mass of the population in European colonies (see Klein 1994). In colonial Bombay, for example, the deteriorating environmental conditions in the last decades of the nineteenth century culminated in a series of bubonic plague outbreaks that lasted from 1896 until World War I (see Klein 1986). The city's predicament at this time emerged out of a mix of *laissez-faire* economic doctrine, social indifference among the city's elites, and an administrative inability to coordinate processes of modernization for the benefit of the city as a whole – a dynamic that would play a significant role in spurring the development of nationalist political sentiments during the early decades of the twentieth century. Similarly in Lagos, Nairobi, and other colonial cities, public health failures in the twentieth century became a spur to demands for independence, yet in the post-colonial era urban conditions have continued to deteriorate (see Gandy 2006a).

A further dynamic behind persistent health inequalities in the cities of the global South is that apart from dramatic exceptions such as the Surat plague of 1994 or the resurgence of the deadly *falciparum* strain of malaria during the 1990s, the public health crisis facing slum dwellers does not directly endanger middle-class residents (see Chaplin 1999). Even newly emerging threats such as extreme drug resistant tuberculosis or XDR-TB primarily present a threat to the poor, those in overcrowded living conditions or people whose immune systems are already compromised through exposure to the HIV virus. Severe disparities in public health can persist because of the array of technological, scientific, and architectural innovations that enable wealthy households to insulate themselves from the environmental conditions of the poor. These public health inequalities – emboldened by the distortions of marketized health care and medical research – are creating the corporeal equivalents of gated communities. These "islands of health" can use their disproportionate political and economic power to demand the eradication rather than the improvement of urban slums. The middle classes in many post-colonial cities have proved particularly adept at capturing state services and effectively disenfranchising the poor. The recent history of many cities in the global South militates against the kind of progressive political alliances that galvanized processes of sanitary reform in European cities during the second half of the nineteenth century. The current neo-Haussmannite agenda of large-scale slum clearance marks an effort to forcibly reshape contemporary cities and enhance the role of "premium spaces" as part of a globalized dynamic of property-led urban redevelopment. With the rise of slums as the "norm" rather than the "exception" across much of the global South, established models and trajectories of urban change are increasingly dislocated in relation to material realities, so that public health is now at the epicenter of a global crisis in neoliberal modes of urban governance.

The Politics of Death

The public health politics of the colonial era rested on a distinction between modernity and its other: when fiscal parsimony and administrative negligence undermined the provision of adequate health care or sanitation, dual discourses emerged, based on the idea that the persistence of squalor and poor living conditions were cultural rather than political in origin. Elite enclaves became subject to a different set of public health discourses from the rest of the population, whose living conditions steadily deteriorated. These dualities have not only persisted in the post-colonial era but actually widened through the vast growth of *favelas*, shanty towns, and slum settlements. The contemporary politics of public health is marked by a process of inclusion and exclusion: there are people who reside inside the global economy and who have access to adequate health care and those who exist outside the system. The Italian political philosopher Giorgio Agamben has elaborated on this distinction between "inside" and "outside" under modern systems of governance to reveal the persistence of what he terms conditions of "bare life" within even the most sophisticated legal and political systems (Agamben 1998). The contemporary exclusion of the world's poor from adequate medical care is thus a form of state-sponsored violence in which millions are denied even the most basic human rights. These "wasted lives", to use the sociologist Zygmunt Bauman's phrase, represent a literal as well as metaphorical process of permanent and deadly exclusion for the poor, the marginalized, and others who have no value within the global economy (Baumann 2004). But what kind of political and economic dynamics lie behind these widening disparities in public health and the restriction of access to even the most basic medicines?

A striking manifestation of this systematic exclusion of the poor from medical care is provided by the Bush administration's efforts to stymie access to affordable retroviral drugs. A dramatic standoff in 2001 between the global pharmaceutical industry and public health activists in South Africa, following the import of cheap generic retroviral drugs manufactured in Brazil, led to the historic Doha Declaration on intellectual property rights and public health (WTO 2001). Generic drug production in countries such as India, Brazil, and Thailand has succeeded in bringing down treatment costs per patient from $10,000 to $300 a year, yet the World Health Organization (2005) has revealed that fewer than 1 in 20 people who need retroviral treatment in the developing world are currently receiving it (WHO 2003d). In order to widen access to affordable drugs, the current production of generic medicines will have to be massively expanded, but the Bush administration and its corporate allies in the pharmaceutical industry have been working assiduously to undermine the potential impact of the Doha agreement (Klein 2003). The US government has been negotiating bilateral trade deals with countries such as Chile and Thailand in an effort to dissuade them from the production of cheaper drugs (Boseley 2004). Tensions exploded into the open at the Bangkok AIDS summit of 2004, where lobbyists on behalf of the US government put forward a series of specious arguments in relation to sub-Saharan Africa: they asserted that the costs of drugs have been lowered, yet discounted brands remain at least twice as expensive as generic drugs; and they claimed that generic drugs undermine profitability and hence the incentive for new research (which is, in any case, overwhelmingly focused on the bloated market for prescription drugs in the US) (Sulston 2003; Angell 2004).[7]

Of the $15 billion pledged by the Bush administration in the fight against AIDS, most of this money will be focused on 15 selected countries willing to abide by bilateral trade deals to prevent the production of cheaper generic drugs, and also on those countries willing to stress the centrality of abstinence as a strategy for AIDS prevention under pressure from the religious Right. It should also be noted that some of the most vocal critics of US policy, among them France, currently make a derisory financial contribution to global efforts to tackle HIV/AIDS, so that the inadequacies of US policy must be viewed in a wider context of Western negligence toward the public health needs of the world's poorest countries (Alagiri et al. 2002). The US government has sought to highlight the inadequacies of healthcare infrastructure in developing countries as a further justification for the diversion of attention from the costs of drugs, yet primary healthcare services have themselves been undermined by the structural adjustment and trade policies promoted by Western financial institutions and their corporate backers. The global politics of AIDS is therefore caught in a neoliberal vicious spiral in which it is impossible to disentangle the needs for social and institutional reform in the worst-affected regions from the challenge of widening access to available treatments. The deliberate restriction of access to drugs or vaccines in order to protect the profits of the pharmaceutical industry is also paralleled by the tardy global response to the threat of avian flu: suggestions that the poorest and most vulnerable countries such as Cambodia and Vietnam should be able to produce generic vaccines have been fiercely resisted. Whilst some Western countries have been quietly stockpiling the Tamiflu vaccine in preparation for a serious outbreak, the areas at the epicenter of the disease in South-East Asia lack even adequate resources to monitor its spread (see Davis 2005).

If anything, the situation facing people whose lives are threatened by less-high-profile killers than HIV such as tuberculosis or malaria is even worse. The ambitious Roll Back Malaria campaign launched by the World Bank in 1998, for example, has proved ineffective, underfunded, and subject to extensive medical malpractice. An outcome of policy failures is the growing drug resistance of the deadly *Plasmodium falcifarum*, which has led to rising levels of mortality from malaria – particularly in Africa, where there is continued use of cheaper but much less effective drugs such as chloroquine and sulfadoxine-pyrimethamine. The World Health Organization and the much trumpeted Global Fund for AIDS, Tuberculosis and Malaria have been singled out for criticism by failing to undertake policies that can possibly meet long-term objectives for improvements in human health (Attaran et al. 2004; Boseley 2006b). The increasing prevalence of co-infection between HIV and tuberculosis, in combination with the advance of drug-resistant pathogens, threatens to overwhelm fragile primary healthcare infrastructures and lead to further cycles of community breakdown and economic decline. Furthermore, the spread of slums, industrialized agriculture, and the collapse of public health services in the global South is creating the conditions in which new and perhaps even more dangerous pathogens may emerge, as evidenced by the threat of avian flu (see Davis 2005). There is an emerging political ecology of disease in the twenty-first century in which the relationship between globalization, urbanization, and pathogenic organisms is being recast, with potentially devastating consequences.

Conclusions

Public health pioneers of the past, such as the German bacteriologist Robert Koch, were not only scientists but also political advocates for social change. Koch recognized that advances in disease epidemiology involved not only the better scientific understanding of the role of pathogens but also a full investigation of the social, economic, and environmental circumstances in which disease can spread through human populations. Improvements in health care were perceived as part of a nexus of reforms ranging from better housing and nutrition to an extension of the franchise to ensure that the poor had adequate political representation. The contemporary politics of public health needs to be considered, however, in relation to wider discourses on security and human welfare that are quite different from those of the nineteenth century. In the place of a recognizable system of nation-states, we are now increasingly confronted with a much more fluid and multi-layered set of institutional structures within which power is widely dispersed. Rather than political rivalries between states, which characterized much of the modern era, we now find the emergence of new kinds of political networks. Early efforts to foster greater international cooperation, such as the creation of the World Health Organization, point to an alternative lineage of global governance and scientific collaboration that holds significant implications for contemporary efforts to coordinate national responses to public health threats. The current Western preoccupation with the threat of international terrorism, for example, has distracted attention from the much more real threats to human well-being created by poverty and ill health. The vast resources – both financial and logistical – now being poured into "security" contrast with the inadequate funding and poor coordination provided for the UN Global Fund for HIV/AIDS, Tuberculosis and Malaria. The increasingly unilateral and self-interested stance of the United States illustrates the stark tensions between attempts to build a coordinated international approach to health care and the continuing centrality of national interests or global institutions that explicitly represent the economic power of a relatively small group of nations (Kohlmorgen 2004). We might draw a parallel with the threat of climate change: unless political institutions can respond to the global public interest, then international negotiations will continue to be skewed toward corporate lobbies or the self-interest of individual states underpinned by the ideas of few renegade voices from within the scientific community. Similarly, with the spread of HIV and other pathogens, we have seen how reactionary or even neo-miasmic conceptions of disease epidemiology have played a significant role in delaying or subverting effective action.

The classic debates over the nineteenth-century epidemiological transition have been framed in terms of rival claims for the role of medical interventions and nutritional improvements in contributing to improvements in human welfare. In a contemporary context, however, both these positions fail to grasp the interconnections between globalization and disease epidemiology. In particular, the negative synergies between neoliberalism and reactionary forms of religiosity threaten to accelerate the spread of HIV and undermine efforts to improve women's health. The provision of effective public health measures, like other essential needs such as housing and sanitation, is most efficiently and fairly provided as a public good. The argument is not simply a question of private versus public – since mixed arrangements for service provision can often work quite effectively – but rather one of the ideological underpinning of the public realm and the unique organizational capacity of the state in the field of public administration. The physical reconstruction of the modern city rested on facilitating new ways for private capital to be channeled into urban infrastructure as well as ensuring an expanded role for technical and professional expertise in urban government. A political synergy emerged between the needs of the urban poor and wider concerns with social and economic cohesion, in order to allow generalized improvements in living standards and public health.

Under a fragmentary or "post-secular" conception of public policy, however, the previously established connections between social welfare and the modern city have become progressively undermined. The renewed global threat of infectious disease has become part of a new political landscape of paranoia, driven by the vast and growing diversion of resources into security. The preoccupation with bioterrorism through the use of obscure agents such as anthrax has been accompanied by reductions in research funding for known killers such as tuberculosis. Yet this Western preoccupation with security is largely irrelevant to the daily threats endured by the poor majority, and especially women, throughout much of the global South. The political challenge is to delineate new coalitions of interest that can demand a global transformation in public policy that is in effect the twenty-first century counterpart of the growing working-class demands for better living and working conditions in the nineteenth-century city. The paradox is that widening global disparities in wealth and poverty play a role in fostering the social and political conditions in which religious fanaticism and hatred for the West can flourish, so that any "war on terror" that fails to address the causes of poverty, despair, and insecurity in the lives of the world's poor will ultimately create a more dangerous world for everyone.

ACKNOWLEDGMENTS

This is an extensively revised version of an essay that first appeared in the journal *PloS Medicine* in 2005. I would like to thank Melanie Brickman, Richard Coker, Susan Craddock, Roger Keil, and Gavin Yamey for their comments on an earlier draft.

NOTES

1   On the emerging global public crisis, see, for example, Garrett (2000), Barnett (2002), Gandy and Zumla (2003), and Lewontin and Levins (2003).

2   On the impact of AIDS in sub-Saharan Africa, see Kalipeni et al. (2004).
3   On the rapid growth of slums and worsening access to water and sanitation, see, for example, UN-HABITAT (2003), Davis (2006), and Watkins (2006).
4   Furthermore, in localities with inadequate water supply, these insects can breed in storage containers, or any exposed bodies of water, so that the different public health hazards of cities become interrelated in new ways (see MacKinnon 2007).
5   See Wallace et al. (1995), Tulchinsky and Varavikova (1996), and Wallace and Wallace (1997).
6   See, for example, Evans (1988), Szreter and Mooney (1998), Sheard and Power (2000), and Gandy (2006b,c).
7   In May 2006, for example, there were street protests in Delhi against the pharmaceutical companies Gilead and GlaxoSmithKline, who were trying to prevent production of cheaper generic drugs, with immense implications for health care across the global South (see Ramesh 2006a).

11

Tuberculosis and the Anxieties of Containment

Susan Craddock

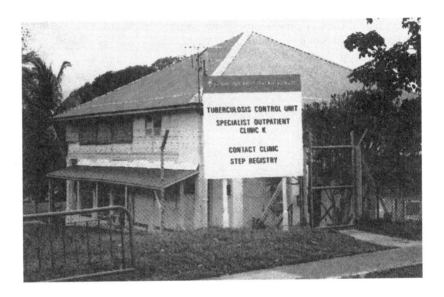

Don't let them know who we are,
Don't let them know where we're from.
Don't let them know what we've got.

Logh, "Ghosts," 2002

The upsurge of tuberculosis in the United States during the 1990s contradicted widespread assumptions that public health campaigns in the middle of the century, and the use of newly available antibiotics, had largely abolished the disease. Subsequent explanations for this ascendance focused on a contraction since the 1970s of municipal public health budgets earmarked for tuberculosis prevention, the rise of urban poverty, and the deterioration of inner-city housing stocks and healthcare services (Lerner 1998; Wallace and Wallace 2003; Draus 2004). As Matthew Gandy points out (Chapter 10), the apparent successes of public health campaigns and the increasing reliance upon effective pharmaceuticals in the middle of the twentieth century deflected attention away from the persistence of underlying social and economic causes of infectious diseases such as tuberculosis. Hence, even the oft-repeated term "re-emergence" became contested, given that tuberculosis in the poorest pockets of US cities never went away but, rather, became easy to ignore within aggregate statistics of improvement.

Though no longer increasing in overall rates, explanations for the persistence of tuberculosis in early twenty-first-century urban America have largely shifted away from a focus on urban poverty and blight, to a focus both on the molecular level, and on immigrant populations and border security in an age of globalization. Like other infectious diseases such as SARS, tuberculosis in major US cities is now predominantly a threat from the outside, but unlike SARS it is perceived not as a product of individual circulations among global cities but rather a sustained pattern of South–North urban migration. The themes that "the new tuberculosis" exemplifies – of an urban disease that is increasingly a product of intensified exchanges of people, technologies, and pathogens – are not necessarily new within public health; as Nick King notes (Chapter 12), public health has a longstanding interest in trying to keep diseases on the "other" side of borders (also see Craddock 2000). Yet these themes nevertheless deserve scrutiny for their new iterations within discourses of biosecurity and genetics, and for the ways in which tuberculosis figures within pronouncements on "emerging infectious diseases and globalization" in high-level public health and policy analyses.

In a 2006 report of the National Academy of Sciences on the impact of globalization on infectious disease emergence and control, for example, workshop participants discussed the impact to infectious disease spread of economic development, trade, and global cultural exchanges, while also acknowledging that highly mobile populations posed disease risks that necessitated a "new but necessary" surveillance. Not all mobile populations pose an equal threat, however. As the authors make clear, "not only are migrants and refugees more likely than the general population to become infected [with tuberculosis], ... they also put others at risk" (National Academy of Sciences 2006). It is difficult, in fact, to find biomedical or health policy literature on tuberculosis control today that does not mention a need for screening and surveillance of immigrant populations, a widespread political sentiment of "border suspicion" that proffers a different view of global mobility than more celebratory accounts of globalization and global cities, and that threatens to generate reactive sentiments of distrust among targeted populations as suggested by the quote above.

In this essay, I examine the centrality of tuberculosis to a profoundly ambivalent set of discourses[1] concerning borders, mobile populations, urbanization, globalization, and the spread of infectious disease. Like SARS and avian flu, tuberculosis exemplifies the contention by Ali (Chapter 14) that networked relations and global forces of all sorts need to be taken into account when examining the spatial diffusion of a pathogen, as well as in tracing its multiple and multi-scaled coordinates of understanding and experience. Unlike AIDS, SARS, or the threat of pandemic influenza, tuberculosis is itself not a particularly feared disease, except in its multi-drug resistant form; rather, the anxieties it currently produces among high-level policy circles stem from its tenacity, its prevalence among low-income countries in a global system of mobility and exchange, and its entrenchment in the US within largely urban and disenfranchised populations of immigrants, the homeless, and the imprisoned. In particular, then, I want to analyze these responses to tuberculosis in terms of their role in reconfiguring public and lay understandings of "diseased populations," the relationship between urbanization, development, and globalization in accounts of tuberculosis containment, and anxieties currently inhering in policy literature over the permeability of international, national, and urban borders. I begin with a brief overview of public health responses to tuberculosis in the early 1900s, both as a way of depicting the continuity of some modes of understanding a tenacious disease, and also to better elucidate differences in contexts, relations, and contradictions within present discussions of tuberculosis transmission and intervention.

The materials I have gleaned for my analysis come from recent articles in biomedical and epidemiology journals, Institute of Medicine reports on tuberculosis, globalization, and emerging infectious diseases, and policy documents from the National Security Council and the Centers for Disease Control. Though the recommendations and discussions contained in these materials are not exhaustive, their visibility makes them influential in the formation of national and international health policy. Given that tuberculosis infected almost 9 million individuals in 2004 and killed the better part of 2 million (WHO 2006c), the adequacy of such policy formations is coming under increased scrutiny (cf., Kim et al. 2005).

Urbanization and the Boundaries of Infection

Public health policy in the US by the turn of the twentieth century was focused upon cities as loci of poverty, disease, overcrowding, and, often, of large and unhygienic immigrant populations. Since the recognition late in the previous century that tuberculosis was infectious, attention had intensified on ways to prevent its transmission, yet this intensified scrutiny also led in most cities to an association of tuberculosis with ignorance and a depraved lifestyle inseparable from profound poverty (Craddock 2000), or immigrant status (Kraut 1994; Markel 1999). In either case, cities were seen as highly disparate in their agglomerations of poverty and wealth, while also revealing of a social and infrastructural metabolism that ensured the diseases of the poor or foreign were constantly threatening to circulate to wealthy neighborhoods through sewers, inadequate sanitation, or the intermingling of bodies through everyday acts of urban commerce and consumption.

Driving perceptions of diseased slums, particularly in cities such as New York and Chicago, was the influx of predominantly poor immigrants into the US in the first decades of the twentieth century, and the rise of vital statistics that showed huge discrepancies in rates of tuberculosis between wealthy and poor urban neighborhoods. Tuberculosis came to be recognized through these statistics as the most important public health problem of the early twentieth century, but its disproportionate presence among tenements and urban slums also pathologized spaces of poverty and their largely immigrant or non-white inhabitants (McBride 1991; Kraut 1994). A primary undertaking for many public health practitioners in the absence of a biomedical cure for tuberculosis thus became the reconfiguration of infectious spaces and bodies in an effort not only to manage disease but to sanitize those urban areas where intermingling of suspect and respectable populations was unavoidable (Craddock 2000).

Backed by the supposedly unerring authority of statistics, a wide range of biomedical and health policy literature is once again pointing to immigrants as the primary source of rising tuberculosis rates in US cities. "After declining dramatically for several decades," claims a National Intelligence Council report, "TB in the first half of the 1990s made a comeback in urban areas and in some 13 states with large refugee and immigrant populations ... Although a massive and costly intervention by state and local authorities reversed the overall infection rate ... TB incidence continues to grow among immigrant populations" (2000, p. 36). In its overview of recent tuberculosis trends in the US, an Institute of Medicine report concludes that TB is fast becoming a disease of the foreign-born given their increasing proportion of cases from 27 percent in 1992 to 43 percent in 1999 (2001, p. 31). By 2003 the proportion rose further to 53.3 percent, with an estimated 80–86 percent of immigrants entering the US during 1994–2003 from countries designated as "high incidence" for tuberculosis (CDC 2005, p. 45). Adding to the alarm is the estimated 10.6 percent of foreign-born individuals with primary isoniazid[2] resistance in 2003, versus 4.6 percent for US-born tuberculosis patients (ibid.). These kinds of statistics have led the National Intelligence Council to proclaim TB, along with HIV/AIDS and hepatitis C, as "the most dangerous known infectious diseases likely to threaten the US over the next two decades" (2000, p. 2).

On the surface, the focus on immigrants and the language of biosecurity in the medical and health policy literatures makes epidemiological sense.

When viewing statistics in any given year over the past decade, the "foreign-born" indeed represent the majority of tuberculosis cases nationally, indicating an apparent need for public health practitioners to target immigrant and refugee populations to mitigate their disease and manage potential avenues of transmission. Yet the reality of both the epidemiology of tuberculosis and its larger social context is more complicated. Even the definition of risk and "high incidence" must be seen as shaped by a confluence of geopolitics, state demographics, public health resources, and social political ideologies, rather than simply as a scientific standard. As discussed in the CDC report on controlling tuberculosis in the US, criteria do not yet exist in the US for designating countries as high incidence for tuberculosis, nor is it really known what such a designation means either in terms of actual risk for individual immigrants or for appropriate control and containment measures. The current list of 14 countries designated as high incidence covers such a broad range – from 33 to 406 per 100,000 population – as to diminish the meaning of the phrase, and even these statistics are not necessarily accurate given significant variability across regions (2005, p. 45). Using country of origin as a measure of risk (i.e., to the US) also overlooks the multiple economic and social factors shaping whether and when migrants acquire active tuberculosis in the US, and whether they acquire their disease before or after their arrival. The CDC report is one of the very few acknowledging that adequate information is lacking to even identify those foreign-born individuals at an elevated risk for acquiring TB, while recognizing that immigrants might be at higher risk once they are resident in the US (ibid.).

Second, new DNA fingerprinting technology enabling precise tracing of case transmission is suggesting that foreign-born individuals are not responsible for the majority of new cases of tuberculosis transmitted within US cities (Chin et al. 1998; Borgdorff et al. 2000; Bloom 2002). In two studies for example, investigators determined that only 8 percent of new cases among a sample population in New York (Bloom 2002) and 2 out of 115 cases among US-born tuberculosis patients in San Francisco (Chin et al. 1998) were transmitted by immigrants. As Bloom bluntly states, "Infection with recently transmitted tuberculosis was not just a Third World phenomenon" (2002, p. 1434). Bloom also refutes the NIC reports' claims that cases of TB continue to rise among immigrant populations by pointing out that only their proportion of the whole has increased against a more rapid diminution of US-born cases, their numbers actually remaining stable in urban areas over the past decade (ibid.).

Statistics and DNA evidence notwithstanding, as implied by Bloom's comment, more than epidemiology is being mobilized in current accounts of tuberculosis in the US. Though never acknowledged within health policy or biomedical reports, it is impossible to extricate discussions of endemic tuberculosis among immigrants from low-income countries from the larger canvas of anti-immigration politics ongoing within the US. Along with charges of resource depletion and job stealing, inflammatory rhetoric of diseased immigrants accessing open borders invariably informs new rounds of presidential and congressional debates over how best to "secure our national borders," to the extent that Congress is now considering a 700-mile-long fence along the US border with Mexico, and the allocation of $1.9 billion to deploy 6,000 National Guard personnel, purchase patrol helicopters, build extra detention facilities, and erect other exclusionary barriers along an ever-permeable and problematic national border (United States House of Representatives 2006b). Where borders are not contiguous, recommendations turn toward strengthening screening processes in countries producing immigrants as well as in the US as a method of creating barriers to infectious intrusion through improved technologies of surveillance. As Nick King attests, "the legitimate observation that certain social groups might have a higher incidence of TB than others can too easily be transformed into fear and stigmatization of 'diseased' ... Third World immigrants" (2003, p. 47).

Less prominent but still present in the epidemiological literature is the understanding that to the extent that tuberculosis is not contained within immigrant communities in the US, it affects equally marginalized urban populations (Chin et al. 1998; Geiter 2001). Having exonerated immigrants from the role of primary tuberculosis transmitters, Chin and his colleagues point out that "the propagation of tuberculosis in an urban community can be largely contained to subpopulations" of HIV-positive individuals, drug users, the homeless, or the imprisoned (1998, p. 1801), thus adding infectious disease to the list of blights already ascribed to these communities and creating a vision of urban life reminiscent of public health depictions a century ago. As reflected in a majority of public policy and epidemiological literature on tuberculosis, understandings conveyed by statistics and DNA tracing have led to recommendations for targeting populations that appear at particular risk of tuberculosis transmission or who sustain higher than average rates within their communities.

On the one hand, targeting of vulnerable populations makes epidemiological and economic sense, as it enables cash-strapped municipalities to focus resources on a limited set of subpopulations (King 2003). It can also be beneficial when communities themselves are engaged in planning and implementing appropriate interventions (CDC 2005).[3] Targeting of individuals can also be effective in mitigating transmission of tuberculosis when it means increasing directly observed therapy (DOT), expanded availability of clinic services (Farmer and Nardell 1998), and testing for latent TB infections (Bloom 2002). Yet the kind of targeting of immigrant and other affected communities recommended by a significant proportion of health policy and biomedical literature has less to do with comprehensive prevention and intervention plans and more to do with containing a largely poor and Third

World threat, however discursively defined, within cities that have received or continue to receive significant inflows of immigrants. Cindy Patton has called this trend of targeting in public health "tropical thinking," for its reverberations with a colonial medicine that similarly confined tropical diseases to well-delineated spaces that were always "there" (the Tropics) rather than "here," a cartography that nevertheless created anxieties in a colonial context under the "compulsions to be in proximity to the primitive" (2002, p. 36).[4]

"Tropical" in this case is not only a locale but a designation, a signal that the Third World is the location of disease while the First World body is the locus of health biologically threatened when boundaries disappear or fail. Current policies that locate tuberculosis in designated Third World zones within First World cities and that focus on screening and surveillance perform a similar function of collapsing prevention into containment that mitigates the threat to a "here" and "us," but that does not necessarily address the root causes and contexts driving tuberculosis transmission within affected communities. Nor does it allow for the possibility that infection can occur outside well-designated boundaries of immigrant status or "developing country" origin. As suggested by studies finding that many immigrants develop tuberculosis five years or more after coming to the US, however, immigrants do not always arrive already infectious, but in fact become vulnerable only after longstanding residence within the US (King 2003).

Much current medical and health policy literature thus resonates with public health policy a century ago in casting blame on immigrants; unlike a century ago, when cities such as New York tackled issues such as overcrowded tenement housing, few seem to be asking how US cities currently support higher rates of tuberculosis for some groups and not others. Inadequate attention has been paid, in other words, to the multiple factors including crowded housing, underemployment, and lack of access to or under-utilization of health care, that over time turn latent tuberculosis in some immigrant individuals into active disease. Instead, there is greater attention to border security and to technologies for deploying at multiple sites to diminish the flow of undesirable populations into the US, whether this is a wall and security forces along a shared border, or improved screening and testing capacities in "high-incidence" countries. To put it another way, targeting at its worst creates profiles of who is likely to have tuberculosis and how to keep them away rather than addressing urban ecologies that ensure a continued presence of tuberculosis in US cities.

Globalization, Development, Containment

Focusing on associations between tuberculosis and immigration points, on the one hand, to a recognition that discussions of tuberculosis must be placed in a larger context of global processes and movements, but it also attests to the anxieties inhering in the outcome of those processes. Explaining the rise of TB in industrialized cities in the 1990s, the authors of the influential IOM report on ending tuberculosis in the US complain that "no longer are populations and the diseases prevalent within them forced by circumstances to remain in the countries or areas where they originate." Instead, "Population movements within and between countries both shift persons from high- to low-incidence countries and cause increased crowding in urban areas, thereby facilitating tuberculosis transmission. Increasing economic gradients increase the allure of wealthier countries for poor people in the developing world" (Geiter 2001, pp. 150–1). Meanwhile, less favored regions of the world are experiencing "worsening economic circumstances, reordering of priorities, and lack of political commitment," which in turn leads to deterioration of public health infrastructure while "at the same time the need for disease control programs and surveillance is increasing" (ibid., p. 151).

The IOM's report is worth quoting at relative length in order to make several brief comments. First, the language of territorial hierarchy is unmistakable here, where borders that previously kept the outcome of profound economic and social inequities geographically distant have dissolved through processes of globalization that are never made explicit, but that form the backdrop of shifting cartographies of health and disease. The unprecedented access to wealthy countries of "poor people" and their pathogens is driving a resurgence of infectious disease in industrial countries unseen for the better part of a century.

It suggests as well the ambiguous yet pivotal role of global cities in the "new" tuberculosis. Though rural or suburban areas are not insignificant in low-wage job provision,[5] cities and their concentration of service jobs constitute the primary "allure" for low-income immigrants and their families. Indeed, what goes unstated in the IOM's comments about population movements is that immigrants arrive in cities not just because of broader global economic inequalities but, more specifically, in part because of the particular requirements of post-industrial service-based economies. In other words, domestic economic restructuring over the past 40 years not only resulted in the export of manufacturing jobs to low-income countries, but also produced an increased demand for low-wage and unskilled labor in urban-based service and construction sectors within the US and Europe. Restaurants, hospitals, transportation services, and dual-income households have all benefited from the availability of low-cost immigrant labor, but the degree to which immigrants benefit is variable. The wages paid in these service jobs, coupled with inadequate social support and healthcare provision, while creating the conditions to foster the kinds of TB rates discussed in the IOM and other reports, also raise questions about defining economic inequality along the

First and Third World divide rather than along the multiple fissures created by inequitable practices of economic globalization.

Third, the stark terms of backwardness versus progress employed by the IOM report are characteristic of a language of development deployed by much of the work within international health policy that deserves more scrutiny than it has so far received (King 2002; Keller 2007). Though a few of these documents recognize explicitly the flaws of Western-centric representations and modes of intervention (Knobler et al. 2006), the majority continue to characterize infectious diseases such as tuberculosis as part of a larger landscape of poverty, overpopulation, and poor governance among developing countries that only Western intervention can mitigate. Though this language is prevalent, a few examples will suffice. The authors of a recent IOM report on the effects of globalization on infectious diseases for instance term the situation a "Malthusian challenge" (ibid., p. 2), while in his introduction to a previous IOM report on emerging infectious diseases, David Heymann of the WHO claims that "With the end of the Cold War, the end of the colonial era, and the decline of Western interest in tropical diseases, the public health infrastructure in many African countries has deteriorated" (2001, p. 30). In their discussion of social and environmental factors behind infectious diseases, Weiss and McMichael claim that "we cannot control our disease destiny," particularly when "overpopulation in relation to environmental resources remains a ... pressing problem in many developing countries, where poor economic and social conditions go hand-in-hand with infectious disease" (2004, p. 70).[6]

The images of helplessness and chaos propagated by this language arguably have constituted the ideological core of development policy-making for decades, and their presence in the international health policy literature has equally negative implications for the kinds of interventions they inform. Integral to this rhetoric is the fact that globalization as an analytic remains so vague in health policy and biomedical literatures that it becomes itself a means of creating boundaries where none exist. As Matthew Gandy suggests (Chapter 10), the mechanics of economic globalization, and more specifically the transnational and bi-national terms by which regional poverty is generated and global inequalities perpetuated, never get discussed. Even a recent IOM report entitled "The Impact of Globalization on Infectious Disease Emergence and Control" circumnavigates the precise politics and contours of current global economic practices and instead describes globalization as "increasingly integrated trade, economic development, human movement, and cultural exchange" (Knobler et al. 2006, p. 2). This kind of simplistic characterization not only glosses the complex and uneven processes of global trade regulations, labor inequities, and austerity programs underlying current global burdens of tuberculosis and other infectious diseases; equally importantly, it plays a key role in supporting those processes.

The distancing achieved by such linguistic elisions effectively then casts blame onto countries for their own poverty and chides their inability to strengthen "deteriorated" public health infrastructures, if the only reason they need strengthening is to deploy screening and surveillance systems that can restore geographical boundaries between the healthy and infectious.

It also means that health policy analysts remain largely content to work with the results of global economic policies that negatively impact health rather than working to shape those policies (Kim et al. 2005). Evaluating the complex regionally specific and multi-scaled factors contributing to increased poverty in many areas, for example, would move analysis away from misguided statements about bad governance and toward more productive efforts at poverty reduction through debt relief, more equitable trade agreements, or better multinational corporate employment policies as part of tuberculosis prevention. A broader spectrum of health policy-makers could also be involved in negotiating technology transfer agreements such as the World Trade Organization's Trade Related Aspects of Intellectual Property agreement (or TRIPS), which currently regulates the terms under which new technologies get disseminated, governs the high prices of new drugs, and in part determines the lack of new research and therapies for diseases such as tuberculosis that have limited markets.[7] In other words, as long as these false boundaries between public health and the political coordinates of globalization are maintained and the language of development embraced, epidemiologists and health policy analysts will continue to actually buttress the very factors contributing to tuberculosis – and to movements of vulnerable populations – rather than intervening in both.

Susceptibility, Immunity, Race

Within the easy slippage from "immigrant" to "ethnic" designations of disease is a parallel trend in recent studies seeking to explain differential rates of tuberculosis along racial lines. The question of racial susceptibility has circulated within debates on urbanization and tuberculosis since at least the early decades of the twentieth century, driven by observations and later proven by statistics that some communities had higher rates of the disease, or that some populations seemed to have less resistance than others to its ravages. As suggested by a physician in the early decades of the twentieth century, the question of susceptibility focused on whether geographical region, urban location, immigrant status, or race was most significant (Cummins 1920). Like the relation between urbanization and tuberculosis, discussions of immunity and race varied between "virgin soil" proponents claiming that immunity was conferred through repeated exposures and not through heredity, to those proponents of a biological susceptibility among particular groups such as black Africans (Cummins 1920, 1929; Dubos and Dubos 1952; Harrison and Warboys 1997). As indicated by Harrison and Warboys (1997), these discussions were durable, but they remained unresolved.

The resilience of "racial susceptibility" debates is indeed reflected in the number of current studies on tuberculosis that utilize epidemiological data, DNA fingerprinting, or genetic variability in humans to posit racial explanations for patterns of susceptibility and transmission. Rather than conflicting with literatures associating TB with immigration, these studies mirror the efforts to define diseased populations and map the contours of susceptibility along historically and ideologically resonant fault lines. In a widely cited study, Stead and colleagues use longitudinal TB test data from nursing homes as well as national statistics showing higher rates of TB among African-Americans than whites to determine that blacks are biologically more susceptible to tuberculosis infection (Stead et al. 1990). DNA fingerprinting studies also consistently find that ethnic designation is a significant variable in the transmission of *Mycobacterium tuberculosis*. In this growing number of studies, depending upon the city, being African-American or Hispanic means having an increased likelihood of transmitting tuberculosis to other individuals (Alland et al. 1994; Small et al. 1994; Chin et al. 1998; Borgdorff et al. 2000).

A third set of studies makes a somewhat more circuitous route toward racial susceptibility by focusing on population-based genetic variations for the potential to confer more or less immunity to *M. tuberculosis*.[8] The rationale for genetic approaches to susceptibility lies in the need to better understand complicated mechanics of tuberculosis transmission and progression to active disease. Why some individuals remain free of infection after repeated exposure, why some never progress to disease, and why others progress rapidly are questions that have remained inadequately resolved and arguably need further illumination if better interventions are to be implemented. The ideal of genetic research is to identify individual-based genes and genetic variations influencing disease risk, yet the logistical and financial impracticalities of this endeavor means the alternative of population-based genetic research (Risch et al. 2002). The controversy starts, however, when populations are defined along geographical and linguistic terms (Cavalli-Sforza et al. 1994; Wilson et al. 2001; Risch et al. 2002). In genetic studies of tuberculosis susceptibility, entire national populations are said to have genetic susceptibility or resistance to tuberculosis based on tests of a few hundred individuals (Bellamy et al. 1998; Gao et al. 2000; Ryu et al. 2000), or alternatively "aboriginal" or "ethnic" subpopulations of a region are examined for similar genetic variability (Cervino et al. 2000; Greenwood et al. 2000; Fitness et al. 2004).

Aside from the fact that these studies so far have been all over the map, so to speak, in their conclusions, their approach in using populations or "ethnic groups" as units of analysis has been criticized by scientists and social scientists alike for assumptions that genetic variability can be traced along geographical or national boundaries. Such assumptions not only rest upon questionable claims of homogeneity that ignore complex histories of population movements and more recent patterns of migration, refugee movements, and reproductive practices, but they also contravene scientific evidence suggesting greater genetic variability among individuals in the same population than between populations (Braun 2002; Duster 2003; Reardon 2005).

Most troubling in this literature, however, is the way in which nationally defined genetic variability maintains the potential to shift seamlessly into racial or ethnic susceptibility. Though this shift so far is not widespread, even two examples provide illustrations of its viability and the roadmap for further claims. In their 1998 study, Bellamy and colleagues researched genetic variation among a cohort in the Gambia, without explaining the choice of West Africa as a base for genetic research. Citing the study by Stead et al. (1990), however, the researchers conclude that "racial variation in the susceptibility to tuberculosis ... strongly suggest[s] that genetic factors are important in the susceptibility to tuberculosis" (1998, p. 640). Subsequently finding that a polymorphism in the NRAMP1 gene, 3′UTR, indicates increased susceptibility to tuberculosis in the 25 percent of Gambians possessing this particular gene variant, these scientists then suggest their results as "in part explain[ing] why American blacks have greater susceptibility to tuberculosis than whites" (ibid., p. 643), given the absence of this gene variant in a majority of Europeans. That a significant majority of Gambians also do not possess this gene variant, that African-Americans do not necessarily trace their ancestry to the Gambia, and that the "strong" research rationale for race-based genetic susceptibility rests upon one author's highly flawed study all points toward the problematic way in which racial category gets mobilized in the service of scientific solutions. Another recent study conducted in Cambodia inexplicably turns to the language of ethnicity in explaining findings that Cambodians both align with and diverge from other population-based studies in their genetic responses to tuberculosis. As the authors conclude, "The novel pattern of genetic associations with susceptibility and resistance to TB detected in Cambodia is consistent with the conclusion that ... selective factors have resulted in the development of ethnic-specific host genetic factors associated with TB" and that such findings should thus "guide TB therapy and prophylaxis in an ethnic-specific manner" (Delgado et al. 2002, pp. 1463 and 1467).

The studies cited above attest to why tensions continue to inhere over the use of racial categories in genetic and other biomedical research despite repeated declarations, including by the directors of the Human Genome Project, that "race" has no biological or genetic meaning. Like similar debates almost a century ago, the apparent irresolution of the "race" question means that studies mapping racial and ethnic categories onto disease susceptibility continue to be undertaken with very little reflexivity about the reason, definition, or context in which these terms are utilized, nor the implications for doing so. As Lundy Braun suggests, "we are left with a wide gap between theoretical understandings of the meaning of race and ethnicity and the use of these understandings by biomedical researchers" (2002, p. 165). One obvious problem with race-based disease susceptibility is the potential for abuse in systems of unequal power relations. Racial category regardless of any basis (or not) in biology is always already a politicized phenomenon functioning within a larger framework of institutional practices and governance, such that widespread understandings of African-Americans or Hispanics (or Somalis or Vietnamese) as either more susceptible to tuberculosis, or largely responsible for its transmission, would not stop at public health interventions. Insurance companies, employers, the military, real estate agents, and other private and governmental institutions could utilize "genetic predispositions toward an infectious disease" as reason for misguided and discriminatory policy formations.[9]

Focus on racial susceptibility as genetically defined also obscures the political economy of racism, rather than race, in shaping disparities in tuberculosis prevalence in US cities today. Ironically, the persistence of institutional racisms and attendant economic and social deprivations are the reasons cited by many scholars for keeping "ethnicity" and "race" as classifications in epidemiological studies of health disparities. Attention to disparities in disease rates and treatment responses, including in tuberculosis, points toward the fact – if not the precise mechanics – of race/ethnicity as a social phenomenon whose pathogenic effects can be mitigated in the short and longer terms through therapeutic interventions, resource allocations, and structural change (Farmer and Nardell 1998). Race and racial susceptibility defined genetically, on the other hand, threatens a return to rigid biological definitions of race that, as recent histories have shown, threaten more damaging effects.

This is not to suggest that all genetic research is harmful. Studies focusing on genetic variations in *M. tuberculosis*, for example, are revealing precise mechanics of transmission among different strains of TB that could prove beneficial in developing new drugs and vaccines (Gagneux et al. 2006). The best genetic research also points out that genetic explanations must always be taken alongside other factors such as social and economic environment in determining the larger picture of disease susceptibility. As Braun suggests, "While genetic predisposition may explain some of the variability in the presence and severity of disease in individuals, the question that has to be addressed is whether genetic predisposition is a useful explanation for racial and ethnic disparities in disease" (2002, p. 167).

Conclusion

Beyond the burden of suffering that TB continues to confer on millions of individuals worldwide, it remains as well a trenchant symbol of contradictory global processes that have benefited some countries and populations through the increased immiseration of others, and in so doing have galvanized transfers of potentially infectious populations. Though national boundaries have long been vulnerable to intrusions of the unwanted, the new rhetoric of tuberculosis, at least within US health policy circles, pivots critically around the conundrum of securing urban and national borders against movements of people and their pathogens in the midst of border erosion in the face of increased exchanges of commodities and capital. In other words, it exemplifies the contradictory architecture of a globalization placing into tension a celebratory rhetoric of open borders promising economic benefits in trade and communication with a profound anxiety over who and what will take advantage of such permeability. Deleuze and Guattari observe that "the administration of a great organized molar security has as its correlate a whole micromanagement of petty fears, a permanent molecular insecurity" (1987, p. 216).

Processes of globalization, while creating a network of supranational connections as well as channels of prosperity (a molar security), have also spawned multiple molecular sites where disease, poverty, and unrest thrive. Put another way, demands on the part of the US and other industrialized countries for better economic access to low-income regions have generated in turn a not-so-petty fear of the destabilizing re-territorializations that such demands have unleashed. The reconfigured geography of tuberculosis is such a re-territorialization according to many health policy and epidemiological studies, a disease that has gone largely from Third World containment to Third World colonization of urban areas in countries such as the US.

The related discourses utilizing genetic research to trace boundaries of transmission and susceptibility around racial status achieve similar goals of delimiting the reach of infectious disease. Rather than furthering any understanding of why some bear heavier burdens of disease than others, however, these studies, by defining populations and race in biological terms in the absence of broader social analysis, merge with the rhetoric on immigration in employing interpretive, historically resonant, and deeply hierarchical linguistic, symbolic, and ideological cartographies in the guise of science to shape assumptions about who is diseased and who is not.

The focus on who is diseased rather than why, in both domestic and global settings, attests not so much to myopia in health policy circles, but to a particular kind of political engagement that generates its own contradiction: by refusing to critique multiple processes of globalization and the effects they have on global tuberculosis prevalence and patterns, policy reports by default condone those processes that perpetuate tuberculosis and achieve very little toward eradicating the disease. Indeed, the notable absence of eradication as an end goal in this literature and the singular focus on containment lend credence to suggestions that infectious diseases are becoming critical components of national security rather than public health concerns (King 2002; Ingram 2005; Cooper 2006). One way through these contradictory anxiety-conjugations of risk would be to see tuberculosis as a political tool for leveraging changes in the more inequitable structures of global practice, rather than blaming those disadvantaged by them. A shift from seeing immigrants or African-Americans as the problem behind urban rates of tuberculosis and toward coordinates of vulnerability in turn would shift discussions away from the language of border security and population containment and toward a language of global bacterial mitigation. Only if these shifts occur are urban and global rates of tuberculosis likely to experience sustained declines.

NOTES

1   I am using "discourse" in a Foucauldian sense here to indicate a particular set of knowledge, ideas, and ideologies (or regimes of truth) that gain legitimacy through the institutional authority of the authors producing it.

2   Isoniazid is a primary first-line drug for tuberculosis treatment.

3   The CDC report is the only major health policy document I have seen that both recognizes the degree to which conditions of risk are unknown in many affected communities, such as immigrant neighborhoods, and that articulates the need to work with such communities in formulating health policies and tuberculosis interventions.

4   Patton uses this designation in the context of AIDS, yet tuberculosis fits just as well within this framework.

5   The meat-processing and packing industry is one example of a rural or peri-urban based employer of immigrant labor in the US.

6   For an excellent critique of the environment–violence–overpopulation–disease nexus, see Peluso and Watts (2001).

7   I say "broader spectrum" of health policy-makers because members of organizations such as Doctors Without Borders have been working for years to broker better terms of intellectual property rights and technology transfers for the benefit of impoverished regions. In addition to the TRIPS agreement, the 1980 Bayh–Dole Act encouraging relations between research institutions and the biotechnology and pharmaceutical industries has also been instrumental in developing market-based rather than needs-based biomedical research into new therapies.

8   Cf., Bellamy et al. (1998), Cervino et al. (2000), Gao et al. (2000), Ryu et al. (2000), Delgado et al. (2002), and Fitness et al. (2004).

9   For examples of similar "race-based" conclusions of physical difference inform-ing dismissal of African Americans from the military in the 1990s, see Duster (2003) in particular.

12

Networks, Disease, and the Utopian Impulse

Nicholas B. King

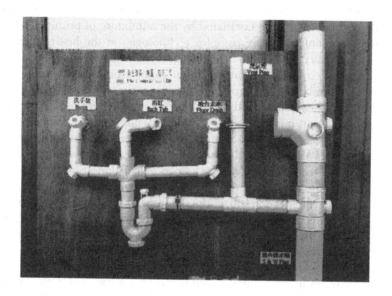

The Utopias are bulletins suggesting the introduction of new elements into social life, new ways of doing things, calling for new training, and requiring new ways of living to which people would have to be accommodated.

Hertzler (1965, p. 264)

Introduction: Eden-Olympia

J. G. Ballard's recent novel *Super-Cannes* (2000) is set in a French multinational business park named Eden-Olympia. Its protagonists, Doctor Jane Sinclair and her husband, are British expatriates who have relocated to a planned community whose residents are under constant surveillance: their movements recorded by security cameras, their behavior tracked by a private security force, and their health closely monitored during regular visits to the doctor in residence.

As Jane Sinclair prepares to take up her new position as Eden-Olympia's resident pediatrician, her husband comments on the apparent health of its inhabitants: "Take a good look at your new patients ... A healthy crowd ... I can't imagine anyone here actually bothering to fall ill." Doctor Sinclair differs, replying: "Don't be too sure. I'll be busier than you think. The place is probably riddled with airport TB and the kind of viruses that only breed in executive jets. And as for their minds ..." (Ballard 2000).

One of foremost oracles of the consequences and contradictions of modernity, Ballard has long been fascinated by the admixture of primitive instinctual urges and unfathomably complex technologies at the heart of modern life. In novels such as *Crash*, *High Rise*, and *The Crystal World*, he observed that dreams of technological utopia often conceal or even conjure human atavism. For Ballard, every apparent utopia – the gated community, the colossal apartment complex, the modern highway system – has a darker, dystopic side. Deep in the heart of modern discipline, chaos roams free.

It is not surprising that in his latest novel, Ballard chooses infectious disease as a sign of the chaotic surplus within the networked spaces of global capital. Doctor to southern France's silicon valley, Jane Sinclair fears that even this gated community, with its daily exercise regimens and private security force, cannot immunize the international business elite against viruses and bacteria. The very postmodern networks that allow them to exercise control over the modern global economy and their own bodies also render them vulnerable to the most primitive microscopic pathogens.

Ballard was not alone in this observation. During the decade prior to the publication of his novel, a small group of American scientists, public health, and national security experts became increasingly concerned with the infiltration of infectious organisms into global networks. They translated their concern into public campaigns around the twin threats of "emerging diseases" and biological terrorism. These campaigns resulted in what I have elsewhere called the "emerging diseases worldview": a coherent vision of the threat that infectious diseases pose to American health and national security, and the best ways of addressing this threat (King 2004). Despite its origins among a small group of American scientists, this worldview has had an immense and enduring influence on contemporary understandings of the international transmission of infectious diseases such as influenza, SARS, and tuberculosis.

Ballard's image of Eden-Olympia provides a fictional allegory for the emerging diseases worldview. In particular, his literary use of transportation and surveillance networks as metaphors for modern control and primitive contamination parallel the scientific and political understanding of networks in this worldview: in each case, networks are real entities laden with metaphorical connotations; and are viewed as both the cause of and a remedy for communicable disease.

Networks of Emergence

In October 1995, the US Senate convened a hearing, chaired by Senator Nancy Kassebaum of Kansas, to examine "the threat and risk of certain old and new infectious diseases on the nation's health" (United States Senate, Committee on Labor and Human Resources 1995). The hearing featured a variety of scientists and health officials testifying about the growing threat posed by the proliferation of global transportation networks.

Geneticist and Nobel laureate Lederberg warned that "the microbe which felled one child in a distant continent yesterday can reach your child today and seed a global pandemic tomorrow" (ibid.). Later, the World Health Organization's James LeDuc articulated similar concerns, telling the committee that "infectious diseases, like the environment, do not recognize national boundaries" (ibid.).

The testimony echoed broader concerns prevalent in the popular press at the time. Just four months earlier, American magazines and newspapers ran multiple cover stories on a deadly outbreak of Ebola hemorrhagic fever in Kikwit, Zaire (now Democratic Republic of the Congo). The apparent ease with which the Ebola virus might be transmitted across international borders prompted the author of *Newsweek*'s cover story to ask, "We want to know whether ebola is headed *our* way. Could it reach critical mass in a Third World capital, then engulf the globe? And what if ebola somehow mutated into an airborne form? Could coughs and sneezes become the agents of mass death" (Cowley et al. 1995, p. 52).

Four years later, Minnesota state epidemiologist Michael T. Osterholm delivered a lecture entitled "Emerging Diseases: An Outdated Concept?" before a good-sized audience at the Boston University School of Public Health.[1] Osterholm began by rhetorically asking whether the concept of "emerging diseases," despite already having a decade-old pedigree, was merely "in favor," or "just a fad." His response to these questions and the one posed in his title was an emphatic "forget it," and he cited as the primary reason the accelerating threat that transportation and trade networks posed to American health and security. Declaring that, "I'm afraid we're at the bottom of the curve ... we're going to see infectious diseases coming back with a vengeance," Osterholm chose compelling, resonant, and alarming examples to illustrate his case. To demonstrate the hazards of international trade, he alluded to both the 1995 Ebola outbreak and a more recent outbreak of West Nile virus in New York City. He speculated that the latter was caused by the illegal importation of exotic birds, and observed that many of the rodents currently being studied as reservoirs of Ebola were frequent legal and illegal imports as well. Raising the specter of two of the most well-publicized viruses of the late twentieth century, Osterholm vigorously argued that better regulation and screening of animals were necessary to protect the public health.

Exotic animals were not the only vectors that Osterholm singled out as particularly threatening to Americans. To illustrate the danger that imported foods posed, he related a cautionary tale in which an outbreak of illness caused by *E. coli* in Minnesota was traced back to unsanitary conditions in a particular Mexican agricultural field. Juxtaposing slides of fresh fruit and produce in a fancy American supermarket with images of Mexican farm workers washing carrots for export in a ditch less than a mile away from an open sewage outflow pipe, he warned that "you don't have to leave Boston to get traveler's diarrhea – it will come to you." In another instance, Osterholm attributed outbreaks of cyclosporiasis in the United States between 1995 and 1997 to the production and importation, initially encouraged by the United States Agency for International Development (USAID), of Guatemalan raspberries.[2] For Osterholm, the globalization of food production and distribution meant that there were "direct implications of developing world food production on your fancy supermarket."

As if the danger of contaminated products were not enough, Osterholm further argued that the bodies of foreigners posed a distinct threat to the health of American citizens. He thus recounted an instance in which an outbreak of measles in the Minneapolis area was traced back to a small area of the upper deck of the local sports stadium. The index case of this outbreak was a member of an Argentine delegation, who had attended an opening night baseball game. The implications of this example were clear: one need not travel to the cosmopolitan port cities of the seaboards to risk exposure to foreign bodies harboring infectious diseases. Simply enjoying an evening of the great American pastime in the heartland of the country might expose one to communicable disease.

Mesmerizing though they were, the anecdotes about food-borne illness and measles were both less compelling and less frightening than his most alarming example: tuberculosis. Declaring that the United States was "a depository of the worldwide TB problem," he warned that the porousness of American national boundaries left the country "like a submarine with screen doors." Observing that the foreign-born accounted for 60 percent of the cases of tuberculosis in Minnesota over the previous four years, he warned the audience that they were now seeing "spillover" from foreign-born into "native-born" populations. Again, the implications were clear: increased travel and immigration threatened to reverse more than a century of declines in tuberculosis morbidity and mortality.

Osterholm was hardly alone in his concerns. During the 1990s, the American public health community increasingly focused on the pernicious health effects that global networks could have on the American polity. Whether because of the increasing international exchange of contaminated foods and products, or the legal and illegal movement of contaminated bodies across international borders, the danger of outbreaks of infectious disease seemed to be on the rise.

Concerns over the health effects of these changes were crystallized in a 1997 report issued by the Institute of Medicine's Board on International Health, entitled *America's Vital Interest in Global Health: Protecting Our People, Enhancing Our Economy, and Advancing Our National Interests* (Board on International Health 1997). Arguing that both international humanitarian concerns and self-interest compelled the United States to address global health, this report identified globalization as an irrepressible agent of transformation:

> Since the end of the Cold War, the world economy has become increasingly interconnected and globalized; increased competition, trade, and communication have brought benefits to people in virtually every country and have created a remarkable degree of mutual interdependence. Yet these changes have also brought risks that frequently cannot be addressed adequately within traditional national borders and have created problems that have spread among nations at an accelerating pace. The movement of 2 million people each day across national borders and the growth of international commerce are inevitably associated with transfers of health risks, some obvious examples being infectious diseases, contaminated foodstuffs, terrorism, and legal or banned toxic substances. (Board on International Health 1997)

As in Osterholm's lecture, the report identified four specific vectors for the "international transfer or acquisition of health risks": the movement of human bodies across national borders; the transfer of contaminated products or foodstuffs across national borders; international variations in environmental and occupational health and safety standards; and the "indiscriminate" transfer of medical technologies (Board on International Health 1997). The Institute of Medicine was by no means the first such body to highlight these particular effects of the globalization of trade and travel. Two years earlier, the Cabinet-level National Science and Technology Council (NSTC) began its report on emerging and re-emerging infectious diseases with a similar warning about the accelerated legal and illegal transgression of national borders: "the modern world is a very small place; any city in the world is only a plane ride away from any other. Infectious microbes can easily travel across borders with their human or animal hosts. In fact, diseases that arise in other parts of the world are repeatedly introduced into the United States, where they may threaten our national health and security" (Buehler et al. 1995).

Networks of Response

The October 1995 hearing also addressed proposed solutions to the problems posed by transportation networks. Foremost among these was the development of mechanisms to rapidly identify, track, and disseminate information about disease outbreaks – in particular, epidemiological surveillance networks. Thus, for example, Osterholm argued that increased funding for such networks – "the basic radar which allows us to understand when we are under attack by microbiologic missiles" – was crucial: "Imagine trying to run O'Hare traffic control towers with tin cans and string. Well, much of what we do in infectious disease surveillance in this country borders on that level of effectiveness ... without the ability to know with accuracy when, where, and why infectious diseases are occurring, we cannot begin to prevent them" (United States Senate, Committee on Labor and Human Resources 1995).

Osterholm was not alone in his recommendation. Throughout the 1990s, scientists and health officials identified surveillance as a fundamental resource for addressing not only natural outbreaks of infectious disease, but also human-created outbreaks as the result of the use of biological weapons by states or non-state actors. For example, in February and August of 1992, the journal *Politics and the Life Sciences* published roundtable articles, with responses, on the implementation of global epidemiological surveillance regimes as a component of biological weapons control. The February issue featured an article by epidemiologist Peter Barss, entitled "Epidemic Field Investigation as Applied to Allegations of Chemical, Biological, or Toxin Warfare." Barss argued that while the institution of international weapons-control agreements was a political process, "investigations of alleged violations ultimately rely upon the results of scientific field studies" (Barss 1992). To this end, Barss recommended the institution of standardized protocols, to be followed by teams of epidemiologists and laboratory investigators from neutral countries, in order to subject alleged violations to "the same impartial standards as any scientific investigation" (Barss 1992). The job of policing international agreements, in other words, required epidemiological surveillance. Barss' comments were supported by the various experts assembled to comment on his article, including virologist Stephen Morse – first to coin the term "emerging viruses" (see Morse 1992) – who explicitly linked weapons convention verification with public health surveillance more generally:

A global capability for recognizing and responding to unexpected outbreaks of disease, by allowing the early identification and control of disease outbreaks, would simultaneously buttress defenses against both disease and CBTW. This argues for expanding permanent surveillance programs ... The coordination of these programs with global health surveillance systems would offer synergistic and cost effective benefits both for global health and for the monitoring of CBTW. (Barss 1992)

Six months later, the journal featured a discussion of an article that further elaborated Barss' and Morse's arguments. In "Strengthening Biological Weapons Control through Global Epidemiological Surveillance," molecular biologist Mark Wheelis argued that while large-scale national biological weapons development programs could be detected through normal intelligence-gathering channels, smaller-scale and covert violations could not. Wheelis recommended the institution of a system of routine, global epidemiological surveillance, which would allow the international community to quickly distinguish between natural and human-caused outbreaks of infectious disease – and thus identify treaty violations. This surveillance network would depend upon basic molecular biological research, particularly identification of the genetic structure of particular pathogens. Wheelis also noted that "such a surveillance system is justified not only by its strengthening effect on the BWC and the GP [Geneva Protocol], but also by the great improvements in understanding of disease ecology and in global public health that it would bring" (Wheelis 1992, p. 181).

The global surveillance apparatus envisioned in the early 1990s would have required training a large cadre of epidemiologists, as well as considerable cooperation for national, state, and local governments and health officials across the globe. This kind of surveillance was described in a 1999 by Walter Reed Army Institute of Research's Julie Pavlin in the following terms: "To facilitate the rapid identification of a bioterrorist attack, all health-care providers and public health personnel should have basic epidemiologic skills and knowledge of what to expect in such a setting. Any small or large outbreak of disease should be evaluated as a potential bioterrorist attack ... Surveillance needs to be more than routine" (Pavlin 1999, p. 528). This form of surveillance is not an activity that emanates from particular institutions, but rather a technology that is dispersed throughout the health-care system: all healthcare activities, from routine interactions between patients and clinicians in an urban hospital to broad surveys of regional and national populations, are points for data collection.

Moreover, this surveillance would rely upon sophisticated networks to collect, process, archive, and communicate information. As biologist Ronald Atlas wrote in 1999:

Rapid epidemiological investigation to identify the nature of the disease outbreak will be critical for limiting casualties in the event of a bioterrorist attack ... Computer networks can aid in epidemiological investigations of unusual disease outbreaks. Rapid recognition of a biological weapons attack will be aided by the creation, at the state level, of high-speed computing networks to analyze

large volumes of data and to communicate rapidly with local and federal
health officials and other government agencies. The Internet provides the
means for a truly global early warning system of disease outbreaks to which
both government and nongovernment organizations can contribute. Disease
surveillance systems must be electronically seamless, with rapid transmittal
of data from clinical settings to local and state departments and CDC.
(Atlas 1999)

More recently, scientists and national security experts concerned about
emerging diseases and biological terrorism have begun advocating "syndromic
surveillance." The goal of syndromic surveillance is to monitor and detect
changes in the distribution of signs or symptoms of disease in a population
that, if they cluster in a recognizable pattern (or syndrome), might indicate
the early stages of an outbreak of disease. This is achieved through the automated collection and real-time analysis of a wide range of health-related
data from a variety of sources. For example, a sharp increase in reports of
fevers and respiratory distress, coupled with an upsurge in sales of over-
the-counter flu medications, might indicate the early stages of an outbreak
of anthrax (Buehler et al. 2003).

The primary novelty of syndromic surveillance lies in its relationship to
expert authority, and its dependence upon computer technology. Traditional
epidemiological surveillance tracks the incidence and prevalence of *disease*,
and thus relies on healthcare professionals to recognize, diagnose, and report
confirmed cases of disease. It also relies on individual clinicians or public
health officials to identify patterns and changes in the distribution of illness
across a population. In contrast, the goal of syndromic surveillance is to
identify potential outbreaks while they are still invisible to healthcare
professionals – ideally, before individual cases of disease have been diagnosed.
This is achieved by electronically collecting data on *pre-diagnostic* health
indicators from a variety of sources, aggregating it into a relational database,
and analyzing it using univariate and multivariate statistical detection algorithms to identify emerging syndromes. Expertise is thus located not in
individual clinicians or public health officials, but rather in electronic databases and surveillance networks.

Small-scale syndromic surveillance networks are already in various stages of
implementation. The Rapid Syndrome Validation Project (RSVP), developed
by the Sandia and Los Alamos National Laboratories in conjunction with the
New Mexico Department of Health, has been in operation in the University
of New Mexico hospital since November 2000. Physicians enter demographic
and symptom patient information onto a touch-screen interface. This
information is transmitted to a server running the RSVP software, which
identifies combinations of symptoms that might indicate one of six syndromes,
including influenza-like illness and adult respiratory distress syndrome. If such

a syndrome is identified, the physician is alerted and the information is forwarded to the State Department of Health (Zelicoff et al. 2001).

Although much of RSVP is automated, it still depends upon physicians to determine whether a patient might qualify for one of the six syndromes, and to actively enter his or her information into the system. Other projects, such as the Real-time Outbreak and Disease Surveillance (RODS) system, bypass physician agency altogether by analyzing data that is routinely collected for other purposes in hospital emergency departments (EDs) and healthcare product retail outlets. Upon arrival at a hospital ED, patients' chief complaint, age, gender, and zip code are recorded by registration clerks or triage nurses; this data is sent on to the RODS server, which determines whether the chief complaint falls into one of seven syndromic categories. A separate National Retail Data Monitor collects information on sales of over-the-counter (OTC) healthcare products from pharmacies and stores, which can then be analyzed in conjunction with the RODS data (Wagner et al. 2003).

Perhaps the most sophisticated example of syndromic surveillance is the series of Electronic Surveillance System for the Early Notification of Community-based Epidemics (ESSENCE) programs. Begun in 1999, the ESSENCE I program automatically collects health data from more than 300 military treatment facilities around the world, assigns symptom clusters to one of seven syndrome groups, and determines whether an outbreak is occurring. This program has since been transferred from military to civilian applications in the form of ESSENCE II, now under development by the Department of Defense and the Johns Hopkins University Applied Physics Laboratory, and funded by the Defense Advanced Research Projects Agency.

ESSENCE II is a prototype system that conducts syndromic surveillance in the Washington, DC metropolitan area, collecting, aggregating, and analyzing a range of clinical data and "non-traditional data sources." These include: school absentee records; patient visits to physicians, clinics, and hospital emergence departments; requests for laboratory tests and confirmed results; calls to 911, poison control centers, and nurse hotline services at healthcare organizations; sales of prescription and OTC medications; electronic claims records; emergency medical services; and reports from veterinarians. The entire process is automated, and analyzed data is made available to health and security authorities through Internet-based interfaces that allow users to display it in the form of graphs or spatial maps, using geographical information systems (GIS) software (Burkom et al. 2003).

Networks as Metaphor and Reality, Problem and Solution

The above examples are given to illustrate two points regarding the role of networks in contemporary understandings of infectious disease. The first is that *networks are* both *objective realities that influence the patterns of disease distribution* and *powerful metaphors for interpreting the causes and significance of those problems.*

On one hand, these examples invoke demonstrable changes in the world that were true in the 1990s and are still true now. During the past several decades, the world *has* become more interconnected: trade and transportation networks have proliferated, and passage through these networks has accelerated; media and surveillance networks have increased in number and sophistication; and all of these developments have produced what sociologist Anthony Giddens terms a compression of time and space (Giddens 1990). Moreover, multinational outbreaks of SARS, avian influenza, and tuberculosis demonstrate that, despite significant attempts to prevent international transmission, travel and transportation networks can still be extremely effective vectors of communicable disease. Local, national, and international health authorities are able to rapidly identify and track outbreaks, using resources such as the International Society for Infectious Diseases ProMedmail listserv, and the World Health Organization's Epidemic and Pandemic Alert and Response network. This increased surveillance has allowed rapid response that likely reduced morbidity and mortality in the recent outbreak of SARS in Southeast Asia and North America.

On the other hand, networks also have considerable metaphoric power when deployed in discussions of infectious disease. Recall Lederberg's example of a microbe that kills a child on a distant continent, then kills one in the United States and seeds a global pandemic in the space of three days; or Osterholm's contention that American borders were like a "submarine with screen doors." Both images convey the idea that movement across global networks is instantaneous and seamless, that time and space have become so compressed that major urban metropolises are effectively right next to one another. In this respect, the idea of a network *amplifies proximity and ease of transmission, while obscuring separation and extant obstacles to movement.* Similarly, Osterholm's examples of *Cyclospora*-tainted raspberries, and travelers carrying latent tuberculosis infections, illustrate a related point: the idea of a network *emphasizes the homogeneity and passivity of its constitutive elements, while obscuring stratification, agency, and context.*

There is of course some truth to each of these points – after all, networks' efficiency depends upon their ability to amplify proximity, reduce obstacles to transmission, and treat each of their constitutive elements as homogeneous and passive. Nevertheless, uncritically assuming that these conditions hold in all circumstances might impede a better understanding of the causes and consequences of disease transmission. For example, assuming that immigrants are passive vectors who transport disease across national borders, rather than active agents whose response to latent infections often depend upon the peculiar stresses of immigration and their socio-economic circumstances at their destination, may oversimplify the complex web of causation that leads to high rates of infectious disease among immigrant communities (King 2002). Emphasizing the role of networks might lead one to favor simple technological interventions in the network itself (such as the irradiation of food products at national borders), rather than social or public health interventions at the nodes that connect those networks (such as, for example, ensuring that Mexican agricultural workers do not work near open sewage outflow pipes). Finally, the ideal syndromic surveillance networks would erase human agency from the assessment and tracking of disease outbreaks, replacing contextual human judgment with threshold-driven computer algorithms.

The second main point that the above examples illustrate is that, in contemporary discussions of infectious disease, *networks are increasingly seen as solutions as well as problems*. Like Ballard's fictional community of Eden-Olympia, in which constant surveillance enhances security but conceals deeper problems, this double-edged understanding of the role of networks is fundamentally *utopian*.

First, utopias suggest a particular view of the contemporary social order. Karl Mannheim long ago argued that, while ideological discourse is directed toward the preservation or justification of an existing social order, utopianism's energies are directed toward social change – even if elements of the existing order are always conserved during this putative transformation (Mannheim 1936). The emerging diseases worldview exhibits a profound attempt to effect social change by presenting either a utopian alternative to, or dystopian critique of, the existing social order.[3]

Second, utopianism epitomizes the peculiar combination of novelty and tradition that is one of the hallmarks of modernity. It belongs to a long lineage of Western prophetic discourse that traces its roots back to the Hebrew prophets, who, faced with profound transformations in the moral order and social and economic fabric of their society, envisioned a reconstructed social order (Hertlzer 1965). Yet, at least since Francis Bacon's *New Atlantis* placed scientific inquiry and technological development at the center of his idealized society, it is also a form that has been closely associated with modern science. Indeed, the great Western dystopian visions of the twentieth century – including Yevgeny Zamyatin's *We*, Aldous Huxley's *Brave New World*, and George Orwell's *Nineteen Eighty-Four* – each placed technological developments in surveillance and biology at the center of their imagined future worlds. As I hope I have shown, the emerging diseases worldview also identifies surveillance and biotechnologies with social transformation.

Finally, utopias direct our attention to issues of *spatiality* in a very particular way. When Sir Thomas More coined the term "utopia," he left its etymology deliberately and famously vague: utopias simultaneously signify both an ideal vision of a perfect society located in the *eu-topos*, or "good-place"; and the impossibility of their material realization, which consigns them to the realm of the imaginary, *ou-topos*, or "no-place." They are at once the "no-place" of desire, a de-territorialized, flexible, and transportable *space*; and the specified spatial ordering of the "good-place," a physical *place* that can be realized through practical planning. Utopias and dystopias present a topological map of contemporary hopes and anxieties, simultaneously projecting the transformation of social relations and political institutions onto specific places and bodies, and using idealized visions of imaginary landscapes to shape modern society through the ordering of its spaces and spatializing practices. By envisioning the world in which they will function and upon which they will act, utopias are a crucial component of the construction of techno-scientific institutions and practices (Redfield 2000).

It is in this respect that the utopian vision found in the emerging diseases worldview differs from previous utopian visions of health. As I have suggested, one can see a transformation in the ways in which it configures space – particularly the spaces of global networks – and the waning importance of territoriality. To return to the ambiguity of the key term: utopia is both the "good-place" and the "no-place" of prophetic discourse. The emerging diseases worldview features a global "good-place" that is, increasingly, a radically transformed "no-place." Now the "no-place" signifies not only the spaces of potentiality, but also the de-territorializing impulses of global capital; now utopia is described not only in terms of the no-place of pure imagination, but also the no-place of imagined purity: the communication networks in which information is circulated in its purest form.

Like Ballard's fictional community Eden-Olympia, the emerging diseases campaign is a dual response to the increasing complexity of the global social terrain: on one hand, it is a recuperation of the imagined "good-place" of a legible and ordered colonial universe; on the other, it is the dream of a "no-place," in which surveillance networks ensure that neither crime nor illness would encroach upon the territory of the technological elite. In Ballard's novel, this utopian vision leads to calamity. Only time will tell how far the metaphor can be taken.

NOTES

1 After leaving his position in the Minnesota Department of Health, Osterholm founded ican, Inc., an Internet-based company that distributes information on infectious diseases to health professionals. He also chairs the Emerging Infections Committee of the Infectious Diseases Society of America and is a member of the National Academy of Sciences Institute of Medicine Forum on Emerging Infections. All quotations and references are taken from notes compiled while the author attended his public lecture (Osterholm 1999a).

2 Osterholm had elaborated on the danger of the "globalization of the food supply" in a 1997 editorial (Osterholm 1997). See also Osterholm (1999b, 2000).

3 Although there are significant differences between the two, utopian optimism and dystopian skepticism share important family resemblances in content and form and are, as Booker (1994, p. 15) argues, "very much part of the same project." Chris Ferns (1999) contrasts the two forms, arguing that utopias stress the disparity between the real present and a utopian future, while dystopias represent periodic inversions of traditional utopias and satires of contemporary society.

13

People, Animals, and Biosecurity in and through Cities

Steve Hinchliffe and Nick Bingham

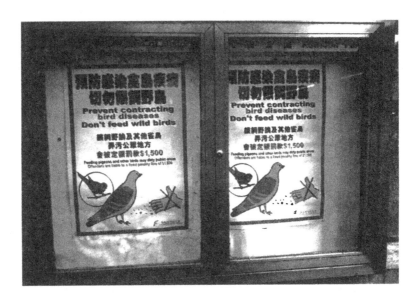

Introduction

As many chapters in this volume have demonstrated, SARS gave stark relief to the connections between urban public health and other places and others' lives (not just human lives). In this chapter, we add to this geography and ecology of disease by noting that cities are not just places where viruses eventually end up and cause havoc. They are not simply dense collections of people that are vulnerable through global networks that connect them to the "pre-modern" agricultural practices of "elsewhere," where people and animals mix tissues and excretions – for two reasons. First, cities are also very much a-modern. Many cities and many parts of cities around the world are no better than their rural hinterlands in terms of services (Davis 2006), and all are full of animals. Second, world cities are rarely, if ever, simply victims of global shifts. They are of course important sites of intensive orderings, where matters as diverse as landscapes and viral forms are organized and distributed. Many chapters in this book rightly point to the uneven quality of life in cities and to the vulnerabilities that are distributed across and within world cities. Thus the interconnections between world cities can produce a particular patterning of viral lives. But we also need to remember that cities are not simply networked; they also network. They are not globalized, but they form focal points where globalization is done.

This combination of the a-modern, living city and the networking effects of cities means that they are places where issues of biosecurity are starting to be realized and played out. Loosely speaking, biosecurity refers to a set of procedures and infrastructures that seek to control and police the movements of living matters. As a topic of concern, it has mainly surfaced in rural locations, partly as a result of the understanding that rural livestock production is the so-called front line in the generation and distribution of zoonotic diseases (Braun 2007). While this is undoubtedly the case, we will argue that biosecurity is also an issue for urban areas, which are rife with living things (humans and animals). Cities, as living places (Hinchliffe and Whatmore 2006) are made up of dense networks of living relations and are therefore as important to the making and breaking of biosecurity as any rural location. Indeed, it almost goes without saying in this book that the dense networks and the concentrations of human inhabitants in close proximity make for high-risk disease ecologies. But it should also be added that cities are, and always have been, full of other animals too. Their role in biosecurity practices needs more attention.

Our main site is Cairo, a city that has long been seen as a colonial site that is both networked and which networks (Mitchell 2002). Our case is the arrival of highly pathogenic avian influenza in winter 2005–6. More broadly, we look at the attempts to control and eradicate avian influenza within Egypt through biosecurity measures. Such measures are channeled through and within Cairo to peri-urban, rural, wild, and domestic settings in which people and birds interact. Our focus on the city does two things. First, we note how Cairo acts as a site for a gathering together of orderings. It is a place of networking that makes and repairs links to other world cities, international governments, international organizations, disease control centers, surveillance operations and so on. Second, we argue that rather than biosecurity being a case of a militarized state imposing orders upon a populace, our urban focus allows us to trace the rough textures of disease "control" networks. Our argument is that cities mark places where the never-finished products of state and society are actually being made and re-made, where expertise is being redistributed through an attempted elimination of certain city–nature formations (Hinchliffe 1999). We conclude by arguing that biosecure states emerge in practices, are always incomplete, and are far from secure.

We start the chapter with a brief introduction to the term "biosecurity." Following this, we outline the avian influenza disease group and then provide an account of Egyptian disease control practices. The chapter ends with a discussion of the fraught relation between networks and control.

Biosecurities

Biosecurity involves lots of things and practices. In terms of its things, a brief review of the uses of the term suggests at least three elements. First, there are the attempts to manage the movement of agricultural pests and diseases, with the aim of protecting *national agricultural productivity*. Second, there are the attempts to reduce the effects of invasive species on so-called indigenous flora and fauna, or the protection of *national natures*. Third, there are the dangers of purposeful and inadvertent spreading of biological agents into the human population. This protection of *human populations* focuses on laboratories that handle potentially hazardous organisms, possible uses of pathogens in bioweapons and bioterrorism, and the possible crossings of animal-borne diseases into the human species (zoonotic diseases).

Biosecurity also involves different forms of security practices. Collier and Lakoff (2006), in part following Foucault (1973, 1977), identify three political logics of security. The first of these, *nation-state security*, has its roots in the establishment of states in seventeenth-century Europe, and involves the will to secure territorial sovereignty. It is premised on a bipolar world of friend and enemy, its spatialization into territorial units, and a militarization of various borders. The latter can be external or internal (the enemy within), with the result that policing borders becomes a matter of foreign and domestic policy. Second, there is the logic of *population security*. With its origins in the social welfare reforms of the late nineteenth century, population security involves attempts to improve overall and individual levels of and access to health and welfare by organizing the purchase of health and social securities. The collectivization of health and social safety nets through public and private insurance and through the organization of health and social infrastructures are the main recognizable instances of population security. Finally, for Collier and Lakoff, there is *vital systems security*. This is a mid-twentieth-century response to the development of extreme emergencies, including most notably the possibility of nuclear attack or other incalculable, and thereby uninsurable, events that lie outside the technologies of formal risk assessments (earthquakes, hurricanes). The logic here is preparedness and emergency planning.

Putting these biosecurities together, we can start to map matters of concern with characteristic responses. And yet, as a reading of Table 13.1 will confirm, biosecurities are not easily separated into single forms or single logics. There are overlaps that require us to look more carefully at biosecurity operations.

Table 13.1   Bio-threats and characteristic responses

Target group/ matters of concern	Conventional bio-agencies	Technology/apparatus
Agricultural integrity and purity	International and national movements of livestock, livestock products and foods with potential to carry pathogens (viruses, prions, bacteria); migrating birds and insects	Border control and policing, surveillance, hygiene regulations, vaccinations; contiguous and mass extermination of animals; insurance of herds
Ecological integrity	Poorly embedded organisms ("non-natives")	Border control and policing, surveillance; extermination strategies
Human health and welfare	Zoonotic diseases, animals and people carrying pathogens that have the potential to produce pandemics; inadvertent and purposeful releases of biohazards	Border control, environmental monitoring, social security, education, detection, algorithms, isolation, surveillance, emergency planning

To elaborate, we can make four related points: First, in practice, a particular thing may not fall neatly into the categorizations outlined above. As we will develop later in the chapter, the current avian flu situation, for example, mixes aspects of the ecological integrity issue (the importation of exotic birds along with seasonal migrations), aspects of the agricultural disease issue (the spread into and within domestic poultry and other bird stocks), and aspects of the human health issues (the risk of infection to those humans living and working with poultry and the wider fears of the development of a human to human transmissible form of influenza from H5N1). Second, as Foucault reminds us (a point repeated in the recent collective work of Rabinow, Collier, and Lakoff) in practice, a form of security is always already multiple, in that it involves at least assemblages, apparatuses, and normativities that, while mostly hanging together, never completely coincide. Third, different logics or orderings do not exist in historic or geographical isolation, replacing one another completely from time to time or varying completely from place to place. Rather (and Foucault is again very clear about this), they are added to one another, sometimes arising in answer to the failing of previous orderings, but always interpenetrating to a greater or lesser extent. Finally, security is probably not best understood as a matter of responding to an already defined threat. Security (as Foucault once again demonstrated only too well) is about the public production of norms, their surveillance, regulation, and enaction (Foucault 1977). Thus, the three forms of collective security detailed earlier (state, population, and vital systems) are never simply a reaction to self-evident hazards, but always at least in part about the constitution of both a particular kind of body politic (self-contained, healthy, and alert, respectively) and a particular kind of bio-insecurity (fear of the outside, hypochondria, and terror of the inevitable, respectively).

What this situation suggests is that one form of security is unlikely to be either pure in form or dominant in terms of effect, and that analytically and politically it is worth exploring the complexities, inter-topological effects, and crossings that occur when biosecurities are put into practice. Some of this work, which would elucidate precise configurations of ways of life (bios), sickness (nosos), and the law (nomos) (Thacker 2005b), already exists, but (much) more remains to be done. Here we work with the multiple practices that make up avian influenzas in order to elaborate on the possibilities once we recognize the contingencies of more than one kind of actor and more than one enaction of disease.

Ordering Avian Influenzas

Avian influenza, or bird flu, is a common enough condition for wild and domestic birds. Indeed, the wide variety of subtypes of influenza virus (all 16 haemagluttinin and nine neuraminidase subtypes of influenza viruses are known to infect wild waterfowl; WHO 2006a) provides a large reservoir of viruses that "perpetually circulate" in bird populations (ibid.). In many cases such viral infections produce few clinical effects (ruffled feathers, reduced egg production in poultry, and little else). However, more pathogenic and lethal forms of avian flu exist that can spread rapidly and approach a lethality rate of close to 100 percent in birds. All are H5 or H7 subtypes with a distinctive set of amino acids in the cleavage site of haemagluttinin. Not all H5 or H7 subtypes are highly pathogenic but, according to the WHO, "H5 and H7 viruses of low pathogenicity can, after circulation for sometimes short periods in a poultry population, mutate into highly pathogenic viruses" (ibid., p. 1). How avian influenza viruses circulate and how they change is a topic of vital concern for bird health. But it is also of concern for many other species too, for subtypes of avian influenza can jump species.

Trans-species crossings of avian flu viruses to humans have been relatively uncommon and have to date and in the main produced only mild forms of human disease. The exception is the H5N1 strain, which had already crossed to humans in 1997 (in Hong Kong, where there were 18 cases) and whose crossings have gradually increased in frequency and distribution in recent years. While individual cases have been tragic and caused human suffering, outbreaks have remained limited in number. Notably, they have all occurred at the same time as H5N1 has been clinically present in nearby poultry flocks, and there have as yet been few, if any, clear cases of human-to-human transmission. All of this suggests that the current H5N1 virus is poorly adapted to its human host. For many, the more worrying danger is that H5N1 or another avian influenza virus will develop the capability to move quickly and effectively through human populations, as it undergoes reassortments (where avian and human viruses "exchange" genetic material during a co-infection of a host pig or human) or through gradual adaptive mutations. While the latter may be detectable through a pattern of relatively small clusters of disease incidence and limited human-to-human transmission, reassortment may give rise to a rapid onset of a pandemic strain whose spread along existing networks could well prove so fast that current detection systems based on syndromic surveillance, or even environmental monitoring followed by bioassay techniques, would be too slow to signal a warning.

The mutability and adaptability of viruses, along with the complexity, intensity, and density of animal–human and human–human interactions makes for a complex political and policy environment (Wilbert 2006), especially in large, densely populated cities. It is to this environment and to the interventions being made in the name of staving off the prospect of urban animal and human disease that this chapter now turns.

Cairo and Avian Flu – Making Cairo Urban

According to many official sources, avian flu is a disease carried by migrating wild fowl, passing to domestic bird life through physical contact, itself a result of poorly secured bird-keeping premises. Any danger of the disease spreading to people is also through direct physical contact, with poorly regulated poultry handling a cause for concern. Where wild and domestic birds exist in close and visceral proximity to pigs and people, the risk of highly infectious diseases crossing species barriers is considered to be at its highest. One WHO document expands as follows:

> Most human cases of H5N1 avian influenza have occurred in rural or periurban areas where many households keep small domestic poultry flocks. The H5N1 avian influenza virus is probably transmitted to humans through exposure during slaughter, defeathering, butchering and preparation of domestic poultry for cooking. (WHO 2006b, p. 2)

Following this simple infection story, an equally straightforward plan of action has emerged. Control is easiest, it is argued, in large commercial farms, "where birds are housed indoors, usually under strictly controlled sanitary conditions, in large numbers. Control is far more difficult under poultry production systems in which most birds are raised in small backyard flocks scattered throughout rural or periurban areas" (WHO 2006a, p. 2). The UN's Food and Agriculture Organisation (FAO) in New York – coordinating the global response closely with both the WHO in Geneva and Global Organisation for Animal Health (OIE) in Paris – followed suit, reversing its earlier policy of encouraging small-scale poultry farming (as a means to development, self-sufficiency, and small business promotion). Instead, it has turned to encouraging secure factory farms.

So as avian flu started to appear more frequently and be more widely distributed from 2003 onwards, a control network was being mobilized in Geneva, New York, Paris, and Hong Kong. The network was informed by and in some senses solidified the main narrative/etiology. So, with the prospect of the H5N1 virus reaching Egypt becoming ever more likely, the government in Cairo took up the disease narrative and started to enact a program of disease control. In the autumn of 2005, the government announced a series of measures: hunting of wild ducks and quail was banned; imports of poultry from infected countries were prohibited; there was to be increased border monitoring; and migratory flocks were to be subject to virological surveillance.

Despite these measures, Cairo's place within a network of abundant international flows generated a sense of foreboding. In a communication made in mid-October 2005 by the WHO's Regional Office for the Eastern Mediterranean, itself located in Cairo, it was noted that "migratory bird flyways pass through the EMR [Eastern Mediterranean Region] on their way between Asia, Europe, and Africa" and "daily dynamic interaction with other countries in the world (expatriate workers, trade, religious visitors, and tourism) could easily result in the introduction of influenza into the Region" (EMRO-WHO 2005, p. 1). The same report made it very plain that states needed to behave as model citizens in order to maintain public (global) health. "What is expected from countries," identifying highly pathogenic avian influenza is "rapidly and appropriately destroy[ing] all infected or exposed birds with proper destruction or carcasses," "functional and efficient influenza surveillance hand in hand with focussed and timely public health measures," "reasonable stockpiles of Tamiflu," "production of influenza vaccines," and "an efficient communication system" (ibid., pp. 2–3).

Having convened a "Supreme National Committee to Combat Bird Flu," with representatives from the ministries of defense, agriculture, and health as well as the WHO, officials were at pains to assure a doubtful and distrusting Egyptian public that all possible safety measures had been taken and that there would be open and transparent reporting of any avian influenza cases. Whether or not this was the case (and with a prestigious African

Nations Football tournament taking place in Egypt immediately beforehand, there were doubts as to the actual timing of events and reportage), the official statement that H5N1 had reached Egypt came in mid-February 2006.

Despite indications that the initial outbreaks had occurred at least in part on factory farms, public officials began stressing the safety of such "highly controlled environments" and suggested that the vast majority of reported cases were occurring in flocks of home raised birds. After banning poultry movements, the main policy response was to announce a cull of all backyard and rooftop poultry, and the banning of live bird markets (where 80 percent of the country's poultry was sold). Echoing the joint WHO/FAO/OIE line, and specifically the words of a senior FAO official who had declared that "The fight against bird flu must be waged in the backyard of the world's poor" (quoted in Grain 2006a, p. 3), the Prime Minister, Ahmed Nazif, announced the ban with the following words: "The world is moving towards big farms because they can be controlled under veterinarian supervision [...] the time has come to get rid the idea of the breeding [of] chickens on the roofs of houses" (quoted in Grain 2006b, p. 1).

This replacement of rooftop and backyard agriculture with industrial poultry production represented a hugely significant intervention into Cairo's urban ecology and the political ecology of Egypt more generally. Urban subsistence production in Egypt generally, and small-scale animal husbandry in the capital in particular, had taken on a new importance over the previous two decades. The reasons for this growth relate in part to shifts in rural land tenure and resultant increases in rural landless laborers, increasing rural urban migrations, and an increase in numbers of urban poor, many of whom were used to keeping livestock. In addition to this growing urban population, reductions in food subsidies from the 1970s onwards, increases in food imports, and the privatization and deregulation of strategic food supplies (see, for example, Mitchell 2002), combined to drive food prices up, and made home poultry production especially attractive. One fairly conservative estimate put the proportion of Cairo households that kept animals at 16 percent, rising to well over 25 percent once the informal settlements and the former villages were included (Gertel and Samir 2000). The keeping of birds – particularly chickens and ducks – was a way of life for people (especially women) in the low-income, densely populated parts of the city, a cheap way of adding expensive animal protein to the family diet (95 percent of this farming was for home consumption). Meanwhile, the home-produced meat was often perceived as being cleaner than bought-in meat, and livestock acted as an economic buffer of sorts in times of increased hardship (ibid.). This living city (Hinchliffe and Whatmore 2006) was not one that matched the ideal city envisioned by modernizers and planners. Indeed, the announcement of the rooftop cull dovetailed with other interventions in city life, and the ongoing rebranding of Cairo as a modern, world city (Mitchell 2002).

Modernity and Biosecurity in Practice

The cull was led by teams of officials from the ministries of health, agriculture, and environment, and enforced by the security forces. Despite this, and despite the issuing of fines for keeping birds and the encouragement to report neighbors who didn't comply with the plan of action, the cull was far from clean or smooth. Some householders hid their birds and refused to let apparently healthy birds join the cull. Compensation levels were unattractive, so sub-clinical birds were rushed to markets in order to realize their best monetary value. When the disease struck, sub-clinical birds were killed by farmers in order to "rescue them" (as people called it) from the disease (Slackman 2006). These dead but infective birds then circulated through markets and into food chains. As chickens were given up to the cull, many households kept their ducks, as these seemed to stay healthy (ducks are good at shielding the virus). The secretion of live household birds to keep them safe and the dumping of diseased birds in canals and waterways by both individuals and the authorities may have risked greater spread of disease. In spring, avian influenza had claimed its first human victim in Egypt (one of six deaths out of 14 infected). There had not been anywhere near enough vaccine or Tamiflu available, and stocks were urgently having to be imported at great expense.

The collapse in home-produced poultry and the fall in demand for Egyptian poultry more generally (35 percent of poultry farms reportedly closed down and one third or 1 million farm workers were laid off), resulted in a 40 percent price hike for fish and non-bird meat (Leila 2006a). Attempts by the government to then import chickens led to street demonstrations, as workers in the poultry industry protested the effect this would have on their businesses.

These practical difficulties in managing the disease in terms of urban food provision, public health, employment, and economies were exacerbated outside the city. Poor information, non-compliance, and a lack of personnel made the cull completely unenforceable in practice in the 20 of Egypt's 26 governorates where bird flu had been detected. As a result, the authorities in Cairo had to declare that backyard flocks could be kept as long as they were healthy and caged.

In early summer, a report by a parliamentary committee asked to assess the government's handling of the situation was highly critical of the ways in which the outbreak had been handled (Leila 2006b). Criticism focused on a number of areas, including a lack of consultation at the planning stage with civil society groups, poor public information, the rash announcement of the cull, which had led to a spreading of disease after infected birds were left on streets and on the banks of rivers, the absence of measures to protect the livelihoods of dealers with infected birds, unhygienic transport of culled bird carcasses to often unsuitable burial sites, and a confused avian vaccination policy (exacerbated by the fact that after expensive supplies of vaccine had eventually arrived from China, its use only served to spread the virus) (Leila 2006b).

Despite these failings, the mass killing of birds had seemingly reduced the problem. New infections had declined by early summer and to all intents and purposes the country was thought to be free from the disease by mid-2006. According to the vice-head of the Poultry Union, success was not due to the preventive measures taken by the government and was simply explained by the extermination of an estimated 34 million birds in the cull. In a few weeks, "Egypt lost 75% of its egg-laying flocks and 50% of all fowl. Since there is almost no poultry in the country, infection rates of bird flu are decreasing" (quoted in Leila 2006b, p. 1).

The decimation and subsequent rebuilding of poultry stocks was far from being evenly distributed. The latter was most evident when the Cairo Poultry Company increased its capital, paid out dividends, and announced plans to build a new 100 million Egyptian dollar slaughterhouse in Noubaria. The new facility would increase the company's output by 350 percent, from the present level of 80,000 chickens slaughtered per day to 280,000, and the company hoped that it would supply 10 percent of the country's poultry consumption (Rasromani 2006).

At this point, it might be argued that even though the method and practice was undoubtedly messy, the results were predictable. Looking beyond the local practices, it might be argued that big capital and government had held sway. Certainly, industrially integrated farming in Egypt seemed to be doing better than household farms. However, it may be that such an outcome is neither inevitable nor incontestable. As the next subsection details, there are other narratives that undermine this sense of an onward march of a modern, technological state.

Overlaps, Interferences, and Netwars

The particular doing of biosecurity in Egypt following the detection of highly pathogenic bird flu, with its military-style cull of bird stocks, would, at first blush, suggest a nation-state security response to a known threat. The attempt was to cleanse the country of the enemy virus and in so doing enact a modernist, urban, and industrial-agricultural landscape. The associated removal of urban and peri-urban livelihoods, and wholesale changes to the political ecologies of livestock, certainly suggest the imposition of martial law and a concomitant curtailing of civil liberties. However, to tell the story in this way would be to overemphasize the "orderly" nature of the process. Securing also involved many other practices, in a variety of locations and with a variety of effects. The result is that to talk of a single logic, or even to talk of a dominant power, is rather premature. It is for this reason that we prefer to speak of biosecuring rather than securitization or even biosecurity. We can make two points here. First, biosecuring involved practices of surveillance and self-regulation that were not simply about territory and securing boundaries, but also about the policing of populations (chickens and people) and the extensions of some liberties (e.g., trade and large corporations) over others (animals, smallholders). Second, as this suggests, securing took place in many locations, involving many different things and objects, many of which were related to other programs of action and other logics (Hinchliffe 2007). Among these were changes to hunting practices, border controls, surveillance and testing, trade restrictions, public information campaigns, vaccination policies, mass culling, market manipulation, corporate restructuring, food imports, reports, parliamentary reviews, and so on. This was hardly the pure and simple establishment of a (sovereign) state of biosecurity, a predetermined and coordinated national response to a known threat. This was the usually trial and error and often desperate attempt to enact different, partially connected, avian influenzas and the associated reshaping of worlds that stretched into, pervaded through, and reached out of Cairo as the central but widely distributed player in a rapidly unfolding drama.

A question to ask at this point is the following: How do these various practices, places, and things interact with one another? What are, to use other terms, the interferences (Mol 2002; Law 2004) or ecologies of action (Hinchliffe et al. 2007)? We can trace four kinds of interference here.

First, places, practices, and things can interfere in ways that support and reinforce each other through operational and ideological cross-fertilizations and cross-subsidies. In the case of Cairo, for example, it would be foolish to ignore how neatly the WHO and the FAO's proclamations on the wild and unregulated causes and consequences of avian influenza chimed with the Egyptian government's longstanding and ongoing attempts to "clean up" Cairo in order to present it as a shining beacon of Africa modern(ist) (for much more detail on this battle, see Mitchell 2002). Cairo's backyard and rooftop flocks became something of a "target of opportunity" (Weber 2005). Likewise, in the name of securing the health of the national body politic, the apparatuses of international agribusiness and Northern biosecurity diktats have meshed to produce a landscape of opportunity. Once the cull policy had been settled, the government had to ease import restrictions on frozen meat and other protein products to make up for domestic shortfalls (especially in the lead up to and during Ramadan, when food consumption increases). The restrictions had previously been part of a plan to reduce the national debt crisis and to encourage more domestic production (Mitchell 2002). In another move that benefited large multinational corporations, commercial

Egyptian farms were restocked with chicks from the US and Europe and, as we have noted, there was now massive commercial potential for an expansion of factory farming in the country.

On the other hand (and second), it is also not difficult to identify how the same events involved activities that might be clear contradictions of one another. It is unclear, for example, how the shift from small producers to commercial factories ultimately aids national sovereignty and biosecurity in Egypt or elsewhere. For what it produces in the name of eradication and purity is at once a whole set of food insecurities (the country is no longer self-sufficient) and quite possibly – as various commentators ranging from academics (Davis 2005) through NGOs (BirdLife International 2006; Grain 2006a,b) to medics (*Lancet* 2006) have suggested – the very conditions of animal density and bio-simplicity that can nourish viral multiplication.

Although perhaps the easiest to point to, and most familiar in terms of conventional social science accounts, reinforcement and contradiction are by no means the only kind of interference that can emerge between different modes of biosecuring. Third, a disease such as bird flu is constituted of other ecologies of action, including confusion (for example, in the relationship between the vaccination and culling programs), concession (for example, when the government were forced to rein back the extent of the cull in rural areas, leaving public information and surveillance in the ascendancy in those parts of the country), adaptation (for example, when the government had to manipulate the market to provide cheap poultry in the run-up to Ramadan), and accommodation (for example, when the complete failure of the Chinese-sourced vaccine became apparent and restocking became a priority).

Finally, we want to note how securing the bio can take the form of a paradox. In Eugene Thacker's work in this area, for example, he notes how a certain, becoming-dominant version of biosurveillance can be characterized as what the US defense industry refers to as "netwars." That is to say, they involve "networks fighting networks, in which one type of network is positioned against another, and the opposing topologies made to confront each other's respective strengths, robustness, and flexibilities" (Thacker 2005a, p. 8). Increasingly, diseases (as well as terrorist organizations) are conceived of as having a network topology, as attempts to produce a distributed mode of existence, one that is self-organizing, mutable, and in process. Such forms of organization are highly resistant to top-down, centralized forms of control and, thereby, networks require networks to fight them. The paradigmatic case has become the relative success of the WHO's efforts to combat SARS (see other chapters in this volume) – involving a "hybrid of computers, communications, hospitals, health advisories, and … medical countermeasures such as quarantine and travel restriction" (ibid., p. 12). Yet as Thacker goes on to suggest, the topological realization of netwars is possibly not radical enough – for in the current design of biosurveillance and disease surveillance networks (DSNs), there remains a logic of control and instrumentalism, one that underestimates the non-human and thereby fails to adjust to the indeterminate characteristics of networks. The challenge, as he says, of establishing sovereignty within a network becomes a necessary paradox, where the need for control is also the need for an absence of control (ibid., p. 13). It may just be that the dynamism and looseness of a disease network, its adaptabilities and accommodations (from the conformations of amino acid cleavages to the hiding of animals) is what gives it strength. This would explain why purifying schemes and conventional surveillance tend to fail. And would suggest that the martial metaphor of a war on disease is not quite right. In terms of taking this forward, a guide might be to ask, with this paradox of control in mind, just as Donna Haraway has done in the past with the immunological body (Haraway 1991) and Annemarie Mol has done more recently with the logic of care (Mol 2008) – whether we might find in these practices any hints that there are other ways of collectively living with disease than imagining that we are perpetually in conflict with it, ways that recognize rather than repress the fragile stabilities involved.

Conclusions

In concluding this discussion of avian flu and its various networks, we will make three points. First, cities are themselves in process and are not simply networked by diseases – they also network and in so doing are dynamic and are being made. The same can be said for nation-states. Neither the urban nor the state are explanations for disease or for its control, they are rather the fragile outcomes of a host of activities and materialities. Cities, states, and diseases are being made in a variety of places, through many different kinds of practices, and with all manner of different things. In the case of bird flu in Cairo and Egypt, the management of disease cannot be described as a nation-state imposing its power or will on society – nor, for that matter, would we suggest that there was a well-formed resistance on the part of society. Rather, city, state, disease, and society are in process in this story – their boundaries and the distinctions between them are not pre-set. To be sure, this does not make our account apolitical – indeed, it is the assertion of new forms of practice and new ecologies of action that may redistribute expertise and knowledge in Egypt (from household food production to large commercial holdings). The analysis here suggests only that this process is not preordained or following some pre-established social order. Rather, the process is dynamic, always heterogeneous, and open to political contestation. Moreover, while we have focused on the practices rather than the ideas of biosecurity in this chapter, our point is not so much that things don't necessarily work out as they were planned (although that is of course part of it), or even that there are, or need to be, local enactments of more global methods. Rather, it is to argue that in the making of a biosecure state there is always an issue of heterogeneity – which we take to indicate that there is always more at stake than that which is to be included in the making of a social order. From the rooftop poultry keepers to the mutable viral forms, there is more to the performance of state than the idea of a modern city form.

Second, and relatedly, rather than inadvertently promoting the programs of the already powerful by suggesting that their schemes are both singular and likely to bear fruit, we would suggest that any attempt at biosecurity is already multiple, made up of a number of modes of ordering (Law 1994). Thus we have talked of modes of securing. We are trying to emphasize a number of things with this term:

- There is likely to be more than one mode of securing in operation in any situation.
- Modes will relate to one another in ways that can be mutually supportive, destructive, indifferent, in conflict, coexist, reduce each other's effectiveness, and so on.
- Each mode is practiced and thereby marks an imperfect attempt at security. Therefore, rather than call them modes of security, they are securings. The resulting state of security will always be, more or less, provisional and subject to change.
- These modes are heterogeneous and distributed over a wide array of actors and things, and don't have a thinking human subject at their center. They are not therefore equivalent to rationalities.
- The potent mixings and interplays within and between people, places, animals, forms, chemicals, embargos, cells, and so on are more than likely to be generative, to produce new conformations.

Our final point is that given this heterogeneity and incompleteness, biosecurity may be as much about surrendering control as it is about jurisdiction over the bios. While it is clearly contentious to argue against efforts to eliminate disease when people's lives and livelihoods are at stake, there is nevertheless a strong sense that when emergency gives way there are reasons to generate broader debates as to the proficiency of current stories, practices, and methods in terms of their ability to address networking diseases.

ACKNOWLEDGMENTS

The authors are indebted to lots of other people and their works, most notably John Law, Annemarie Mol, and others who have inspired us to think again about the multiple and about disease.

Part V

Networked Disease:
Theoretical Approaches

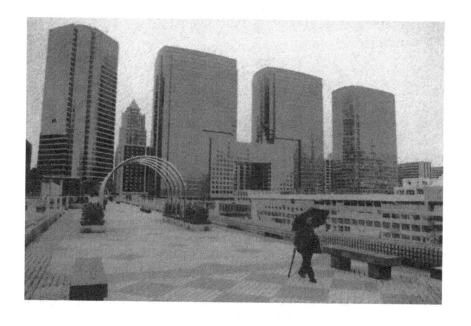

Introduction

S. Harris Ali and Roger Keil

The readings in the previous parts of this volume have raised a myriad of issues involved in the relationship between infectious disease and cities. The contributions in this part take on the task of situating many of these issues into a conceptual framework. An overarching emphasis of these contributions is to conceptualize infectious disease as a phenomenon arising from the convergence of various social and material processes that are linked together in rather nuanced, complicated, and unanticipated ways – ways that are unique to the contemporary era. As such, it is argued that to gain some understanding of an outbreak phenomenon in terms of these processual developments, what is needed are newer conceptual tools and theoretical orientations that are more in line with the circumstances and conditions of our contemporary existence. In this light, several prominent themes may be identified in the theoretical writings of this part.

First, all chapters in this part implicitly acknowledge the role of *dialectic processes* in the dynamics of disease spread and response. Three such processes may be discerned in the readings: the dialectic between the urban and the global, that between nature and society (or the material and the cultural), and the rural–urban dialectic. Second, all contributions stress that a central focus for the understanding of the contemporary infectious disease phenomenon should be the study of *interconnectivities* between people, viruses, and technologies, and how these interconnections are influenced by cultural, economic and political forces. Third, in a related manner, the theoretical works of this part emphasize how these interconnections may be understood in terms of *networked connections,* and in particular, the *flows* that connect up the nodes that constitute a network – whether these are: cities in a network of global cities, hotels and hospitals within the hospitality and health networks of a particular global city, wet markets in a vast food distribution network, computers in a global digital information network, jets in the global air transportation network, or even commodities in a network of commodity chains within a system of global capitalism.

In "SARS as an Emergent Complex: Toward a Networked Approach to Urban Infectious Disease", S. Harris Ali considers how urban–global inter-actions of various sorts can come together to produce unexpected and dis-proportionate effects, such as an urban disease outbreak. Drawing upon recent work dealing with networks, flows, and complexity, Ali develops a "networked disease" perspective that captures the uniquely emergent, con-tingent, and dynamic nature of a disease outbreak as conjointly a social and material phenomenon. He then explores the implications of the networked disease perspective for: (i) understanding the largely successful efforts in con-taining SARS in terms of the accelerated flow of digital, epidemiological, and clinical information in comparison to the relatively slower flow of the virus itself; and (ii) bringing to light new forms of inequality, particularly networked inequality related to unequal access to public health and infor-mational resources in an increasingly networked world.

Bruce Braun further investigates the ramifications of SARS as an emer-gent phenomenon by focusing in on the ontological implications that arise. In "Thinking the City through SARS: Bodies, Topologies, Politics," Braun is interested in looking at the ways in which SARS, as a shared event, prob-lematized our commonsense and taken-for-granted understandings of our bodies, cities, and politics. For Braun, our ontological understandings of the city as a setting in which nature is separated from the human or social were shattered with SARS, as our understandings of lived city life now had to explicitly grapple with an infectious disease that had its origin in a wild animal reservoir (i.e., the civet cat in rural China). This raised awareness of "nature" has vividly brought to the fore the fact that our bodies are porous to the external environment in ways we did not fully appreciate, or at least took for granted, prior to the outbreaks. SARS also raised our awareness of the porousness of cities themselves. That is, under the present conditions of globalization, cities can no longer be viewed as bounded, contained, and sealed containers. Rather, the presence of the SARS Coronavirus (SARS-CoV) brought to the forefront the idea that a city is now porous to all dif-ferent types of flows, including viruses and people. Furthermore, with SARS it was also realized that all of these flows may have their own respective temporal–spatial "rhythms" – for example, the lifecycle of a virus (or the incubation period of a particular virus) or the travel patterns of human beings. Thus, ontologically speaking, it must now be recognized that cities (particularly global cities) are unbounded and polyrhythmic. Lastly, Braun discusses some of the political implications of this new ontology triggered by the changing connectivities of people with other bodies (humans, animals, machines, or large collective bodies such as the state), especially in relation to issues of individual sovereignty and freedom.

Interestingly, the flows and networks implicated in the transmission of the SARS are not limited only to viruses and humans, but as alluded to by Braun, they also involve animals and food, and these also cross the scale of nations and bodies just as microbes and people do. This theme is taken up explicitly in the chapter by Paul Jackson, "Fleshy Traffic, Feverish Borders: Blood, Birds, and Civet Cats in Cities Brimming with Intimate Commodities." Jackson investigates the flows of connection that tie the civet cats of rural China to the lives of those in global cities. As part of these investigations, Jackson considers the more general question of how the commodification of animals for consumption is connected to viral spread – as, for example, not just in the case of the civet cat and SARS, but poultry and avian influenza. For Jackson, understanding these types of relationships requires a consideration of broader issues, such as how food production and consumption are constituted by flows of capital and culture, or the question of how rural food production is related to urban market consumption. In considering how these various flows are interrelated and how they interact, Jackson notes that the southern part of China's Guangdong province is one of the world's leading areas in the manufacture and export of commodities, and if food is one such commodity, then the wet markets of this region represent a significant point of convergence for the intermingling of various flows, thus facilitating inter-species transfer of the virus. At the same time, however, what is often overlooked is that these sites also serve as points of convergence for economy and biology. The global economy and economies of cities must in the final instance rely on resources and food from the rural areas, but this is often not realized. As Jackson notes, resources and food appear in the form of commodities, and a commodity, as Marx notes, is an expression of a social relationship that is disguised or masked in the form of an object (thus those engaged in process of exchange are not aware of the social relationship or connection between themselves as producers; they only see a relationship as an exchange of things – that is, a relationship devoid of the social – the relationship between humans becomes reduced to the relationship between things). The key point is that the commodity only has meaning in a relational context; it must, as Jackson notes, work in a space of flows and a web of interconnections, but what is often forgotten is that viruses navigate these interconnections on the backs of commodities. Thus, capitalism and disease spread are intimately intertwined, and the networks of capitalism and the networks of disease spread are coincident.

It is clear that when flows converge together to produce a disease outbreak, there is much social and political disorder. As such, much of the political action that ensues is understandably directed toward the restoration of order. The common approach to restoring order, or at least to stop the spreading of disorder, is to break the flow of the virus through containment measures such as quarantine and isolation via the surveillance and monitoring of human movements – especially within and through cities – as well as through border closures and the inspection of bodies. These strategic actions, however, have significant political ramifications for governing powers. Philipp Sarasin explores these issues in "Vapors, Viruses, Resistance(s): The Trace of Infection in the Work of Michel Foucault." Sarasin notes that for Foucault the containment measures mentioned above represent opportunities for those in power to expand their control over people. This political control of the human body has evolved to take on different forms over time. Sarasin outlines how Foucault describes this evolution by noting first that, during the time of leprosy in the Middle Ages, lepers would be incarcerated in camps at the periphery of the city. This form of political control of the body was supplanted by a new form exercised during the time of the plague in the seventeenth century. This second form was based on the panopticon model of the internalization of self-control (i.e., discipline). Such a form of political control was in line with the political reality of the day; namely, the advent of liberalism. The political control of the body evolved still further and a third mode could be seen in the measures taken against smallpox contagion in the eighteenth century; namely, the "practice of inoculation" to protect the population through vaccination. With this approach, control measures emphasized security rather than discipline and, with this, an emphasis on statistics and probability distributions. The adoption of the statistical/inoculation practice similarly reflected the political ethos of the day; specifically, in the more fully developed liberal democracy of that time, the exercise of power emphasized the freedom of the individual – and it respected this freedom even for the price of a certain risk of infection in the population.

According to Sarasin, although often overlooked and neglected, what lies at the heart of Foucault's discussions of the political control of the body is the *metaphor of infection* – and this is of particular relevance in terms of understanding the political fallout from disease threats to the city. As alluded to earlier, Sarasin notes that both the infected and infection are taken to be synonyms of disorder. As reviewed above, one way to deal with a situation of disorder is to remove altogether those elements that are held to be responsible for this disorder – as was the case with the leprosy model. Such an approach makes a stark distinction between those who are infected, and therefore labeled as the *threat*, and those who are benign, and on this basis, seeks to completely eliminate the former. The smallpox model, on the other hand, accepts that a threat exists within their midst, but accepts this as a price to be paid for the freedom of all. Sarasin notes that current politics wavers between the leprosy model of complete control and discipline and the smallpox model of partial control and discipline, with an accepted public toleration of some risk. We may, however, be moving toward a convergence in the post-9/11 era, where threats and non-threats are seen in black-and-white terms within the context of the "war on terror" – reminiscent of the leprosy model – while at the same time retaining an overly determined security focus characteristic of the smallpox model. This has significant ide-ological implications in times of a disease outbreak in contemporary times – as seen, for example, by the racialization of SARS discussed by Keil and Ali, or in the onset of a health scare examined by Hooker (both in Part IV above).

14

SARS as an Emergent Complex: Toward a Networked Approach to Urban Infectious Disease

S. Harris Ali

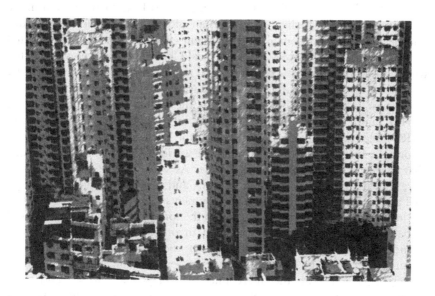

Introduction

According to the traditional model of infectious disease causation – namely, the classical epidemiological triad – a disease outbreak can only occur provided that there is an environment in which an external disease agent is able to come into contact with a susceptible host. The coincidence and interaction of factors related to the agent, the host, and the environment therefore implicitly implies that a disease outbreak is an *emergent* phenomenon. In this chapter I take as a starting point the notion of emergence to develop a Networked Disease approach that conceptualizes contemporary outbreaks and epidemics as socio-environmental phenomena uniquely defined by today's global networks and global flows. To develop this Networked Disease approach, I draw upon elements of complexity theory, Actor-Network Theory (ANT), the "network society" perspective and environmental sociology. What these perspectives hold in common is an emphasis on contingency, emergence, and dynamism. It is argued that because of recent social and environmental developments, such aspects can no longer be ignored in the analysis of modern urban disease outbreaks. Consider, for example, that compared to epidemics of the past, the SARS epidemic of 2003 was notably unique in certain respects. First, the unprecedented speed with which the disease spread highlighted the significant mobility and dynamism associated with contemporary disease outbreaks. Second, the manner in which the SARS Coronavirus (SARS-CoV) spread – through the global cities network – is also unique to our era (Ali and Keil 2006). Such a mode of transmission also highlights how urban–global interactions can produce unexpected, disproportionate, and emergent effects such as those implicated in the spread of the SARS-CoV from rural China to global cities across the world. And third, the nature of the social and political responses elicited by the disease at the urban and global levels were quite different in comparison to the past. This is seen, for example, by the World Health Organization's (WHO) unprecedented action of issuing travel advisories against certain SARS-affected global cities, as well as in the unprecedented degree of collaboration between scientists around the world to identify and genetically characterize a new virus in record time. As we shall see, these responses were in part due to new communications and information technologies, as well as recent social and political developments that define our era – that is, the influences of neoliberal ideology and the forces of economic and cultural globalization. In sum, it is argued that in order to capture the uniquely defined characteristics of the transmission and response to SARS, special attention needs to be focused upon emergent, contingent, and dynamic aspects associated with the interconnectivity of people, viruses, and technologies. The incorporation of these considerations into analysis will, in turn, require new methodological orientations and tools such as the Networked Disease approach that is to be developed here.

Emergence, Networks, and Complexity

As a possible solution to the realist versus social constructionist quandary, John Hannigan (2006, pp. 148–53) proposes that analysts of environmental phenomena adopt an emergence model of nature, society, and the environment in which the relationship between the social and material is viewed as both interactive (fluid) and material. This analytic orientation has the advantage of enabling us to capture some of the key defining elements of many of the environmental health phenomena we currently face. In several ways, this perspective is especially suitable to the analysis of emergence. First, this is because it focuses attention on the inherent ambiguous or uncertain qualities of emergent phenomena. This would include, for example, the identification of the unintended consequences of technological interventions into nature noted in Ulrich Beck's (1992) risk society thesis (especially, insidious risks such as those having chemical or nuclear origins). Second, an emergence model will draw attention to the emerging social structures that may form in response to environmental health threats. These may include, for example, new social movement organizations, epistemic communities of scientists, and community groups. Third, the emergence model has the advantage of enabling environmental health phenomena to be analyzed in terms of the flows that come together to give rise to the phenomena in the first place. An emergent flow approach is therefore consistent with the "disaster incubation" approach, which seeks to understand how social and biophysical processes converge in an unnoticed manner to produce a disaster (for the application of disaster incubation theory to the analysis of a waterborne disease outbreak, see for example, Ali 2004). In light of the above, the first task in the development of an emergence model is to identify those flows that converge together to give rise to the emergent outcome. Following from this is the task of understanding the actual dynamics and implications of the networks that emerge from the convergent flows. The first of these tasks is more basic and involves the identification and description of the relevant flows and may be addressed through application of actor-network theory. The analysis and characterization of the flows and emergent network is much more complicated and may best be approached through complexity theory. Let us briefly discuss each of these approaches in turn before turning to the illustrative case of SARS in a more detailed fashion.

As originally proposed by Bruno Latour (1987, 1988, 2005) and further developed by others (e.g., Callon 1986; Law 1987, 1999; Murdoch 1997a,b, 1998; Manning 2002), an actor-network is essentially an emergent and dynamic complex that forms when numerous social and material elements become linked together in particular ways. Indeed, from the ANT perspective the world is essentially comprised of diverse networks of association or linkages. Each type of network is comprised of various nodes (e.g., social institutions, technologies) that are connected to each other through flows of various types (e.g., money, information, people, devices, animals, etc.). The process of tracing how the linkages of an actor-network come about are central to the inquiries of ANT. By tracing how the SARS-CoV traveled across the world (i.e., tracing the network connections), and taking into account what particular actor-networks were drawn in by its presence at particular sites, we will be able to, at the very least, gain an accurate descriptive characterization of the SARS outbreak(s) – thus taking the first step toward analyzing this infectious disease as an emergent phenomenon. To a certain extent, this task is made easier in the specific case of a disease outbreak. This is because public health efforts to contain the outbreak are aimed at breaking the chain of transmission through quarantine and isolation. In turn, such an approach relies on the method of contact tracing where data concerning those who have had personal contact with an infected case are collected. Epidemiological data of this type can be used to trace the chain of transmission, thus enabling analysts to chart the spread of the disease through mapping processes. In terms of the conceptualization of an outbreak as an emergent phenomenon, such mapping of the disease represents only the most basic of descriptions. To move beyond this purely descriptive framing toward a more comprehensive account requires a more detailed investigation into the nature of emergent networks and flows – that is, an inquiry process that lies at the heart of complexity theory.

The objects of study for complexity theory are those systems that adapt and evolve as, they self-organize through time (Urry 2005). The question then is, how do you study and characterize such systems? Complexity theorists address this question by focusing on certain system characteristics or properties. First, the *dynamic* qualities of a system are studied because a system is first and foremost conceptualized as a configuration of constantly interacting parts. The dynamism of the system is generated on the basis of iterative feedback loops of various kinds (between the parts of the system) that will naturally result in a constant state of flux. Second, the emergent qualities of a system receive explicit attention as critical foci of research investigation. Complexity theorists assume that the characteristics of the system cannot be explained by reductionist approaches that consider only the properties of the system's constituent parts in isolation. In other words, a complex system has *emergent* properties. Consequently, a system is in a continual process of spontaneous emergence (Thompson 2004). Third, a complex system is said to exhibit the property of *non-linearity* because it is disproportionately sensitive to small changes in internal and external conditions – particularly with respect to the initial conditions. Consequently, a system will undergo various types of unpredictable changes, such as avalanche effects where an apparently stable system suddenly collapses (for example, a pyramid of sand that will unexpectedly topple when one more sand grain is added), or exhibiting patterns of spontaneous self-restoration and punctuated equilibria (Urry 2005). The classic example of a non-linear effect is the "butterfly effect," where the very small perturbations in air pressure caused by the flapping of a butterfly's wings on a calm day result in unanticipated changes in the initial conditions of a weather system. Such actions, it is argued, may set off a chain of events that amplifies effects on other parts of the weather system (again in unpredictable ways), thus ultimately precipitating an extreme weather event, such as a tornado. Complexity analysis therefore brings to the fore the necessity of studying different patterns of path-dependent development, where the current state of the system is based on past events.

Although originating from the efforts of physical scientists to study complex natural systems, recent efforts by social scientists have expanded the notion of "systems" to include both natural and social constituents, thus enabling them to adapt complexity theory to the analysis of socio-material phenomena. For example, John Urry (2004) uses complexity theory to analyze the "system of automobility," where the car and the driver together – the car–driver – are considered to be a node in a network of automobility that is constantly moving and changing. In this networked system of automobility, material (and environmental) features of the car are inextricably bound to the social and institutional support system that encourages and facilitates travel by automobile (including, for example, the fossil fuel economy, the highway infrastructure, and so on).

Law and Urry argue that the forces of economic and cultural globalization have produced a current social reality that has become increasingly complex, elusive, ephemeral, and unpredictable. As a result, the social realities of "globalization" have transformed, as they are now "less about territorial boundaries and state and more about connection and flow" (2004, p. 403). For example, the contemporary global networks of finance, tourism, information, military power, and terrorism have introduced uniquely defined instabilities that are fleeting, ephemeral, and geographically distributed in such ways that they are suddenly proximate. Such unstable outcomes may be thought in terms of the processes of disembedding and re-embedding that Giddens (1990, p. 21) contends is one of the defining aspects of contemporary globalization. According to this line of argument, social relations are "lifted out" of their local contexts and then restructured across indefinite spans of time and space. Instabilities are further reinforced through the rapid and diverse mobilities of peoples, objects, images, information, and wastes. The complex interdependencies between, and social consequences of, these diverse mobilities also highlight the importance of considering the emergent, dynamic, and non-linear properties of socio-material systems (Urry 2000). And it is for these reasons that Law and Urry (2004) make the case that complexity theory is better suited to meet the new and unique challenges involved in the study of contemporary social and environmental phenomena.

Tracing the Spread of SARS

The first case of what is now referred to as SARS was an individual from Foshan, Guangdong province, who had eaten a meal that consisted of a "wild cat" (i.e., the palm civet) in November 2002 (Zhong and Zeng 2005). A cluster of cases amongst family members and hospital workers exposed to this individual soon followed. Around the same period, workers and food handlers in the wet markets of Guangdong province were also stricken with this mysterious disease of unknown etiology (Guan and Sheng 2003). By December, SARS had appeared in two other cities of the province, and on January 21, 2003, an expert team of provincial and national health officials went to investigate these outbreaks (Knobler et al. 2004). The team recommended that a case reporting system be established to monitor the spread of the disease, but their report did not receive adequate attention from hospital officials in the province, as many were away due to the Chinese New Year celebrations. Furthermore, because much travel occurs during this festive season, the opportunities for the SARS-CoV to spread were greatly enhanced (Knobler et al. 2004). The community spread of the yet to be identified virus was also influenced by the new political economic realities of China – dimensions not usually considered in those analyses based on the classical epidemiological triad (see Ng, Chapter 4, and Baehr, Chapter 8).

Spiess (2004) notes that reform efforts to facilitate China's transition to the market economy resulted in the dramatic downsizing of the state sector. As a result, large numbers of displaced workers were forced into the embryonic private sector, where they no longer had the healthcare coverage they once had as state employees (private insurance schemes were yet to be deployed). Consequently, over 75 percent of the population did not have health insurance, and stories started to abound about long line-ups forming in front of hospitals that were demanding payments up front before they would treat SARS patients. Although the government responded by announcing a "medical aid fund for low-solvency patients and farmers" (Spiess 2004, p. 65), the medical treatment problem was compounded by the presence of a vast "floating population" of an estimated 80–150 million peasants who had previously drifted from the countryside to prosperous urban centers throughout China. Because these individuals lacked the legal residency status needed to stay in the city, they were denied education and medical care, while being forced to live in cramped urban ghettoes under the constant fear of arrest and deportation. After the true extent of the epidemic was revealed by government officials, this segment of the population understandably fled the city to return to their native rural towns, thus increasing the possibilities for pathogen spread into the country's vast hinterland. By late May 2003, the SARS virus had spread to 5,000 people spanning over 20 provinces in China (for accounts of the spread of SARS in China, see also Abraham 2004; Kleinman and Watson 2006). Globally speaking, the spread of the SARS-CoV began in February 2003, when an infected doctor from Guangdong province infected 11 guests at the Metropole Hotel in Hong Kong, whereupon the disease spread to other cities including Toronto, Singapore, Hong Kong itself, and Hanoi. By late March 2003, there were 1,320 confirmed cases, with 50 deaths throughout the world (Murray 2006, p. 20).

One of those infected by a traveler from the Metropole Hotel was the Hanoi-based WHO infectious disease expert Dr Carlo Urbani. Dr Urbani officially alerted the WHO about the threat of this highly infectious disease but, tragically, succumbed to the disease himself soon thereafter (Knobler et al. 2004). In response, on March 12, 2003, the World Health Organization (WHO) issued a worldwide alert on this new infectious disease that they named SARS. From this point on, public health officials in the various affected cities quickly began the labor-intensive tasks of contact tracing, surveillance, and organizing quarantine for those infected, while a global network of scientific researchers quickly immersed themselves in the tasks of determining a case-definition to assist the contact tracing and in identifying and characterizing the causative agent of the disease itself. At the same time, various local, regional, national, and global organizations were mobilized to respond to the disease threat itself, including, for example: local hospitals and public health agencies, ministries and departments of health, as well as emergency management departments at various levels, the World Health Organization's surveillance and infectious disease agencies, airports, hotels, and restaurants in the tourism sector, and schools.

SARS and the Global Health Response

During the earlier stages, information about the outbreaks was unofficially transmitted through e-mails, Internet chat rooms, local media outlets, and the electronic reporting systems of the Global Public Health Intelligence Network (GPHIN) and Pro-Med (Knobler 2004). On the basis of information obtained through these channels, on February 10, the WHO officially contacted the Chinese government to verify the information they were receiving through these other sources. Attempts at maintaining some level of secrecy about the extent of the outbreak were altogether abandoned by the Chinese government on February 11, 2003, when the Chinese Ministry of Health formally informed the WHO about the mysterious disease outbreaks in Guangdong province. The Chinese government was quickly criticized by the global public health community for not identifying the outbreak quickly enough, as well as for not communicating any available information through official channels (Heymann 2004).

By mid-March, the WHO-supported Global Outbreak Alert and Response Network (GOARN) established a virtual network of 11 leading infectious disease laboratories from across the world. These laboratories would communicate and share information through a secure website and daily teleconferences. In an unprecedented manner, temporarily putting aside competitive aspirations, the world's scientific might was united in its efforts to fight one disease (Stohr 2003). One month later, three laboratories within the WHO network had independently identified a novel coronavirus as the causative agent of SARS (Peiris and Guan 2005). And, as one medical international medical specialist notes, before the advent of the Internet, such a process would likely have taken months (Omi 2005).

The rapid identification of the SARS-CoV, its reservoir, and the subsequent delineation of its genetic code – all within a one-month period – was hailed by the WHO as the hallmark of global scientific collaboration and highlighted the importance of international informational networks, and especially the Internet, in global infectious disease response (Heymann et al. 2005). In the terminology of ANT, such platforms as GPHIN, GOARN, and Pro-Med, on which the informational networks were based, served as *obligatory points of passage*; that is, sites through which flows must pass through during their journey through the emergent actor-network. The funneling of information through these specific types of networks was obviously important for the nature of the SARS response at the public health and medical levels. For this reason, a premium was placed on relevant information of various sorts, including epidemiological, clinical, and laboratory data such as data gathered from the contact tracing carried out by local public health agencies and hospitals. Such data were compiled by the WHO from sources around the world, and in this regard, the WHO's Executive Director of Communicable Diseases noted that:

> I think that it would be fair to say that this is the first global outbreak where there was a 24 hour availability of information and information was continuously coming in through networks of doctors, of clinicians, of virologists, of epidemiologists. And that information provided the evidence on which day to day evaluation of recommendations could be made and changed. In other words, first off there was just a recommendation to be careful. Second there was a recommendation to screen passengers because SARS was spreading internationally. And when that didn't work there was a recommendation to avoid travel. And finally they worked. So this was evidence-based information available in real time to make the recommendations. (Interview, WHO official, Geneva, September 28, 2005)

SARS and Complexity

The global outbreak of SARS can be conceptualized as the emergent outcome involving the convergence of at least three specific types of flows: viruses, people, and information. It is in analyzing the movement and interactions of these flows that we may attain a clearer understanding of the dynamic, emergent, and non-linear properties of SARS as a networked system. As the brief review above reveals, there were specific networks associated with the spread and response to the SARS-CoV respectively.

In terms of the spread, mounting evidence indicates that the SARS-CoV originated in the palm civet cat reservoir (Guan et al. 2003). The crossover of the virus from this animal to humans most likely occurred in the "wet markets" and restaurants of Guangdong province, as supported by the fact that roughly one-third of the earliest cases of the disease were found to be in those who handled, slaughtered, sold and/or prepared the civet cat for consumption (Guangdong Province Center for Disease Control and Prevention, unpublished data, cited by Breiman et al. 2003). In terms of network theory, therefore, the wet market represents a nodal point where two types of flows – humans and animals – converged. Furthermore, it is worth noting that the wet market may be thought of as a liminal node that exists at the interface of rural and urban flows. Such liminal nodes are of significance to spread of new and emerging diseases, because they represent those points at which human beings first come into contact with previously untouched nature, including contact with new viral species living in animals and insects (Abraham 2004, p. 7). The potential for a particular nodal site to act as a "tipping point" in the spread of a disease may increase by social conditions and circumstances. For example, the socially informed hygienic practices associated with butchery in the live animal market may have resulted in pools of blood and remnants that served as ideal breeding grounds for viruses such as the SARS-CoV (Wang and Jolly 2004; Zheng et al. 2004). At the same time, changing cultural preferences in consumption may have also played a triggering role in the SARS outbreak. It has been noted that the growth of the affluent class in China has led to an increased demand for meat, thus leading to increased activities in wet markets (Bell et al. 2005; Omi 2005; see also Jackson, Chapter 17). What these changing social conditions illustrate are the important roles that contingency and path-dependency play in transforming a nodal point of a network in such a way as to increase the potential for disease spread. It is in reference to such an insight that the scientist who discovered the SARS-CoV as the causative agent of the SARS makes the following remarks:

> A disease outbreak such as SARS probably happened many times before, but what would have happened is that it would have affected a few people in a village; a couple of people would have died and it would have burned itself out then. But now, what's the situation? We now have these animals brought together in these big markets because there's a huge demand for exotic foods. So, it's not one type of animal, may be in a small village market. Now, we are having hundreds of them. The size of markets has increased; the interaction of the human population has increased. Okay, so the amplification in the markets is one factor. (Interview, Hong Kong, December 30, 2005)

The contingent yet path-dependent aspects of the SARS emergent complex are also apparent in the manner in which the viral and human flows traveled through the global cities network as well as within particular global cities themselves. Urry (2005) notes that today, one of the characteristic features of globalization involves the ephemeral nature of ever-changing social and material relations due to global fluids, as illustrated by, for example, world money, social movements, digitalized information, the anti-globalization movement, international terrorism, and smart mobs. According to Urry (2005, p. 246), although global fluids may travel along various predefined routes, they may also unexpectedly escape these pathways on occasion, thus leading to unanticipated effects and adding to the emergent, dynamic, and non-linear qualities of the phenomenon in question. This would be seen, for example, when a person who is unaware that he or she is infected inadvertently spreads the disease – as was the case with the travelers from the Metropole Hotel.

The unpredictable, dynamic, and non-linear nature of the spread of SARS was amplified in the case of this particular disease for several reasons. First, the accelerated speed of airline travel coupled with the two to ten day incubation period of the SARS-CoV meant that infected, yet unsuspecting and asymptomatic individuals, could elude screening measures (such as thermal scanning at airport entry points) and inadvertently spread the disease (Keil and Ali 2006). Second, SARS involved what is known as the "super-spreader" phenomenon, where an individual with enhanced infectivity will infect a much higher number of people than would normally be expected. This was seen for example, in the spread of SARS amongst the 11 guests of the Metropole Hotel from one infected "super-spreading" individual (CDC 2003a; Gostin et al. 2003). The presence of a super-spreading individual in a crowded airport, airplane, or the capillary system of a city will undoubtedly lead to multiple and unpredictable routes for a virus to travel. Third, as the SARS-CoV spread through the global cities network, the probability of transmission is much higher due to the higher population densities of major urban centers – as evidenced, for example, by the suspected environmental spread of SARS to over 200 people in the Amoy Gardens apartment complex in Hong Kong.

Finally, it should be noted that the dynamic and non-linear effects associated with the diffusion of the SARS-CoV are even further exacerbated by the role of chance circumstances, such as the particular living and familial arrangements of an infected individual. For example, although Toronto and Vancouver were affected nearly simultaneously in March 2003 by a SARS-infected traveler, by June, Toronto had more than 209 probable cases, while Vancouver had only four (Meyers et al. 2005). The difference has been attributed the chance circumstances related to the differing contact patterns and familial circumstances of the infected individuals. Specifically, the Toronto case involved an individual who was the matriarch of a large extended family, and who had contact with an extensive number of family members and friends, while the Vancouver case involved an individual who lived alone with his wife, thus limiting the opportunity for spread (Meyers et al. 2005).

SARS and the Network Society

Spaargaren et al. (2006) suggest that one important avenue of research that could be pursued in their proposed "sociology of flows" perspective would be a focus on the social relations and networks that give rise to, or accompany, environmental flows. In this context, the aim would be to identify and analyze the new networks, arrangements, and infrastructures that both constitute and govern different sorts of environmental flows. Such an analytical emphasis on emerging social structures is also found in Hannigan's (2006) emergence model of environment and society. Taking the cue from these perspectives, we can see that perhaps the most noteworthy aspects of the global response to SARS was the development of one such emerging social structure – namely, the emergence of an international network of scientists who shared epidemiological, clinical, and laboratory data in a concerted effort to contain the disease. As discussed above, the network of collaborators was extremely effective on several fronts: in identifying the causal agent of SARS; in developing a universal case definition for this disease; in the worldwide epidemiological tracking of the disease; and in genetically characterizing the disease – all in an unprecedented span of one month (Heymann et al. 2005). What can account for such success in the case of SARS? The answer lies in part in the nature of the networks implicated in the disease spread and response. To understand how this is so, I turn to Manuel Castell's (2000) work on the "network society."

Castells (2000) argues that globalization and information technologies have triggered a new type of institutional configuration or constellation that has resulted in a new kind of time–space organization of social practices. Such organization is predicated on what Castells refers to as the "space of flows" – a space comprised of the material infrastructure and virtual components that enable sustained real-time interactions between people over vast distances. Castells further contends that with the advent of the Internet, the "space of flows" has increasingly become more and more influential, to the point that it now dominates or replaces the traditional logic of the "space of places", where social organization was historically rooted and dependent upon purely localized experiences because of the necessity of having to contend with the obstacles of traversing large distances over long periods of time. In a network society organized along the space of flows, geographical proximity is no longer an element of space, because interaction based on the exchange of information can occur instantaneously. A further implication of the space of flows is that "time is timeless," in comparison to the space of places, where social practices are still based on clock time (that is, time is organized on the basis of the rhythms of nature or as social constructs of a culture). As will now be discussed, these distinctions in the operations and operating logic of the space of places versus the space of flows have significant implications for the manner in which the global SARS response unfolded.

The environmental sociologist Raymond Murphy (2004) notes that extreme environmental events and acts of nature may act as a stimulus for "improvised response"; a type of action that Hannigan (2006) sees as integral to the development of emerging social structures. This is because under the conditions of an extreme event, existing certainties wash away, making it possible for new actions and formations to develop, at least temporarily. Thus, in the case of the SARS, the urgent and compelling need to respond to a potentially global pandemic prompted usually competitive scientists from around the world to put aside narrow career interests and collaborate and share data via the formation of newly formed information networks.

The manner in which the SARS information network formed also exemplified a certain networking logic. It is a characteristic of networks that when one node is not responsive (or not functioning), then it no longer contributes to the movement of flows. Such a node in essence is no longer part of the network. When this occurs, alternative routes spontaneously develop to circumvent the damaged node, thus restoring the flow. Such a dynamic unfolded when the Chinese government refused to officially share information about SARS with the global public health community during the earlier stages of the outbreak. In reaction to these circumstances, the flow of information concerning SARS in China occurred through the establishment of unofficial channels, such as public health websites and personal blogs on the Internet. The role of the Chinese government as a node in the global public health information network was therefore by-passed. Networked developments such as these help illustrate how the spaces of flows comes to dominate the space of places in the modern era.

A second example in which the global SARS response can be understood in terms of the distinction between the space of flows versus places is to consider the speed at which viruses and people spread relative to the speed of information travel. Rosa (2003, p. 4) notes that one of the impacts of globalization is seen in the development of accelerated societies, in which acceleration penetrates every nook and cranny of societal development, including technological acceleration, the acceleration of social change, and the acceleration of the "pace of life" (cited by Jensen 2006, p. 332). And as alluded to above, jet travel has accelerated the speed at which viruses can now traverse the globe. Nevertheless, the speed of flows through mechanical and biophysical systems is limited by physical parameters, such as the maximum speed at which aircraft can travel or the rate at which viruses are able to multiply (i.e., the imposed limits of the basic reproductive number and incubation period of a particular virus). These limits are minor in comparison to the speed at which information can travel in the digital age (i.e., in essence the speed of light). This difference was used to an advantage during the global SARS response, since the sharing of information via the instant time of computer networks vastly outpaced the biologically defined time of viral reproduction and travel. For this reason, whether one is to speak of the accelerated speed of viral traffic between global cities via aircraft, or the viral traffic involved in the interpersonal contacts of those infected (i.e., the transmission rate of the disease), the latter speeds are no match for the speed of information exchange via digitalized information networks. As a consequence, by "outpacing" the virus, the scientific establishment was able to break the chain of transmission of the SARS-CoV quite handily – an outcome that was no doubt assisted by the presence of other fortuitous factors. For example, one characteristic of SARS was that a person was most infectious at that point when he or she was the most ill. The likelihood was therefore much higher that a SARS-infected individual would admit him or herself to a hospital (and be subsequently identified and quarantined or isolated there) at the exact time he or she had the greatest potential to initiate a community outbreak. Unfortunately, this also meant that the spread of the disease was largely nosocomial; that is, largely confined to healthcare workers (NACSPH 2003).

SARS and Networked Inequality

It should be noted that although the effects of the dominance of the space of flows over the space of places contributed to the success of the global SARS response, such dominance may also mask certain issues related to the unequal distribution of resources required to effectively respond to diseases in the Network Society. Mol and Spaagaren (2006, p. 69) note that within a sociology of flows perspective, new inequalities may be defined in terms of relative *access* to resource flows. In the context of the present discussion, "access" refers to both direct access to the flows of a particular network as well as the ability to influence the flows in terms of speed, direction, intensity, and so on. Thus, Mol and Spaargaren (2006) note that access to information flows via the Internet, to flows of capital, or to the skills of people moving around the world will distinguish those better-off individuals, groups, and cities from their marginalized equivalents. In light of these insights, it is quite fortunate indeed that, in the case of SARS, the space of places – as manifested in the flow of viruses and peoples through and in the global cities network – coincided with the space of flows. That is, because the SARS viral traffic implicated global cities, the information and technology infrastructures and resources needed for an effective response were already in place and accessible. Furthermore, the fact that the outbreaks occurred in cities of great economic significance most likely politicized the outbreaks more than would otherwise have been the case. This would ensure, for example, that any possible access problems would be quickly addressed. In line with this, one WHO officer notes that:

> Certainly Hong Kong, Singapore, Toronto ... these are, you know, well developed cities where people are coming and going all the time and it carries a different connotation because of that ... And because these places are very important in terms of economics, important in terms of global movement of people and goods, this became a very politicized outbreak. People were alerted to the danger and people actually thought, well, I'm quite likely to go there, I might need to go there, and so we were very quickly being put under a lot of pressure to provide information on travel safety, on safety of goods, and those kinds of questions, which given that it was a completely new disease, are quite difficult to answer until you've got a bit more information. (Interview, WHO Headquarters, Geneva, September 27, 2005)

As such, the rapid reactions and responses by global public health officials (and the world community in general) to SARS may not have as readily occurred had the viral traffic pattern implicated cities of less influence in the global economy. Such issues of access inequality will likely be particularly important issues of concern with reference to future epidemics, because the emergent, dynamic, and non-linear characteristics of a disease outbreak may mean that next time, the disembedding and re-embedding mechanisms of an infectious disease may implicate cities of the global South.

Concluding Remarks

The global outbreak of SARS was the emergent product of a complex of flows involving viruses, peoples, and technologies. The interactions between these flow types was unpredictable and non-linear, largely because of the large and diverse number of factors that could influence the interconnectivity and directions of these flows in any number of directions, including, for example: changes in culinary preferences and socio-economic conditions; airline travel paths and speed in association with the incubation period of the virus; the phenomena of "super-spreaders"; and the contact patterns and familial arrangements of those infected.

In light of the above, the SARS outbreak as emergent networked phenomenon appears to exhibit all the properties of a complex system (such as dynamism, emergence, and non-linearity), and therefore appears to be quite chaotic and unpredictable. Despite this, however, the global response to SARS was generally successful, a fact that I have argued was due to certain foundational developments of the network society. The hallmark of this response was the rapid formation of a virtual network of international scientists who joined forces to identify the causal agent of the disease, develop a universal case definition for the disease, and characterize the genetic code of the virus – all within the span of one month. These impressive results highlight the significance of the space of flows over the space of places in the contemporary era, as informational exchange could occur at a faster rate than that of viral diffusion. When considering future outbreak scenarios, however, questions regarding the efficacy of the response remain. This is because of issues related to access to networked resources. As the international spread of SARS occurred largely through the global cities network, access to such resources was not problematic, but this may not be the case if future outbreaks occur in less developed cities.

15

Thinking the City through SARS: Bodies, Topologies, Politics

Bruce Braun

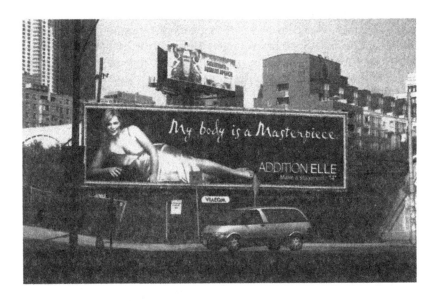

Something in the world forces us to think. This something is an object not of recognition but of a fundamental encounter.

Gilles Deleuze (1994, p. 139)

SARS as Event

The arrival of the SARS Coronavirus (SARS-CoV) in Toronto in early March 2003 prompted both a public health crisis, with 213 confirmed cases and 44 deaths within four months, and a crisis in the public health system, which was shown to have a number of chronic problems, from inadequate information systems and overworked staff, to lack of surge capacity and unclear structures of governance. In the weeks and months following the outbreak, these problems received a great deal of attention in the media and in a series of highly visible public inquiries (see Naylor 2003; Campbell 2004). In this sense, SARS was an event that placed the matter of public health in Toronto in sharp relief, illuminating its social, cultural, and political dimensions, and the strengths and weaknesses of the institutions charged with governing the health of the city's residents.

In this chapter I wish to understand SARS as an event in a somewhat different manner, not only as a problem calling for solutions at the level of law, the state, health policy, and hospital design, but *as a problem for thought itself*, as an event that perplexes us, unsettling our commonplace understandings and categories through which we apprehend the world. If SARS posed a problem for thought, it may well be our "good sense" about cities and urban life that it most insistently unsettled, by challenging how we understand the bodies that inhabit them, how we imagine their complex spatialities and temporalities, and how we perceive cities as political spaces in which bodies are always in the process of formation.[1] My objective here is to *think the city* through SARS by pursuing three intersecting lines of inquiry, each of which presents conceptual, political, and practical challenges to the field of state rationality we know as public health. In the first instance, I will suggest that SARS, along with the presence of other zoonoses, brought to light a set of absent actors – animals, microbes, airplanes, sewage systems, respirators – that had been banished to the margins of our conceptions of urban life, even as they actively contributed to how urban lives were composed and lived.[2] One of the more interesting aspects of the SARS pandemic is that it challenged us to locate animals *inside* the fabric of apparently "social" collectives. The most commonly told story of SARS, after all, begins with horseshoe bats and civet cats in China, which over the course of the epidemic came to be understood as intimately connected to the social and political lives of humans in places such as Singapore and Toronto.

Like other zoonotic diseases, SARS thoroughly scrambled the boundaries of the city and the bodies in it, displacing the human body into a set of wider "molecular" geographies that stretched far beyond its immediate environs (Braun 2007). In important respects, the SARS crisis had the same effect on our understanding of the city itself, bringing it into view as an *unbounded* and *polyrhythmic* space, rather than a fixed location in abstract space. *The unbounded body corresponds to the unbounded city.* This comprises a second challenge to our "good sense" about urban life. As we will see, thinking the city through SARS, and infectious diseases more generally, may call for *topological* understandings of city spaces and the bodies that inhabit them, such that geographies of health and risk come to be seen in terms of a continuously shifting skein of networks, at once local *and* global, biological *and* political, each with its own spatiality and temporality. Such an anti-essentialist corporeal geography suggests that health and illness be viewed not as qualities that belong to bodies *per se*, but rather as the *emergent effects* of the biological, political, and economic networks that compose them and that position different bodies as more or less vulnerable or secure.

Finally, the event of SARS revealed the city to be an intensely *biopolitical* space, in which the biological life of humans (and animals) was included in mechanisms and calculations of power. This insight is far from new; public health, after all, has long taken the vitality of the nation's body as its concern (see Foucault 1978; Gandy 2006b). What may have changed, however, are the geographies and political rationalities of the biopolitical city. Viewing the city through the lens of infectious diseases provides a window onto this. On the one hand, it allows us to consider the *everyday* ways in which power penetrates bodies (through the engineering of space or the instilling of habits), as well as the manner in which certain bodies are included within the biopolitical city only through their exclusion; that is, by the withdrawal of the state's protection. On the other hand, we will see that with globalization, biopolitics is no longer about the *internal* spaces of the city alone, but is increasingly part of global projects of "biosecurity" that understand the mutability of biological life and the folding of time and space as problems for political reason. In such projects states of emergence are translated into states of emergency, and biopolitics becomes increasingly a global diagram of power in which all bodies are caught up, but within which some are sheltered from risk, and others exposed to it.

If the first two lines of inquiry suggest an urgent need for rethinking our ontology of cities, the last line of inquiry restates this ontology in a political register, asking how, and with what effects, the networks that compose "health" and "risk" have become matters of concern and objects of government.

Political Physics: Urban Bodies and their Composition

The body never coincides with itself.

                                                    Brian Massumi (2002)

Among the most dramatic aspects of the outbreak of SARS in cities such as Hong Kong, Toronto, and Taipei was the sudden appearance of certain objects and practices: surgical masks on streetcars, "social distancing" at public events, or the avoidance of public spaces altogether (such as airports and hospitals, or, in Toronto, stigmatized Chinese restaurants). This was mirrored by the entry into common parlance of otherwise obscure technical terms – "aspiration," "respiratory droplets," "negative pressure rooms" – which collectively traced the outlines of the body in terms of an anxious geography of circulation and exchange at the molecular scale.

Each of these objects and practices made explicit in public life something that epidemiology and microbiology has maintained for some time: that far from self-contained and discrete entities, bodies are by their nature promiscuous and unruly; they continuously exchange properties with other bodies, whether human, animal, plant, or machine.[3] In significant ways, SARS brought residents in places such as Toronto to a greater awareness of their bodies as unbounded and precarious entities, and a greater understanding of cities as complex and unpredictable biosocial spaces. Many found this knowledge disconcerting, and registered their unease through precautions aimed at regulating the body's movements and exchanges. While uncertainty and fear declined as the virus became better understood, the event as a whole unsettled residents' "good sense" about the cities in which they lived. Not only were places such as Toronto revealed to be *global* places, a matter to which I'll return, but they also came into view as inherently *biological* spaces, composed not only of buildings and streetcars, money and commodities, but of living matter of all sorts, articulated in complex spatial and temporal configurations.

It is with the unsettling nature of the biological city that I wish to begin, for it suggests two, equally urgent, lines of inquiry. The first asks why, at the beginning of the twenty-first century, it jars us to think of the city in biological terms. After all, it was less than a century ago that urban reform movements in Europe and North America thrived on explicitly "epidemiological" or "bacteriological" understandings of the city, and sought to transform urban spaces and the behavior of individuals accordingly (Gandy 2006c; see also Osborne 1996; Craddock 2000).[4] The second asks a more philosophical question: If the SARS crisis revealed our ontology of urban life to be inadequate, what might a more adequate ontology look like?

Cities as social spaces: genealogies of erasure

Let me begin with the first question. How are we to make sense of this separation of the "biological" from the "urban"? When we consider cities, why do they appear to us as complex social and political spaces, but rarely as complex biological spaces? A comprehensive answer would have to follow several strands, both ideological and material, and here we can only begin such an effort. A familiar refrain proposes that in Western thought, at least from the time of the Industrial Revolution, the "city" has been opposed to "nature." Arguably this distinction reached its apogee in nineteenth-century Romanticism, but its influence has undeniably been felt in modern environmentalism and numerous twentieth-century anti-urban movements, which shared a common understanding of cities as unnatural or artificial spaces, and viewed urbanization as a fall from grace akin to humanity's expulsion from the Garden (see Williams 1973; Cronon 1994). Against the soil and vegetation of the country were juxtaposed the steel and concrete of the city; against the fertility of rural fields, the apparent sterility of city streets. Within these narratives cities marked our transcendence *over* nature, or gave witness to our disregard and destruction *of* nature, but they had nothing to do with the *presence* of nature, for urbanization had decidedly brought nature to an end (Hinchliffe 1999). Indeed, that geographers and social scientists today still tend to study cities solely in terms of social or economic processes, while biologists eagerly cast their eyes to fields and forests beyond the city's bounds, is only one indication of how deeply engrained this dualism has become.

We can locate other, more mundane, explanations in historical transformations of urban space. In his work on Paris and New York, Matthew Gandy (1999, 2002) has traced how urban planning and renewal during the twentieth century increasingly removed from sight many of the technical systems and physical processes that constituted the social life of cities. Sewage lines and water mains were buried, as were conduits of every kind, such that the city – at least that which was above ground and visible – appeared to be increasingly divorced from the biological processes of human existence, and from the myriad technological objects that made social life possible (Kaika and Swyngedouw 2000; Kaika 2005). While cities in the West remained intensely biological spaces, they no longer *appeared* as such to the residents walking their streets. All manner of biophysical matter still coursed through urban space, often at ever-greater volumes and speeds. Yet, after the initial excitement of the first large capital works projects passed, these circulatory systems, and the matter that flowed through them, became part of an invisible city whose workings no longer were a central part of public or political discourse.

These were hardly the only changes to city–nature formations that occurred in this period. At least in North America, the same decades saw ordinances that limited the keeping of live food animals in the city, or that expelled slaughterhouses and feed lots from the urban landscape, deepening the apparent "denaturalization" of urban spaces (Philo 1995). This sense was enhanced further after World War II, when it seemed to many that the so-called war with infectious diseases had finally been won, and that progress had relegated the bacteriological city to the dustbin of history, or at least safely sequestered it far away in the "developing" world (King 2002; Cooper 2006). This "victory" was in part due to the very same technologies, infrastructures, and zoning that hid the biological city from residents, although it was an effect too of the widespread use of antibiotics and vaccines, which allowed human bodies to increasingly appear separate from the extracorporeal systems that composed them.[5] With the growth of genetics and biotechnology in the years that followed, this impression was only deepened, as health and risk were increasingly located *inside* the body and "chronic" diseases, such as cancer and heart disease, moved to center stage.

These developments were deeply paradoxical, for, to paraphrase Latour (1993), the body *appeared* increasingly autonomous only through massively increasing the retinue of non-humans mobilized in the name of its vitality. Far from preceding these dense networks of living matter and corporeal technologies, the vital properties of bodies were formed and sustained *through* them. Yet despite this, the centrality of the biological to the urban was rarely noted; except in the form of parks, gardens, and house pets, or in the guise of the "uncanny"' – the broken water, smells wafting up from manholes and sewage outlets, sightings of "wildlife" in backyards and alleys, or the discomfort of an untimely head cold with an unknown cause (Vidler 1992; Gandy 1999; Kaika 2005) – the world of living matter no longer seemed particularly relevant to our urban existence.[6]

Cities and bodies-in-formation: toward a new ontology of urban life

The significance of the SARS crisis, then, was not only that it revealed problems with institutions of public health; it also revealed inadequacies in our ontologies of urban life. But what might a more adequate urban ontology entail? And what concepts might help us in such an endeavor?

I will return to the biosocial character of cities in a moment. First, let me propose that in the wake of SARS we might do well to understand the city as a *machinic assemblage*. This admittedly strange term, borrowed from Deleuze and Guattari (1987), seeks to capture a sense of the city not as the site of entities and spaces whose qualities are known in advance, but as a complex set of material forces that have emergent effects (see Latham and McCormack 2004). The city is "machinic" in that the forces and relations that constitute it continuously call forth new and novel forms.

This is an abstract concept, but we can develop it in a logical fashion by returning to the field of public health, and to the event of SARS. Arguably the central concern of public health since its inception in the eighteenth and nineteenth centuries has been the vitality of human bodies. More to the point, public health has concerned itself with bodies not as they are known in the clinic or laboratory, but as they are constituted in the spaces of everyday life; that is, with *lived* or *practiced* bodies, in all their movements and interactions. This insight is crucial, for what we learned from the SARS crisis – an insight already latent within public health – was that the "good sense" of the body that we had inherited from humanism was inadequate. In the early months of 2003, it quickly became evident that bodies do not form an autonomous or prior ground upon which social life is founded – as much social thought and political philosophy presumed – but are always *in the process of formation* through their connections to other bodies, whether institutions, machines, water, air, plants, or animals. To borrow a concept from the seventeenth-century philosopher Benedict de Spinoza (1994 [1677]), SARS reminded us that the body is a composite entity rather than a discrete thing, and that bodies, in the words of Nigel Thrift (2006, p. 464) are "integral with the world outside them," extending "beyond the obvious integuments of their 'internal physiology' in persistent and systematic ways."

Metaphysics is not usually where we turn to think about public health, or urban geography, but the relational ontology that Spinoza developed, and which later writers such as Nietzsche and Deleuze further elaborated, is helpful in a number of ways. Not only does it enable us to think about the city as a site of bodily composition, but it calls attention to *how* bodies are connected to other bodies and with what effects. Not all connections are of the same value, nor do these connections remain constant over time. Moreover, as we learned from SARS and other zoonoses, connectivity presents us with a paradox. On the one hand, connections are necessary for bodies to persist. We must eat and breathe to live: without connections – without folding the body's exterior into its interior – we wither away, literally losing all capacity to act. These connections are myriad – water mains and telephone lines, urban gardens and supermarkets, restaurants and drug stores – and they are simultaneously organic, technological, economic, and political. The geography of the body-in-formation is remarkably complex. On the other hand, connections can render bodies vulnerable. Viruses and bacteria, for instance, or urban technologies such as electrical grids or speeding cars, all threaten to de-territorialize the body in catastrophic ways. In short, the same networks that enable or increase the vitality of bodies also expose the body to forces that threaten its present composition. We experience this double-sided nature of networks with each trip to the supermarket, where food products are labeled and marketed in terms of the presence of desirable properties that *enhance* the body and are sought after, and in terms of the absence of undesirable properties whose presence *threatens* the body, and are thus warded against. As we learned from mad cow disease, which has quickly become a morality tale for the integrated networks in which we live, life and death are *both* network effects, which is one of the reasons why food networks have become such important sites of political contestation.

Conceived in this way, bodies – and urban life more generally – can no longer be restricted to the "social," for as SARS and other zoonoses have made clear, cities are composed of a shifting skein of networks that mix together the biological, chemical, technological, and political. Rather than the site where humanity has most successfully separated itself from nature, the city is perhaps best seen as a "post-human," "more-than-human," or even "inhuman" space, in the sense that the human – as a coherent entity – does not precede the technological and socio-ecological networks that comprise cities, but is instead composed in them, emerging as the effect of what we might describe as the "ontological choreography" of urban life.[7] There are not cities in one place, and nature elsewhere: there are only city–nature formations (Hinchliffe 1999).

It is with this in mind that we can most fully appreciate the return of animals to our conception of cities (see Wolch 1996; Wolch and Emel 1998; Philo and Wilbert 2000). But it may be necessary to widen our sense of *how* the animal is part of social life. It is not enough to think of the animal as an "out-of-place" remnant of the wild among us, or to embrace the animal as our companion and thus understand human–animal relations solely in emotional terms. These are surely important, but what SARS taught us is that the animal is not simply an "other"; it is part of a dynamic biological world *with which our bodies continuously swap properties*. Alongside stories that stress the importance of interaction with animals for the emotional development of children, it is now common to read stories about the "risks" associated with animals, even the pet that shares your home or bed. With newfound attention to zoonoses, our relation with animals is defined not solely in terms of alterity, or ethical responsibility, but also in terms of "enfoldings"' of living matter (Hinchliffe and Whatmore 2006). The animal is *in* us, not simply before us. Indeed, despite the appearance of the city as a "social" space, animals have always been part of its corporeal life and its ethical–political communities. They have continuously circulated through its spaces, in the form of dairy products, meats, clothing, even pharmaceuticals, not to mention waste and viscera. They have surrounded us as house pets, rodents, birds, foxes, and feral cats. And they have formed complex human–animal assemblages, at times aided by insects, viruses, and bacteria that trace lines of connection between them all. What is unique about the present may only be the specific *qualities* and *geographies* of these human–animal assemblages, as food networks have become more global and as the intensely "visceral" work of food production has been spatially segregated from urban life in such a way that has fostered the impression of cities without animals.

The Biosocial City as an Unbounded or Polyrhythmic Space

This leads us to a further set of issues. While SARS, BSE, avian influenza, monkeypox, and a myriad of other zoonotic and food-borne diseases give testimony to the enfolding of humans and non-humans, they also demand that we consider the many ways in which these complex city–nature formations are stretched across time and space, to the point at which today many of the networks that comprise urban bodies circle the globe. It is not enough to displace the body into the spaces of the city; we must rethink the spaces of the city itself.

The second fundamental challenge issuing from SARS, then, concerns our conception of the *space–time* of cities and the bodies within it. As quickly became evident during the SARS crisis, the vitality of bodies in the everyday spaces of cities such as Toronto is related to activities in distant places. Animals may be part of our intimate urban relations, but SARS taught us that they do not need to be near in *absolute* space for this to be the case; proximity is an effect of connection, not distance. It is widely believed that SARS-CoV is endemic in horseshoe bat populations in Guangdong, China, and that it jumped species to civet cats in late 2002, either on farms where the two live in proximity, or in the province's live animal markets (Lau et al. 2005). It is in these markets where the first cases of human infection are thought to have occurred, and from which the virus spread to Hong Kong, and then rapidly to numerous global cities through air travel. While the specific vectors of transmission are still debated, the rapid spread of SARS – and the apparent vulnerability of populations distant in absolute space – has dramatically challenged "bounded" understandings of cities, and demanded that we recognize cites as complex *topological* spaces with multiple spatio-temporalities that are at once local and global.

But what does it mean to think of cities topologically, and why should this matter if our concern is the health of the populations in them? We are accustomed to thinking about bodies and urban space in ways that privilege the geometrical space of the grid (in which things have fixed locations "in" space), and in ways that privilege linear understandings of sequential time. SARS at once exceeded and unsettled these conceptions of space and time, for not only did it reveal that human existence is more than "social," it also taught us that the spatialities of bodies were "stretched" along the length of networks and that "proximity" was a measure of the body's position within them. That these networks are always multiple (such that the body is fractured and discontinuous rather than singular and unified), and that each network "folds" or "crumples" space (so as to scramble commonsense conceptions of the near and the far, as well as political rationalities organized around these spatialities), only complicates further the body's composition (Serres and Latour 1995; Bingham and Thrift 2000). Each network also carries a distinct temporality and velocity, such that many *different* pasts cohere in the *same* present, and such that disjunctures exist between the relations constituting any entity or event. The spatio-temporalities of the body are therefore multiple, which is to say that the body has no single form, but is composed within a shifting set of forces and relations.

This is admittedly an odd way of thinking about bodies and spaces, since within "good sense" they appear to exist as "things-in-themselves," apart from the heterogeneous associations that enable them to "hold together" or "endure." Yet, with SARS it became much easier to understand the body in these terms, since the virus had the effect of *fracturing* the body, revealing it to be a contingent effect of the skein of networks that composed its vitality: live animal markets in Guangdong, hotels in Hong Kong, transcontinental air routes, suspended water droplets in airplane cabins, hospital emergency wards in Toronto, not to mention the restructuring of public health services, new medical technologies and the particular spatial orderings of law. If this skein of networks is the body's *ontology*, then the space–time of the body is nothing less than the space–times of the multiple networks that compose it. In short, bodies and cities are not only "more-than-human," they are also "polyrhythmic" (Amin and Thrift 2002; Smith 2003).

As noted by others in this volume (see, for example, Chapter 2 by Rodwin, Chapters 3 and 9 by Keil and Ali, Chapter 4 by Ng, and Chapter 5 by Teo et al.), this presents obvious challenges for public health. While public health frequently focuses on local practices (hence, the proliferation of "local" health authorities), topological space confounds the local and the global. This was duly noted during the SARS crisis, when it became apparent that, at least in an epidemiological sense, "wet markets" in Guangdong, China potentially were as proximate to classrooms at York University or streetcars on Yonge Street, as were butcher shops on Spadina Avenue, or farms in rural Ontario. This presents a quandary for such rudimentary public health practices as health surveillance, for not only are these networks complex and multiple, they do not coincide in any direct way with political boundaries, and thus with the sovereign power of individual states.

Arguably, we have only begun to grasp the complexity and dynamic nature of these networks. Not only do the local–global networks within which matters such as "health" are addressed rarely hold still, but this is increasingly said of molecular life itself, which is today seen to be characterized as much by mutation and reassortment as by order and stability.[8] Indeed, global health officials (WHO, CDC) have stressed that humans are not the only ones actively reconfiguring global networks. The very nature of viruses – their ability to mutate, delete, reassort, and recombine – means that quite apart from our activities, non-human actants are *also* scrambling the networks of which we are a part. A single reassortment can change the whole topology of human–animal relations, shifting a specific network overnight from being a condition for *life* to carrying the potential for *death*. In Eugene Thacker's (2005a) words, within these "spatio-temporal multiplicities," things are "continuously churned up," forming "unexpected combinations."

We find additional challenges in the disjunctive spatio-temporalities of intersecting biological and technological networks. There is always a gap, for instance, between the moment when a body is infected and when patients present symptoms. It is thought that with certain SARS cases the incubation period may have lasted as many as 12 days. International flights are measured in hours. Hence, while still pre-symptomatic, an infected body can travel the world undetected. This was complicated further by the difficulty in diagnosing the SARS-CoV infected body, since the symptoms that the body presented were shared with infections caused by other pathogens (Hon et al. 2003). At least initially, detection at early stages of infection was difficult, a problem exacerbated by a second temporal gap between the emergence of the disease among humans in November 2002, and the first generation of diagnostic tests, which were not available until April 2003.[9]

We can extend this spatio-temporal problem further, since the SARS-CoV infected body also has its own unique rhythms that are mapped across the body in different ways at different times. Diagnostic tests are designed to detect the presence or absence of viral RNA. With SARS-CoV, viral RNA was detectable in the respiratory tracts of a substantial proportion of patients within the first four days of infection, but was *not* detectable in stool or urine samples until days 5 to 7. Later in the progression of the disease, this corporeal geography of viral RNA shifted, as viral loads were redistributed across the body's topography. Finally, viral RNA positivity – a measure of viral quantity within the body – had its own rhythms, with rates of RNA positivity peaking 10–12 days after the onset of illness. In some patients the virus could be in detected in secretions for more than 30 days, although no longer able to be cultured after the third week.[10] This may in part explain why hospitals became critical, and often risky, spaces for patients and health workers alike, since patients were often at the stage of greatest viral shedding only *after* they were admitted. In short, the *viability* of the virus had its own geographies and temporalities, and the peculiar nature of these meant that certain bodies – in this case healthcare workers – were at more risk than others.

The geography of SARS, then, was not simply one of bodies (in the singular) and the viruses that infect them, but rather *a shifting geography of pathways and nodes*. In turn, the challenge for public health was nothing less than devising strategies that could in some way conform to, anticipate, or intervene in, these polyrhythmic assemblages.

SARS and the Biopolitical City

Understood in these terms, it is not difficult to see why zoonotic diseases have in recent years received considerable attention in the media, within the medical community and among state agencies. Indeed, some have argued that globalization has transformed the twenty-first-century world into what Dr Bernard Vallat, the Director General of the World Organisation for Animal Health (OiE), has called a "global biological cauldron" with increased risks of catastrophic pandemics.[11]

In such a condition, public health – or "health security" as it now often called – necessarily involves the building and cutting of networks, a fact that may lead us to moderate apocalyptic warnings of global pandemics. To be sure, networks are "dangerous" – with modern air travel viruses can circle the globe at breakneck speeds – but the networks that compose urban lives also include elements that *mitigate* against a global pandemic. We too often forget this. Indeed, the density of such networks – the connections between individuals and health providers, for instance, or the dense networks of medical technologies, bioinformatics, laboratories, diagnostic devices, antivirals and vaccines, even cell phones and email – are as central to our body's ontology as the length and speed of viral networks that link bodies in Toronto with those in rural China. These networks have the potential to *increase* the capacities of bodies, rather than merely threaten their ability to persist. Hence, as Eugene Thacker (2005a) brilliantly puts it, "health security" is today increasingly about networks fighting networks. In the case of SARS, for instance, the WHO quickly established a global network of 11 laboratories that shared results in real time via a secure website and daily teleconferences. On the website were posted microscopy pictures, protocols for testing, and ICR primer sequences (Stohr 2003). The network identified the coronavirus, conclusively named it as the causative agent of SARS, and contributed to the development of diagnostic tests. As Heymann and Rodier (2004) note, this virtual network not only provided rapid knowledge about the causative agent, mode of transmission and other epidemiological features, its real-time information also made it possible for the WHO to provide specific guidance to health workers on clinical management and protective measures to prevent its further spread. Indeed, the most significant fact about SARS may not have been its quick spread, but that its spread was halted at record speed (Demmler and Ligon 2003).

The point here is not to fall back on Whiggish notions of progress, or to assume that *more* technology is the answer to health risks. Nicholas King (2002) rightly warns us against such assumptions. Rather, it is to avoid one-sided narratives that understand global networks solely in terms of a threatening mutability or an inexorable and exponential expansion of risk, since such accounts can quickly become the justification for unexamined extensions of sovereign power in the name of "security" (Braun 2007). As soon as we present the future not just in terms of a "state of emergence" immanent in the biosocial networks that constitute the present (an ontological claim about the nature of time and space and the virtualities of biosocial matter), but also as a "state of emergency" (a political claim about threats to the social and political order), we run the risk of validating the exercise and expansion of sovereign power without democratic accountability. To say that public health is about networks – about *tracing* networks, and about *constituting networks that cut other networks* – takes us instead to the question of how such networks are constituted, with what effects, and with what sorts of openings to the future. That many of these networks are contentious should not be surprising, since they raise pressing and still unresolved questions about intellectual property, privacy, accountability, and state sovereignty, and since they seek to foreclose certain biosocial futures in favor of others.[12]

None of these practices are innocent; they allow for some forms of life and not others. More important, they bring us to a key point: that public health operates in a *biopolitical* register, which is to say that at the end of the day it seeks to bring "life" into the realm of political calculation.[13] This takes us to a third and final way in which the event of SARS challenges our conception of the city. With SARS, we begin to see all the ways in which the city is a biopolitical space, a space in which our biological existence is related to our political existence in particular, power-laden ways.

Here I will limit my comments to two observations. First, it has been common in discussions of infectious disease to raise concerns about "civil liberties," with the questions typically phrased as follows: At what point does the state have the right to limit people's movement, their right of association, or their free speech? Is the state authorized to restrain individual freedoms in the name of health? What constitutes a valid exception to the rule of law, and who decides? These debates frequently focus on the practice of quarantine, which has historically been an effective way to cut chains of transmission, or at least buy time for public health responses by slowing the spread of disease. The problem with quarantine, however, is that it is immensely difficult to reconcile with notions of individual freedom and democratic deliberation, since it is an explicit extension of sovereign power.[14] As such, the SARS crisis brought Torontonians face-to-face with the relation between sovereign power and law, and the capacity of the Canadian state to determine and limit "rights."

Leaving our analysis here, however, allows for the impression that it is only at *exceptional* moments, and in *exceptional* practices, that power is exercised over the body. Indeed, debates over quarantine generally accept a central premise of liberalism: that in the absence of states of emergency, individuals are authors of their own lives, and the city is merely a collective space in which, during "normal" times, free individuals gather. The event of SARS helps us place in question such abstract notions of the "individual" and "freedom," and understandings of democracy that assume that right precedes power. In the first instance, SARS revealed the individual to be a multiplicity rather than a unity, and as much an effect of the play of external forces as the author of them. As important, the SARS crisis called attention to the many ways that the "practiced" body, and the networks that constitute it, are always already targets of political rationality, and thus how the state continuously seeks to organize the conduct of individuals. As became clear in a range of different cities during the SARS crisis, the state, and public health officials, were less concerned with limiting freedoms than they were concerned with producing *governable* bodies; that is, individual subjects who would *choose to manage their biological lives in particular ways.* This was perhaps most evident in the countless advisories issued by local, national, and international organizations, or in attempts to educate people about "preventive measures." Residents of cities such as Hong Kong, for instance, were told to "build up good body immunity" through proper diet, regular exercise, and adequate rest, or by reducing stress and avoiding smoking. Likewise, they were encouraged to "avoid touching the eyes, nose and mouth," told to "not share towels" and to "open windows to improve ventilation," and advised that sick children "should not be taken to school or childcare centers." Schools were given lists of preventive measures, bus drivers told how to maintain and sanitize their vehicles, and adults encouraged to learn how to wear masks properly to maximize their effect (see Leung and Ooi 2003).

None of this advice was new. Indeed, as an element of state rationality, public health has always been a biopolitical exercise, concerned with managing "life" in such a way as to optimize, even increase, the powers of the state's constituent body. To borrow from Nicholas Rose (2006), public health long ago took the "clinical" body of nineteenth-century medicine and located it within a series of extra-corporeal systems – flows of air, water, sewage, germs, contagion, familial influences, moral climates, and the like – and thus in a sense accepted and made its concern the sort of topological understanding of the body that SARS again brought into public discourse. The target of public health policies has never been the body in relation only to itself, but bodies in motion, in relation to other bodies, to food, and to animals, and even those animals in relation to each other. What SARS brought to light, then, was not only the exceptional exercise of sovereign power, but also the ways in which power continuously suffuses urban space and penetrates subjects' bodies in the mundane practices of everyday life.

This does not mean that biopolitical practices today are merely continuous with those of the past. With SARS, we witnessed the development of new surveillance practices, the utilization of new social marketing tools to target specific "at risk" populations, the development of novel design proposals for hospitals and airports, and a number of new spatial practices recommended for healthcare workers (see, for instance, Affonso et al. 2004). Moreover, with the ascendance of neoliberalism, biopolitical regimes have seen important shifts. Reforms to public health at the local and national scales have increasingly shifted the burden of managing the biological life of populations from national governments to local authorities (often in the form of unfunded mandates), and from the state to individuals, whereby individuals are increasingly compelled to "manage" risks through making "wise choices" (see Rose 2006; Rose and Novas 2004, Heath et al. 2004). In this respect, SARS revealed in stark outline the limits of health policies organized around "individual responsibility," and the consequences of state disinvestment in public health (Keil and Ali, Chapter 3).[15]

The most significant difference, however, may be found in the merging of *biopolitics* with *geopolitics* (see Braun 2007). With the focus on SARS, avian influenza, mad cow disease, Ebola, and other zoonotic diseases, biological life has been refigured as inherently unpredictable and human life placed firmly within its chaotic molecular geographies. On the other hand, globalization has been said to increase these virtual risks, such that biological events elsewhere are continuously implicated in the future of "health security" at home. The problem here is less the recoding of biology in terms of its inventiveness than the ways in which this has become a justification for new, extra-territorial forms of sovereign power, validated through the language of "risk" and "security." As Cooper (2006, p. 120) perceptively notes, within security discourse, the target of public health "is no longer the singular disease with its specific etiology, but *emergence itself*, whatever forms it takes, whenever and wherever it happens to actualize" (see also Dillon 2003; Thacker 2005a).

This merging of the biopolitical city with geopolitical strategy is evident in the global extension of surveillance networks which, in Nicholas King's (2002) words, seek an "unending picture" of global populations, now including domestic and wild animals. But it is also evident in a whole range of new biopolitical practices whose objective is the management of the biological lives of *distant* people, from attempts to reorganize and police "wet markets" in China, to the training of new classes of paraprofessionals in Thailand with expertise in human–animal relations, to various incentives and legal instruments to compel peasants to "conduct their conduct" in particular ways (Braun 2007). These new biopolitical and geopolitical forms, by which power "takes hold" of the lives of distant strangers, are understood and justified by institutions as diverse as the WHO and the World Bank through the rhetoric of "global goods," although it is far from clear whose "good" is taken to be global.

Conclusion

Each of these biopolitical practices deserves to be analyzed on its own terms. The larger point, however, is that as the securitization of biological life presents itself as the answer to the shifting and overlapping biosocial networks continuously recoding bodies, biopolitics increasingly leaves the city behind and becomes *global* in its reach.

With this insight, we can perhaps bring together the various ways in which SARS and other zoonoses have challenged our conception of the city and the vitality of the bodies in them. On the one hand, the SARS crisis taught us that bodies are "composites" and that cities are "machinic assemblages"; that is, SARS enabled us to see the city as a complex "post-human" or "more-than-human" space in which individual bodies are in continuous constitutive relations with other bodies, whether human, animal, or machine, or larger collective bodies such as the state. The vitality of the body is in large part determined in and through its connections. Accordingly, public health increasingly takes "connectivity" as central to its concerns. On the other hand, SARS revealed that the networks that constitute urban life are at once multiple and stretched across space and time. If the body is understood in terms of the "enfolding" of living and non-living matter, such enfoldings point to the *topological* nature of bodies and spaces. This presents public health with new challenges, for "health" can no longer be understood as a "local" matter – since the networks that constitute the body's ontology are often global – and can no longer presume that the constituted "body" is a static entity, since the networks that compose healthy or unhealthy bodies are neither singular nor stable.

Finally, the SARS crisis made clear that public health names an *ontological politics* (Mol 1999), in so much as it is about constituting bodies through constructing or disrupting networks. These networks are at once biological, technological, political, and economic, and they are at the same time local *and* global. But this leaves us with more questions than answers, for it is not at all clear how "health security" in a globalized world is to be defined, by what practices it is to be achieved, or whose health is to be privileged. As has become clear in the difficulties faced by health officials responding to avian influenza outbreaks in countries such as Indonesia, attempts to produce "global" health security are often greeted by skepticism, or actively resisted, by local communities, who fail to see how *their* health is being secured. What, then, does it mean to govern networks, and in whose name is this to be done? Which networks are to take priority? And where does, or should, sovereignty lie within these integrated networks in which distant bodies are stitched together?

NOTES

1 Deleuze (1994) argued that thought proceeds by way of the event precisely because the event exceeds, unsettles, or destroys "good sense," refusing to allow the world to return to the same.

2 Zoonoses are diseases that are transmitted from animals to humans, or from humans to animals. Although they have recently attracted immense attention, they are far from new.

3 For a discussion of how images of the body have changed in late-twentieth-century medical and popular discourse, see Martin (1994) and Rose (2006).

4 The remaking of the "bacteriological" city was, of course, markedly uneven, both within the West, where certain neighborhoods and residents were abandoned rather than included, and in colonial cities, where the "bacteriological" city was often limited to European sectors (see Gandy 2006c).

5   Triumphant declarations about the eradication of infectious diseases were as much a measure of the increasing segregation of postwar cities than their changed epidemiologic condition. Infectious diseases did not "return" to the city with SARS; among disadvantaged communities, often abandoned by the state and unseen by affluent suburban residents, diseases such as tuberculosis maintained a continuous presence throughout the twentieth century (see Farmer 1999; Gandy and Zumla 2003; Draus 2004; see also Craddock, Chapter 11). Indeed, it merits comment that interest in infectious diseases among urban scholars has increased at the same time that central cities have seen new cycles of investment. As affluent residents have occupied trendy lofts and markets, they have once again come in contact with migrant workers, the working poor, and the homeless, for whom the biological life of cities has never stopped being an everyday concern, and for whom the reduction of health and social services has arguably only increased their precarious position.

6   We could doubtless locate many other causes for the erasure of the biological, such as the triumph of *Homo economicus* in economic and social geography in the 1960s and 1970s, or the cultural turn of the 1980s and 1990s, each of which in its own way further removed the unruly materiality of the city from the concerns of urban scholars.

7   I borrow the term from Cussins (2005).

8   In the case of avian influenza, much has been made of "genetic drift" and "genetic shift," two processes by which viruses such as H5N1 may mutate into forms capable of human-to-human infection.

9   Even with reverse-transcriptase polymerase chain reaction (RT-PRC) methods, rapid confirmation was not possible during the pre-symptomatic or early stage of infection.

10   On temporalities of SARS, see Meltzer (2004) and Cheng et al. (2004).

11   Public comments at International Symposium on Emerging Zoonoses, Atlanta, March 22–24, 2006.

12   As I write, debates are raging about the public or private nature of information gathered in these networks, with entities such as the Centers for Disease Control in Atlanta resisting public circulation in order to protect intellectual property rights.

13   We owe the term "biopolitics" to Michel Foucault (1978 [1976]), who argued that in the eighteenth century political power increasingly came to concern itself not with decisions over life and death, but with the *management* of life; that is, with ordering and enhancing the vital or productive processes of human existence.

14   It is precisely the link between quarantine and individual freedom, and the "abuse" of state power, that is the central theme of the film *Outbreak* (1995).

15   One of the consequences of SARS – and other infectious and food-borne diseases – has been new calls for state investment in public health infrastructure and workforces. For others, however, the state's failure to adequately respond to such so-called "natural" disasters has provided the basis for calls for further disinvestment, on the grounds that the state *failed* to protect its citizens (for a discussion in relation to Hurricane Katrina, see Peck 2007). For these critics, the proper response to state failure, then, is not to reverse the weakening of state capacities, but to accelerate it.

16

Vapors, Viruses, Resistance(s): The Trace of Infection in the Work of Michel Foucault

Philipp Sarasin

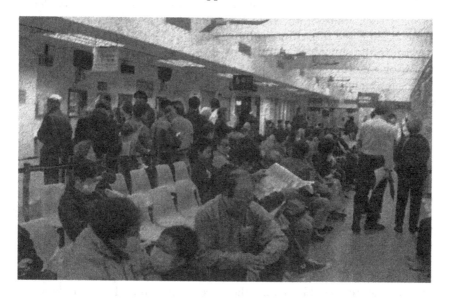

In this chapter, I want to demonstrate that the discourses and practices of the "new normal," which are associated with life in our networked cities of the world during the contemporary "war on terror" and political epidemic control, may be better understood against a specific conceptual background: I will show on the basis of the work of Michel Foucault how a critical theory of power discusses and employs the theme of infection and metaphors of infections. Such a conceptual discussion can lay the groundwork for understanding today's patterns of spatial technologies of power, which we have seen proliferate in a world haunted by re-emerging infectious diseases as diverse as HIV/AIDS, SARS, and tuberculosis. The concept of "infection" is complex, even ambiguous and alluring. During antiquity, infectious diseases were traced back to a "contagion" that was thought of as something incomprehensible and unknown, something that had to be sent from someone, an agent that came from "outside" (Temkin 1977). "Miasma" was the word that the Greeks used for contaminated air, and from the eighteenth century until well into the second half of the nineteenth century, it referred primarily to the "vapours" of the soil (Riley 1987). To date, the term "infection" has not lost its latent surplus of meaning. Although we no longer suspect the gods as the senders of bacteria and viruses, even in modernity infectious diseases were seen in many ways as an external threat, sent by an "enemy" or introduced to our territory by foreigners. The political language of modernity – reaching into postmodernity – has a tendency to equate political enemies or ethnic and "racial" aliens metaphorically with the threat of infection, or directly with infectious germs (see Bein 1964; Anderson 1996; Russell 1996; Stern 1999; Weindling 1999, 2000; Gradmann 2000; Jansen 2003; see also Moore 2000; Naimark 2001). This did not only happen in the context of the SARS epidemic in different places across the globe, but also in the context of the fear of "Islamic terrorism," which has especially haunted American politics since the late 1990s. Ever since the end of the Clinton era, terrorism has been equated with "bioterrorism." The anthrax letters of October 2002 also seemed to confirm this assumption (see Sarasin 2006).

Strategies to ward off the threat of infection have, since antiquity, been integral to the technologies of power. These strategies were almost always spatial strategies, and they are intimately linked to the construction of states, territories, and cities. Not accidentally, as we will see below, writers such as Foucault have trained their eyes on metaphorical city states to instruct us on the changing models of infectious disease in and through the urban worlds in which they have occurred. Border closures and quarantines, control of commodity exchange, meticulous monitoring of the movement of people, and inspection of their bodies can be useful measures to prevent the spread of epidemics that could threaten the lives of thousands. They are, however, also always tempting ways for power to expand the control over its subjects. If, for example, the boundaries of a nation are metaphorically equated with the boundaries of the "body politic" and protected against all kinds of "infections," then the threshold between the medical–epidemiological and the metaphorical–political concepts of infection has already been transgressed in a dangerous way. This is what has happened significantly after 9/11, more precisely in the National Security Strategy of the United States (White House 2002), wherein distinctions become apparently superfluous and politics, epidemiology and epidemic control become one: terrorism, infectious diseases, bioterror, and border control to prevent illegitimate traffic – the flipside of "legitimate traffic," in other words, against clandestine immigration over the Mexican border – collapse in one short paragraph into an "opportunity" for stricter control of infection at the borders of the body of the nation.

Analogously, the fight against terrorism is at times explicitly interpreted as a fight against a "viral infection." In a speech to the American Congress in July 2003, Tony Blair interpreted the connection between poverty, dictatorial regimes, and fundamentalist Islam as the milieu in which "a new and deadly virus is emerging. The virus is terrorism ..." (BBC 2003). This pattern of thought – conceptualizing Islamic terrorism as a virus – was very explicitly elaborated in the summer of 2005 by Paul Stares and Mona Yacoubian, from the quasi-governmental US Institute of Peace in Washington, in order to develop a strategy of action for the fight against terror based on the epidemiological control of pandemics: They suggest that terrorism should be understood as a "virus" that leads to "infection." According to the authors, this approach would have a range of advantages:

> First, it would encourage us to ask the right questions. What is the nature of the infectious agent, in this case, the ideology? Which transmission vectors – for example, mosques, madrassas, prisons, the Internet, satellite TV – spread the ideology most effectively? ... Second, an epidemiologic approach would help us to view Islamist militancy as a dynamic, multifaceted phenomenon. Just as diseases do not emerge in a vacuum but evolve as a result of complex interactions between pathogens, people, and their environment, so it is with Islamist militancy ... Third, it would encourage us to devise a comprehensive, long-term strategic approach to countering the threat. Public health officials long ago recognized that epidemics can be rolled back only with a systematically planned, multi-pronged international effort. (Stares and Yacoubian 2005)

Here again, by means of a few metaphorical operations, politics mutates in a dangerous way into epidemic control – political opponents and microbes become indistinguishable.

No philosopher of the twentieth century placed the human body in the center of his work and presented it as a historical object like Michel Foucault (see Sawicki 1991; Jones and Porter 1994; Peterson and Bunton 1997). In the *Birth of the Clinic* (1973) it is the dead body through which the individual becomes identifiable; in *Discipline and Punish* (1977) the body becomes the subject of disciplining, which ultimately targets the soul, but needs to subject the body to its rules in order to enforce the automatisms of obedience. A year later, in *History of Sexuality*, it is the "sexuality" of the body that permits its individual normalization and constitutes the starting point for the regulation of the "population." The later concept of "concern for self" is equally targeting the body and the soul. The soul has now been assigned to aesthetically and ethically shape the self-aware subject.

Related to these classical Foucauldian themes focused on the body and the subjects is a line of argumentation that, while it runs through large parts of Foucault's work, remains mostly implicit and unnoticed: the trace of infection, a trace of minor references, and hints about both actual and metaphorical infections. With Foucault, we can learn about the relationship between power and infection, because his ideas of power and modern governmentality are based on three "models" that, in an idealtypical way, were focused on the three classical infectious diseases leprosy, plague, and smallpox. The present text is at first nothing but a short passage through Foucault's work in order to reconstruct the trace of infection, which for us is of both theoretical and practical interest. Interestingly, in the context of this book on urban networks and disease, Foucault's models of power, as derived from models of infectious disease, are associated metaphorically and historically with (more or less metaphorical and mythological) cities of the past: Thebes, the medieval cities, and early modern Paris. At the end, I will argue that, with Foucault, one is able to defend a concept of liberalism that can directly be derived from this trace.

Fevers of Madness

Foucault's first major book, *Madness and Civilization*, published in 1961 (in English in 1965), begins with leprosy: "At the end of the Middle Ages," so the first sentence says, "leprosy disappeared from the Western World" (p. 3). Certainly, it did not disappear completely, but the many leprosaria emptied and their goods were bequeathed to the poor. However, the structures of exclusion, according to Foucault's argument, remained: "Often, in these same places, the formulas of exclusion would be repeated, strangely similar two or three centuries later. Poor vagabonds, criminals, and 'deranged minds' would take the part played by the leper [...]" (p. 7). Foucault's – contested – thesis of the "Great Confinement" of the deviant underclasses and, first and foremost, of the insane since the mid-seventeenth century is modeled on leprosy. The leprosaria were the immediate model for the handling of this newly perceived illness, and the fear of infection has accompanied the history of madness ever since. The insane were confined just like the lepers before them, their voices falling silent behind the walls of the asylum. It was Foucault's concern to let the history of the displaced and repulsive "Other" of reason reappear, because that history had until then "never made an appearance" (Foucault 2004, p. 93, translated by A.A.).

After the "Great Confinement" of the seventeenth century, there was another crucial transition in this history of insanity in the Age of Reason. This transition departed from the Enlightenment practice of confining insanity, which, in the spectacle of its raving madness, revealed itself as pure "non-reason," and thus as the mirror image of enlightened reason. Instead, insanity was liberated from its chains by psychiatric reformers Philippe Pinel in France and William Tuke in England, squeezed into the psychiatric classifications and moral constraints of the patriarchal clinic, and the insane were forced to proclaim the new nosological truths of the nineteenth century (Foucault 1965, ch. 4). To identify the transition as such was conventional. The liberation of the insane from the dungeons of Bicêtre and Salpêtrière by Pinel in 1793 is, after all, not only one of the founding myths of psychiatry, but of medical humanism in general. But what leads Foucault to read Pinel's act not as a genuine liberation, as the philanthropic beginning of psychiatric medicine? He will argue that the psychiatric framework of classifications is hardly any better than the chains and dungeons of the eighteenth century. But this is not the point. Foucault discovers instead that the "liberation of the insane" is a retroactive myth, because it had nothing to do with what the alienists at the end of the eighteenth century had in mind. The real history evolved differently. "Suddenly," says Foucault, "in a few years in the middle of the eighteenth century, a fear arose – a fear formulated in medical terms but animated, basically, by a moral myth" (Foucault 1965, p. 202). A fear of what? Foucault writes:

> People were in dread of a mysterious disease that spread, it was said, from the houses of confinement and would soon threaten the cities. They spoke of prison fevers; they evoked the wagons of criminals, men in chains who passed through the cities, leaving disease in their wake; scurvy was thought to cause contagions; it was said that the air, tainted by disease, would corrupt the residential quarters. (1965, p. 202)

At the end of the Ancien Régime, this epidemic, which originated in the hospitals and mad-houses, threatened "entire cities [...], whose inhabitants would be slowly impregnated with rottenness and taint" (Foucault 1965, p. 204). No wonder, then, that in 1780 the origin of an epidemic that spread through Paris was traced back to the Hôpital general; there was even talk of "burning the buildings of Bicêtre," which was subject to a "putrid fever." Not only the mad-houses, but also regular hospitals, were perceived this way: With the mingling of the sick and their transpirations in the over-crowded rooms, doctors saw them as a place where the disease could not develop in a "natural" way; for the poor they were a place to die and, at the same time, a dangerous seat of infection that threatened society (Foucault 1973). The metaphor of infection allowed society in the second half of the eighteenth century to put the vague peril of looming evil into words. However, it was not at all meant just metaphorically:

> There appeared, ramifying in every direction, the themes of an evil, both physical and moral, that enveloped in this very ambiguity the mingled powers of corrosion and horror. There prevailed, then, a sort of undifferentiated image of "rottenness" that had to do with the corruption of morals as well as with the decomposition of the flesh, and upon which were based both the

repugnance and the pity felt for the confined. First the evil began to ferment in the closed spaces of confinement. It had all the virtues attributed to acid in eighteenth-century chemistry: its fine particles, sharp as needles, penetrated bodies and hearts as easily as if they were passive and friable alkaline particles. The mixture boiled immediately, releasing harmful vapors and corrosive liquids. [...] These burning vapors then rise, spread through the air, and finally fall upon the neighborhood, impregnating bodies and contaminating souls. Thus the idea of a contagion of evil-as-rottenness as articulated in images. The palpable agent of this epidemic is air, that air which is called "tainted," the term obscurely suggesting that it is not in conformity with the purity of its nature, and that it acts as the communicating element of the taint. (Foucault 1965, p. 203)

Leprosy continued to be the epidemiological model for this phantasm of infection. But, unlike in the Middle Ages, "the house of confinement was no longer only the lazar house at the city's edge; it was leprosy confronting the town" (1965, p. 202). Louis Sébastian Mercier, cited by Foucault, calls it "a terrible ulcer upon the body politic: Even the air of the place, which can be smelled four hundred yards away – everything suggests that one is approaching a place of violence, an asylum of degradation and infortune" (1965, p. 202).

At the beginning of the modern history of insanity was an unrest, which began prior to Pinel and which had nothing to do with the humane desire of the medical profession to cure insanity: "If a doctor was summoned, if he was asked to observe, it was because people were afraid – afraid of the strange chemistry that seethed behind the walls of confinement [...]" (Foucault 1965, p. 206). Foucault takes the contemporary phantasms literally: The danger of infection was the true reason for the liberation of the insane, the true origin of the many medical reforms of the time of the revolution. The liberation of the insane by Pinel and Tuke appears as an effort to "purify" and "neutralize" the houses of confinement. This is "to reduce the contamination by destroying impurities and vapours, abating fermentations, preventing evil and disease from tainting the air and spreading their contagion in the atmosphere of the cities" (Foucault 1965, p. 206). Here appears one of the "grand" themes of Foucault: What it means to create order, and against what order is enforced. The opposite of order appears as madness, which enters the stage as an epidemic. The infected and infection are synonyms of disorder.

Impurity as a Genealogical Principle

From a cursory perspective, the trace of infection disappears in the work of Foucault in the late 1960s: The semantic of contagion and fever that shaped an important argument in *Madness and Civilization* appears neither in *Order of*

Things (1966) nor in his methodological book *Archaeology of Knowledge* (1972 [1969]). This changed with the publication of *Discipline and Punish* (1975). To the extent that Foucault now wanted to analyze structures of order outside of all discursive conditions, the contrast of outside and inside, of order and infection, reappeared in his work in a more pointed way. *Discipline and Punish* puts power again at the center of the analysis and describes it along the model of an infectious disease and resistance. Discourse analysts are concerned with the reconstruction of rules that guarantee the identity of an epistemic object such as madness or sexuality in a scientific discourse. As "happy positivists," they substitute the "analysis of accumulation" with the "theme of transcendental foundations"; that is, the analysis of the accumulation of statements that constitute an epistemic object (Foucault 1972, p. 125). Genealogy, in turn, does not analyze foundations in the sense of a Hegelian philosophy of history. It rather discovers behind the masks of identities the "recognition and displacement" of the Self as an "empty synthesis," its heterogenesis, "numberless beginnings," "a profusion of lost events," "errors, false appraisals, and faulty calculations" (Foucault 1984a, p. 81). Whereas discourse analyses reconstruct rules and thereby tend to construct a purified field of what can be said and what is excluded, genealogy is based on impurity as its true principle.

Foucault was maybe never more Nietzschean than in these lines of "Nietzsche, Genealogy, History." In any case, he was never as decidedly historical and genealogical than in the text of 1971 (see Foucault 1984a). Because genealogy as a radicalized historiography serves primarily to dissolve the idea of an ahistorical essence of things: "it is to discover that truth or being does not lie at the root of what we know and what we are, but the exteriority of accidents" (ibid., p. 81). It shows that "there is 'something altogether different' behind things: not a timeless and essential secret, but the secret that they have no essence or that their essence was fabricated in a piecemeal fashion from alien forms" (ibid., p. 78).

Especially with regards to the seemingly ahistorical "identity figures" of the "Self" and the body, the genealogical proof of historicity leads to the denial of this kind of identitarian essence of humans: "Nothing in man – not even his body – is sufficiently stable to serve as the basis for self-recognition or for understanding other men" (ibid., pp. 87–8). Foucault uses Nietzsche (and implicitly his reference to the hygienic theories of the nineteenth century, which understood the human and the body as dependent on the conditions of the environment) to substantiate this radically nominalistic position (see Sarasin 2001).

We believe, in any event, that the body obeys the exclusive laws of physiology and that it escapes the influence of history. But this too is false. The body is moulded by a great many distinct regimes; it is broken down by the rhythms of work, rest, and holidays; it is poisoned by food or values, through eating habits or moral laws; it constructs resistances. (Foucault 1984a, p. 87)

Foucault learned from Nietzsche that the historicity of the body lies in its susceptibility to infection – Foucault calls it "poisoning" – and, conversely, in its ability to develop resistances, to change physically through the modification of what we today call the immune system. Because the body is exposed to certain "regimes" – dietary regimes – which since Galen are classified under the rubric *sex res non naturales*, there is, according to Foucault, no stable essence to humans, nothing unchangeable, that would connect all humans in a transhistorical and transcultural way. The infection with "poisons," food (Nietzsche's obsession: see Janz 1981), and "values", and the resulting development of resistances, appear to be the real basis for the historicity of the body. Because it is susceptible to infection, it is "impure," and because it is impure, its appearance, its current form in its various manifestations, can be genealogically deconstructed just like that of common artifacts.

In other words, "impurity" turns out to be the central genealogical principle, because genealogy traces ideological statements of identity, essence, development, and totality back to the many "dispersed," "random," and "erroneous" figures that are foreign to the stated identity, but of which it is made up. At the same time, impurity is the characteristic epistemological metaphor of genealogy. The genealogist radically and consciously blurs the distinction between epistemological object and subject. An "aseptic" and "pure" historiography is one, according to Foucault, that refrains from taking sides and surely believes to be able to proceed in an impartial and objective way (Foucault 1994, pp. 538–645).

The Plague and the Disciplines

Foucault applied this modified perspective in a broad historical study in his book *Discipline and Punish*, in 1975 (see Foucault 1979). One of the central questions of the book is how it was possible that in a time in which individual liberties were proclaimed, the heads of the kings rolled, "humane" prison sentences replaced the bloody criminal law based on physical retaliation, and power ceased to threaten with death, the disciplining of individuals and their subjection to the mechanisms of power did not decrease, but in fact increased: the fabric was more tightly knit, the responsibilities anchored deeper in the subjects, the productivity of the bodies increased. This was obviously an urgent genealogical question for Foucault, because of his perception of the societal conditions in France in the 1970s. Foucault's answer to this question is essentially that with the architectural structure of the panopticon, which was designed in 1887 as the ideal institution of surveillance by the English philosopher of law Jeremy Bentham, a mechanism unfolds in society, a "principle" through which individuals are being meticulously disciplined under the visible surface of the proclamation of liberties.

This grim vision of a totally administered society was the idealtypical accentuation, and, at the same time, the preliminary historical culmination of a series of techniques of governing that had begun with the exclusion of lepers into asylums at the fringes of the cities in the Middle Ages. Commenting retrospectively on his work on the exclusion of the insane, Foucault says that, "if it is true that the leper gave rise to rituals of exclusion, which to a certain extent provided the model for and general form of the great Confinement, then the plague gave rise to disciplinary projects" (Foucault 1977, p. 198). The regulations of the plague that he cites construct a system of complete control of all borders and crossings within the city and demand the rigid confinement of the citizenry into their homes: "It is a segmented, immobile, frozen space. Each individual is fixed in place. And, if he moves, he does so at the rise of his life, contagion, or punishment" (p. 195). This is thus the plague model: "This enclosed, segmented space, observed at every point, in which [...] each individual is constantly located, examined and distributed among the living beings, the sick and the dead − all this constitutes a compact model of the disciplinary mechanism" (p. 197). But the plague is itself a model − a counter-principle of order, a "festival" of disorder as it had been imagined in the literature of seventeenth-century low-brow comedy, a festival of "suspended laws, lifted prohibitions [...], bodies mingling together without respects, individuals unmasked, abandoning their statutory identity and the figure under which they had been recognized, allowing a quite different truth to appear" (p. 197). In other words, then, the plague is a model of impurity that dissolves the masks of identity.

This "dream" of the plague as the collapse of order was countered by the authorities of the seventeenth century, so Foucault, with the "political dream" of discipline. This is a vision of the "penetration of regulation into even the smallest details of everyday life through the mediation of the complete hierarchy that assured the capillary functioning of power" (p. 198). Foucault does not speak of cities in which the plague had actually broken out, but of the "the utopia of the perfectly governed city," for which "the plague (envisaged as a possibility at least) is the trial in the course of which one may define ideally the exercise of disciplinary power." Just as jurists and state theoreticians imagined a state of nature, "rulers dreamt of a state of plague in order to see perfect disciplines functioning" (p. 199). This confirms the recurring juxtaposition of infection and order in Foucault's work. The administrative "dream" of a state of plague therefore also reflects the limits of power threatened by infection, milling crowds, and disorder: "Behind the disciplinary mechanisms can be read the haunting memory of 'contagions', of the plague, or rebellions, crimes, vagabondage, desertions, people who appear and disappear, live and die in disorder" (p. 198).

It is exactly this fear that is the driving force behind Bentham's panopticon: an annular building consisting of individual cells with no contact between them, but directly visible from the central tower, where one supervisor is sufficient to induce in the inmate a "state of constant and permanent visibility" (p. 201). The panopticon has one central purpose: to prevent contact among confined individuals so that communication, association, and infection are equally prevented. This shows that from the perspective of power, communication and the mingling of subjects are as big a threat as infection itself. As has been continuously claimed in the West, with the plague in mind, infection is simply the dangerous merging of unequal bodies and the uncontrolled transgression of borders. Since the "Black Death" of the fourteenth century, for which the blame was immediately pinned on the Jews, the lepers, the Arabs, the "Sultan of Babylon," and so on, the plague has become the metaphor for the looming evil, the deadly menace, the foreign bodies that threaten the social body.

"Universally Destructive Viruses" and the Smallpox Model

Foucault rarely speaks of microorganisms as a real and genuine threat. He rather uses them primarily as a metaphor or model. In 1976, following his book on punishment, he discusses the regulation of the population with the newly introduced concept of a "bio-politics" or "bio-power" (Foucault 2003, p. 243). The threat of microorganisms to human life appears here as an uncontrollable counter-principle to the biopolitically constituted power and its regulatory interventions into the life of the species. In the *History of Sexuality*, Foucault writes:

> It is not that life has been totally integrated into techniques that govern and administer it; it constantly escapes them. Outside the Western world, famine exists, on a greater scale than ever; and the biological risks confronting the species are perhaps greater, and certainly more serious, than before the birth of microbiology. (1990, p. 143)

This brief comment shows that Foucault, despite all the metaphorization of infectious diseases, was aware that humans live in a generally precarious and insecure position *vis-à-vis* microorganisms. Foucault was unsure at the time what this meant for humanity. The "biological risks" of microorganisms that "confron[t] the species" were clearly an "Outside" of power, a kind of counter-principle, but they appear as simply deadly – no more "festival" of disorder and collapsing identities. However, the critical gaze of the genealogist on biopolitical power remains caustic: In fact, what Foucault seems to say here is that the danger of infectious diseases to humans has only increased with the rise of microbiology since the end of the nineteenth century. It was thus only logical that he farsightedly warned in a lecture in March 1976 that microbiology armed with genetic engineering is itself the biggest possible danger to humankind, a threat that can only be compared to nuclear war, when, in fact, "it becomes technologically and politically possible for man not only to manage life but to make it proliferate, to create living matter, to build the monster, and ultimately, to build viruses that cannot be controlled and that are universally destructive" (Foucault 2003, p. 254). This was truly contemporary and current thinking. Since the first successful experiment with recombinant DNA at Stanford University in the early 1970s, microbiologists, epidemiologists, and keen military experts have begun to wonder what – military, epidemiological, medical – consequences the production of non-natural hybrid organisms could have. The global scientific community of molecular biologists and geneticists agreed at the conference of Asimolar in February 1976 that experiments in genetic engineering have to meet high safety standards – but in so doing they also exposed the fact that the so-called misuse of genetics will from now on be a latent threat for humankind.

The genealogist and analyst of power who modeled its appearance after a pattern of infectious diseases did not pursue the study of biopower. He, in fact, abandoned the concept of biopower altogether at the end of the 1970s. This conceptual turn, which can be subsumed under "governmentality," was in turn not insignificantly shaped by an infection model: the smallpox model of power. To a certain extent, it was the answer to the hanging question of how the potentially increased threat of microorganisms in modernity can be conceptualized in relation to power.

Foucault's conceptual shifts, which became apparent in the lectures on *History of Governmentality* that he held in 1978–9, were significant. Essentially, his concern was essentially to discard the plague model of power, as he increasingly realized that power and the rule of the state cannot simply be understood in terms of a universalized pattern of the panopticon – as if modern societies were completely controlled plague cities under total surveillance. The – primarily economic – freedom of the individual appears in his analysis of modern governing rationality in a new way, as something irreducible, "as something fundamental": Modern governmentality is a form of rule that "can only be exercised through the freedom of the individual" (Foucault 2006, p. 79, translated by A.A.). This freedom is the limit of power; the freedom of the individual is not given *a priori*, but is a product – in fact, a calculation – of liberal power. It cannot, however, be bypassed and it constitutes a limit to power. Without free subjects whose "desire," or rather whose self-interest, has positive effects for society as a whole, modern society cannot be understood. An analysis that fails to recognize this is wrong.

In order to highlight this historical change – but also the change in his own thinking – Foucault reminded his audience of the example of "leprosy, which stands for a type of power which is characterized as separation of the binary type between those that were sick with leprosy and those that were not." The second example is that of the plague, which stands for a type of power that "literally covers the cities with a network of control" – in short, "a system of the disciplinary type" (Foucault 2003, p. 24). And now we have the new model, "the smallpox or the practice of inoculation."

Contrary to the disciplining form of defense in the context of the plague, the authorities of the eighteenth century reacted to smallpox primarily through statistical observation, by measuring the factual occurrence of cases, and empirically by trying to protect the population from contagion through vaccinations. In the context of liberal governmentality, a risk management that is based on these perceptions of the problem must not – and that is the important point here – go so far as to turn to disciplining individuals, because this would undermine their freedoms, which constitute the foundation of the system. Therefore, according to Foucault, "if one governed too much, one did not govern at all." A state that is too strong destroys its own objectives – it must respect the relative "impenetrability" of society (Foucault 1984b, p. 242) even at the price of a certain risk of infection. This does not mean that Foucault is simply singing the praises of liberalism. He rather tries to understand how modern power uses the freedom of the individual and its relative "impenetrability." He wants to show that in relation to the freedom of the individual there emerges a "security dispositive" to counter the risks arising from the freedoms in the context of an entire population. Contrary to the disciplinary dispositive, which aims at adapting individuals to a certain norm, the security dispositive is based on a statistical notion of normality: normality in the sense of the existence and occurrence of cases and their distribution curves in a population. The security dispositive does not try to "discipline" these cases, but to understand their "nature" and their movement, and to correct for the resulting risks.

Smallpox Liberalism

Reading the multi-layered and in some aspects also contradictory work of Michel Foucault, one necessarily runs the risk of constructing one's own lines of argument, which cannot be reconstructed from other perspectives. This may be also true for the reading of Foucault that I have proposed here. I believe I have shown that some of Foucault's most important arguments are based on an epidemiological logic, and that it was no coincidence that Foucault, for instance, dedicated his seminar at the Collège de France in 1978 to the history of vaccination practices (Foucault 2003, p. 25). Nevertheless, the question of the significance of the trace of infection in Foucault's work remains open. On a rather theoretical level – and strictly concerned with the structure of Foucault's thinking – I consider two elements as central. First, infection as an illness of the body, as a threat of decomposition and death: Foucault has, perhaps like no other philosopher since Nietzsche, attempted to connect his arguments to the body and to use the body as a site of "truth," as a site where things get decided, where they really happen, where relations of power become real, where promises have to be kept, and where false appearances are revealed. Will the body die or not? Will it starve? Will it survive an infection? Will it be excluded, confined, disciplined, controlled, put under surveillance? Is it possible to vaccinate it? The body is the site where the struggles over truth are ultimately fought out; in Foucault, the body does not represent anything, it is not just a "sign" or a "medium," but that strategic, "most material and vital," site that power has used and occupied (Foucault 1990, p. 152). The second important element here is the relation between the principle of infection and the aspiration of power to bring about order: mingling crowds versus surveillance, association versus separation of individuals in cells, scandalous chatter and uncontrolled discourses versus the order of discourse and the "discursive police," "impure" genealogies versus a "sterile" history, and so on. It almost seems that the "entire" Foucault can be reconstructed along this line of argument. The fact that this line and thereby the trace of infection resolve completely is evidence of the genuine turn in his thought at the end of the 1970s.

This brings us to the question of the political analysis that becomes possible with this Foucauldian "toolbox." In the context of contemporary infectious diseases (such as SARS) and their social ramifications, and social or political phenomena that are fantasized as "infections" (such as terrorism), Foucault's analyses of power based on the plague and smallpox models gain in importance. The smallpox model of power, as conceptualized by Foucault, is essentially based on the fact that power gives up the dream to completely eradicate the pathogens, the intruder, and the germs, to control society "in depth" and to discipline the movements of all individuals. This basically means that power rather coexists with the pathogenic intruder, is aware of its occurrence, collects data, compiles statistics, launches "medical campaigns," which can perfectly take on the character of standardization and disciplining of individuals – but discipline, or even complete discipline, cannot be a reasonable objective of liberal power in modern times. When this is its goal, though, when power wants to return from the smallpox model to the plague model, it becomes totalitarian. In other words: The liberal state must respect the freedom of the individual, even at the cost of a certain risk of infection. The smallpox model shows that modern societies can live with the risk of infection without immediately devising the essentially racist alternative "us or them" – "us" or the microbes, "us" or the "terrorists." Current politics, however, clearly seems to waver as to whether it should stick to the liberal smallpox model, or switch to the plague model of complete control and discipline. But the smallpox model would teach us that we could indeed live with terrorism (just as we are *de facto* living with infectious diseases) – as a form of political criminality – which needs to be combated by the police with the full rigor of the law and as a tactical problem for postmodern societies.

Translated from the German by Ahmed Allahwala

17

Fleshy Traffic, Feverish Borders: Blood, Birds, and Civet Cats in Cities Brimming with Intimate Commodities

Paul Jackson

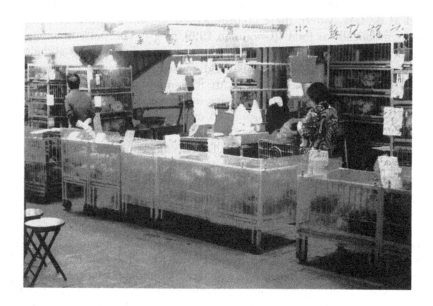

The structure of food production and consumption form an elaborate network intermingling flows of capital and culture. Probyn (1999, p. 216) argues that a major obstacle in understanding food "is its enormity, and the ways in which it spills into every aspect of life." Yet Frederick Kaufman, in *Harpers*, provides a fine journalistic account of tracing the food linkages in the kosher certification process:

> Markets may atomize and globalize, manufacturers may specialize within specializations, but unlike the rest of us, the rabbis have not drifted into bewilderment. They are watching the fragments, and they are counting.

Now, consider that a single bite of a Frito-Lay brand certified-kosher barbecued potato chip delivers dehydrated starch from Idaho, dehydrated onions from China, dehydrated garlic from India, and a bit of paprika from Spain, all of which must be certified kosher. "A simple product has ten, twenty ingredients ... Twenty certifications behind the certification, you see? I don't think anyone understands the globalization of the food market as [the rabbis] do. (2005, p. 77)

The diffused network around commodities leads to interconnections that are intensely produced, politically contested, culturally dependent, and intimately personal. For food there are two sets of metabolic relations that are simultaneously social and material: "*on the land*, where agricultural nature and its harvest are co-produced and co-evolve with social labour, and *at the table*, where these co-productions are metabolized corporeally and symbolically as food" (Goodman 1999, p. 17). This polar understanding of food – land and table – is key to understanding food as a chain of relationships, particularly, as will be discussed, in terms of commodified relationships. Yet these relations are becoming increasingly unmoored from both land and table by intensive industrialization. What deadly disease properties has food incorporated or spawned en route to the urban markets?

Food and disease are biological materials that imbed in, and transmit through our bodies. While Probyn (1999, p. 216) stresses the "the brute physicality of food," in turn the brute physicality of disease cannot be ignored. Food-borne diseases raise the temperature on the "feverish borders" where the "fleshy traffic" of meat is patrolled. Widely discussed, food is an intimate commodity – perhaps *the* most intimate commodity.[1] As a commodity, food is extremely leaky and "quasi" – as it is tangled into a variety of fields and domains, from natural to cultural to technological. Meat holds a special place in the menagerie of intimate commodities. The co-mingling of disease and food allows the imagination to wander into the realm of wild meat, congealed death, and animated monsters. Food and disease have "inherent tropic qualities ... from metaphor to materiality" (Appadurai, in Crewe 2001, p. 632) that lend themselves to panache in both theory and images. However, disease should not be seen as a construct, or theory, or a metaphor; the reliance on these devices arises from deep-seated fears and insidious nature. Susan Sontag (1990, 3–4) writes that, "it is hardly possible to take up residence in the kingdom of the ill unprejudiced by the lurid metaphors with which it has been landscaped." Yet there are dangers in using disease metaphors – what Sontag calls cheap shots – in that declaring neoliberalism is like a virus is very easy, but not very helpful. This doubly erases the violence and deaths from viruses and economic restructuring.

The SARS Story: From Butcher to Barbeque

The intimate commodity sometimes becomes a public debacle. While severe acute respiratory syndrome (SARS) virus was not framed as a food-based disease or food scare, SARS was allegedly a transnational disease ultimately related to food, whose viral origin was traced back to the harvesting and consumption of wild civet cats, specifically, in a wet market that traded in lucrative wild meat commodities in Foshan, China. The SARS virus was found in a group of masked palm civets and a raccoon dog. From these animals a new coronavirus emerged and caused the first pandemic of the twenty-first century. The wet market was found in the southern province of Guangdong, in what Mike Davis (2005, p. 58) has described as a "postmodern Manchester" – the world's leading area in the manufacturing and export of commodities. Mei Zhan (2005, p. 37) states that the people of Guangdong province and Hong Kong are "famous for their bold appetites for exotic animal foods." Yet the first reported SARS patient wasn't a consumer, but a wet market animal handler. Later investigations found significant SARS antibody levels in animal dealers (Yu et al. 2003). After the link had been made, civet cats were pulled off the market. As wet markets were seen as the source of the disease, the markets were shut down throughout Asia (Zhong 2004). At the height of the SARS outbreak, the Chinese Government banned any animal that could not be farmed. While there were some wild civet cats, interestingly the majority were commercially farmed. Correspondingly, all the wild animal markets were banned; when the SARS crisis didn't subside, the Chinese government announced the slaughter of 10,000 civet cats (Zhan 2005, pp. 34–5). Accordingly, the food culture in China has shifted, with increased hygiene surveillance – cleanliness is strongly advertised and promoted publicly.

The role of the super-spreader from Guangdong to Hong Kong, then to the rest of the world, has been widely documented. Curley and Thomas lay the responsibility for the SARS epidemic as a failure of China's "internal inadequacies," which unwittingly created a "human security threat of regional and global proportions" (Curley and Thomas 2004, p. 29). China allowed spillover into other nations. China's failure is framed as a lack of implementing "street-level" policies that coordinated different organizations; but individuals were also blamed for not "pulling in the same direction," thus destabilizing the nation-state (Curley and Thomas 2004, p. 20). There were international attempts to counter this destabilizing health crisis. The World Health Organization, in light of their global alert, implemented precautionary measures and delineated bounded geographical areas known as "hot zones." These territorial responses involved the creation of barriers in flows of people: banning of flights, refusing visas, health checks, and quarantine (Curley and Thomas 2004, p. 22). While framed as a global disease, SARS affected specific cities depending on their connection to super-spreaders. One such city was Toronto. In Toronto, SARS converged with another food-based disease in a circus of spectacles.

One notable manifestation of the spectacle of SARS and Toronto was the rock-benefit derivatively named SARS-stock. The event took place in July 2003 and was the convergence of a multitude of relationships on a certain site, Downsview Park (Canada's first urban national park). SARS-stock was permeated by an immense variety of flows that folded in a variety of borders around the convergence of two food-based diseases: SARS and mad cow (also known as BSE, and in humans called Creutzfeldt–Jakob disease). SARS-stock was part of Ontario's long-term plan to lure tourists back to the city – hard hit by the WHO travel advisory that resulted in a loss of nearly US$400 million due to the subsequent decline in tourism (Gibson and Jean-Louis 2003). SARS-stock was a "benefit" and symbol for healthcare workers in Toronto, two of whom died as a result of workplace infection. Additionally, thousands of hotel and tourism workers who had been laid off as their industry slowed down were also involved in SARS-stock. Close to 200 hotel workers volunteered at SARS-stock to flip burgers and turn sausages. The championing of beef was due to a recent outbreak of mad cow disease. The BSE scare – involving the transfer of prions (proteins) across species and allegedly to humans in the consumption of beef (see Hinchliffe 2001) – touched down in Western Canada, causing borders to be shut to Canadian beef products at the same time as SARS. Politicians from all levels of government also got involved in promoting Canadian beef at SARS-stock. The North American Association of Ribbers and Smokers was created and set up a quarter-mile strip of nine competitive barbecuers from Canada and the US in an event called "Beef Without Borders" (CBC 2003b). There was a national balancing of food involvement with SARS-stock; beef was brought in from Western Canada, potatoes and oysters from Eastern Canada, and with the addition of Native Canadian sourced water, a strange national food solidarity was articulated. The politics of SARS-stock is reminiscent of an AC/DC song – a "dirty deed done dirt cheap." The appropriateness of the response, the pomp and spectacle, did not promote the health of Toronto. The phrase "bread, not circuses" is the quick retort to this event. A question arises: Why were they peddling potentially at-risk beef at an event for health professionals and the health of Toronto? The politically mobilized scales of the crisis – urban and national – diminished the effort of those on the front lines, such as nurses, who worked hard to minimize the spread of the disease. Additionally, there was the marginalization of Asian communities and neighborhoods that were stereotyped – they became *de facto* pariahs in Toronto, a city that prides itself on inclusiveness. In regards to the global pariahs, should China be blamed for SARS? In a highly connected world with increasingly porous borders, what becomes clear is that "viruses, bacteria, and various kinds of plants and animals have never respected national borders" (Pirages and Runci 2000; in Curley and Thomas 2004, p. 19). This level of porousness in borders, nations, scales, urban regions, and bodies is a key issue. Theoretically, the borders between wild and domestic, meat and commodity, consumption and body, rural and urban must be unpacked, for the flows of disease do not respect these divisions.

Wild/Meat

In recent disease outbreaks, animals have taken on a new role. Mei Zhan (2005, p. 38) states that the "civet cat, in particular, became a protagonist in the origin stories of SARS." Orientalist representations of wildness and the exoticness of Chinese bodies were connected to what is, and is not, "appropriate" to eat, leading to the incredulity and disgust from the West. For Zhan, the term wild is "both vague and all encompassing," in that:

> "wild" was no means reductively "natural", nor could it be structurally defined in opposition to "domestic" or "farmed" ... "wild" was marked with a set of heterogeneous meanings specifically and intimately related to, if not produced by, human consumption ... We also need to pay critical attention to the enmeshing of civet cats and other "wild" creatures deep within everyday life ... during a medical, social, and political crisis of potential global scale that the "wild" took on contingent and contested forms through a variety of actions that were once biological, political, legal, historical, social, transnational, and visceral. Elusive and heterogeneous, the "wild" emerged as a temporary point of convergence in discourses of SARS. (2005, p. 35)

Control of disease can be seen as the extermination of microscopic wildness. This wild discourse has returned with avian influenza. Maps of migratory bird flyways are regularly circulated in newspapers and on websites. Qinghai Lake, the largest lake in China and also the crossroads for waterfowl flyways, is now closely monitored, since 6,000 wild birds died of H5N1 in 2005. At Qinghai Lake, a stopover for hundreds of thousands of birds, the virus replicates in their intestinal tracts and the excrement enters the water supply, which is then consumed. Different strains of diseases exist in the same population, but also in the same bird (Zackowitz 2006). Yet this is not a new development. What is new is that this ecological system is intersecting with agricultural production systems and the metabolism of cities. While this migratory disease ecology lasts for about a month, there is the possibility of these wild birds infecting domestic livestock.

While the term wild is vague, these bird populations are an unmonitored reservoir for diseases. Zoonosis is generally understood to refer to the transmission of infectious diseases between humans and wild/domestic animals (Slingenbergh et al. 2004, p. 467). The general consensus is that 75 percent of all emerging diseases of the past two decades – Ebola, BSE, Nipah virus, Rift Valley fever, monkeypox, and SARS – are due to an animal pathogen crossing the species boundary into a human host (Brown 2004a, p. 435). These trans-boundary diseases increasing involve free-ranging wildlife. Human encroachment on wildlife habitats (and wildlife encroaching on human habitats) puts pressures on the wildlife/human/domestic animal interface. One danger is that humans are biased, preferring to study themselves and ignoring disease in animals until the disease jumps the species barrier. Control of emerging diseases therefore must involve all hosts in a multidisciplinary and cross-species analysis (Cleaveland et al. 2001, pp. 992–8). Understanding these inter-species relations has consequences in how we envision global connections, and ideas of containment and responsibility.

Interestingly, all recent diseases of zoonotic origin are associated with a specific geography. Avian influenza and SARS have a Chinese origin, AIDS and Ebola came "out of Africa," mad cow disease is a product of Britain; "[r]ich or poor, north, south, east or west, the lesson is that novel infectious disease can appear anywhere" (Weiss and McLean 2004, p. 1137). Avian influenza should not be blamed on Guangdong, for there have been 13 outbreaks of an influenza variant in North America in last seven years (Monke 2004). For avian influenza there is the strict patrolling of the borders of wild and livestock; when the threat of infection increases, livestock is ushered indoors – paradoxically intensifying the risk factors. But Brown warns that "this microbial perfect storm will not subside. There will be no calm after the epidemic, rather the forces combining to create the perfect storm will continue to collide and the storm itself will be a recurring event" (2004, p. 436). This microbial storm watching should not be a surprise since, according to Beck, nature has "boomerang qualities" that bounce back in the face of industrial capital (in Crewe 2001, p. 630). While understanding the role of zoonosis in this storm is key, I must concur with Zhan (2005, p. 37) that the media representation is perhaps more important than the scientific debate: "the story of 'zoonotic origin' did not blame nature itself for the SARS outbreak; what went wrong was the Chinese people's affinity with the non-human and the wild." This affinity allowed the virus to move between Chinese bodies by the visceral act of consumption. Chinese consumers were blamed and treated with disgust for flirting with wild nature, being too intimate. But before the wild is to be consumed, meat must be transformed into commodities.

Meat/Commodity

Commodities, and commodity chains, have been under intense scrutiny for some time now. More than just economic units of exchange, limited to sites of consumption, means of production, or the product of labor, commodities leak across these understandings. On top of this, food must be cut away from the general commodity literature. Yet a further slice should be made for meat in particular, as Robbins (1999, p. 419) explains:

> If meat seems to matter more than many other food commodities, it is perhaps because of the unusually wide range of dramatic and visceral meanings that flesh can possess. It can be embodied life force, palpable class power, congealed death, or an elixir of health. Meat is the product of violence associated with privilege but also the by-product of an increasingly distributive economy associated with a flood of goods to meet the needs of many.

Highly desirable meat – produced by violence into congealed death – allows disease to flourish. Noel Castree (2001, p. 1519) asks a key question: "what imaginative geographies both of ourselves and of distant others are entailed in any attempt to make visible the geographical lives of commodities?" Rather than creating a biography of just the meat commodity, one can look at the geographical *lives* within or around a commodity – literally and viscerally. What little specters of death are transferred within those biographies and what new microscopic lives arise from the congealed death of meat? More importantly, what lives are held in the balance when we ignore the leakiness involved in commodities?

SARS and bird flu are similar from this perspective. Both emerge from the harvesting of meat, and it is suspected that both diseases are transferred to humans at the site of production in the commodity chain. These diseases can trace trails in the kingdom of the ill "reworking ... meaning along different sites in the chain" (Leslie and Reimer 1999, p. 402). Commodity chain analysis allows a structure to be elaborated. To focus on the complex webs of relationships, but also the leakiness in geography and the materiality around nature, food and the city emphasize the unique spatialities of products and chains (Leslie and Reimer 1999, p. 411). Yet if commodities are reduced to an object of pure exchange – detached like the trading of frozen concentrated orange juice on the stock market – the labor, gender, and visceral-ness of food and disease fall to the wayside, resulting in both muted politics and silent risks. Chains vary widely, depending on how products are constructed by varying logics; how discourses and knowledges are distributed and traced (Leslie and Reimer 1999, p. 405). Food commodities must "touch down" in a geographical location.

Food, as a "provising" system, is dependent upon organic material at both ends of the chain. These organic properties, understood as biology and nature, are located both in the land (production) and diet (consumption). Biology "tempers" the political economy of food systems in terms of risk, perishability, seasonality, sustainable production, and labor (Fine and Leopold 1993). This biological temper of food brings to the fore the geographical limits of food chains or the corresponding technological fixes that are required to extend the reach – such as preservatives, freezing, or packaging, generally associated with transnational or industrial food production. From these technological innovations, "the European metropolises ballooned on globally pilfered flesh and fuel, their populations grew ever more distant from the flux and the volatility of the biophysical world" (Clark 2002, p. 116). Presently, oceans cannot separate the volatility of disease; and cities subsisting on pilfered flesh are increasing in number.

Mike Davis declares that the "superurbanization of the human population ... has been paralleled by an equally dense urbanization of the meat supply" (2005, p. 84). In what some are calling the global Livestock Revolution (Delgado 2003), the rapid urbanization of the South is resulting in a growing demand for meat. This Livestock Revolution is enmeshed in what Stassart and Whatmore call "fleshy traffic." Stassart and Whatmore (2003, p. 449) speak to the metabolic exchange in the consumption of flesh from animals that underscores the porous border of our body – imagined to be sealed and contained. Health risks around meat emphasize the "troubling spectres of fleshy mutability that haunt the shadowy regions between field and plate" (ibid.). Fleshy traffic and microbial traffic (McMichael 2001) are intimately linked. The mutability of the meat/flesh comes from livestock intensification. Avian influenza must be distinguished here from civet cats that are luxury goods and that are farmed in much smaller numbers. The fears over avian influenza are based on the large-scale, industrial character of the Livestock Revolution. The traditional small-scale animal production that dominated the Asian region is being abandoned, or marginalized for lack of competitiveness.

The industrial origins of this Livestock Revolution can be found in chicken broiler system that emerged around the 1950s in the southern United States. Broiler chickens became as a fully integrated system of complex processes operating as a single, coordinated entity (Boyd and Watts 1997, p. 192). The character of that regional production complex exhibited flexible and just-in-time manufacturing qualities. The logic of the system was based around the commodity-specific attributes of chicken biology (Boyd and Watts 1997, pp. 194–206). This production system has been was unmoored and exported throughout the world. The corporate agro-food giants of livestock production can exist almost anywhere, completely unmoored from farming. Now systems of warehousing, feed, and poultry are just different forms of inputs and outputs. Workers are reduced to custodians and processors. This Livestock Revolution in the South is supported by advances in biotechnology and life sciences from the North – such as aggregation of production, biosecurity, vaccination, and multiple-stage production systems (Slingenbergh et al. 2004, p. 473). Boyd's history illustrates that broiler chicken industry pioneered this "poultry science" through industrial techniques such as intensive confinement and continuous flow in animals. Throughout the history of the poultry industry, there was the constant battle with disease – testing was institutionalized by the 1950s. There was the continual effort to contain the biology of chickens and the diseases that sprang forth from industrialization. Boyd says that since nature is unpredictable, "any program aimed at the systemic intensification of biological productivity will almost inevitably be confronted with new sources of risk and vulnerability" (Boyd 2001, p. 634). Disease is inherent to the industry. The emergence of livestock diseases and associated zoonotic infections are related to: the intensification of animal production; a "static" environment in which disease can spread; transmission throughout the entire livestock food chain; and the specific ecological characteristics of the disease (Slingenbergh et al. 2004, pp. 470–1). But the space in which these risks and vulnerability intersect is the new development.

The Green Revolution was necessarily tied to suitable land; however, the Livestock Revolution is more footloose. The connections between land and feed have been severed. Location is to be as close to markets as possible, therefore in urban and peri-urban sites that sometimes lack adequate infrastructure. There is a relationship between production and the geographical distance to the nearest megacity due to the perishable nature of animal protein products – processing, distribution, and retail must be immediate. The greater demand for meat, in concert with rising human populations (with rural–urban migration and the economic pressure on land in expanding cities), and the productivity of urban livestock commodities have increasingly become a lucrative business. So while the intensification of livestock has happened, the associated biotechnologies, vaccines, and refrigeration have not been completely instituted (Slingenbergh et al. 2004, pp. 471–8). This is supported by Tu et al. who, while investigating the civet cats for antibodies, found in 41 civet farms in Guangdong province that had fewer than 100 animals, that no "biosecurity measures were used in farms or markets, and no veterinary examination or accreditation was required for civet farming or trading" (Tu et al. 2004, p. 2246).

But how can these industrial forces, that congeal meat into a commodity, be understood with more nuance and intricacy. Kirsh and Mitchell explain how, for Marx, capital as a social relation becomes "frozen" in a commodity through technologies. Commodities are dead labor, "work ossified and made concrete in the shape ... [and] as divisions of labor deepen and become more technical," a commodity becomes more complex and more variegated. The broiler chicken has become a "final, ossified thing … a conglomeration, a stitching together of any number of discrete processes, often occurring over vast stretches of space and time" (Kirsh and Mitchell 2004, pp. 696–7). But when disease is ossified into the commodity, the dead labor can both destroy the laborer and the system of exchange. Dead labor can carry death. Meat is congealed death in both the violence and the processing of production that allows disease to flourish. But in another way, as Bridge and Smith say: "Relieved of their traditional role as the 'dead world' of economic cargoes and anthropological artifacts, commodities – and their circulation – have gained new life" (2003, p. 257). Literally, in the case of disease: commodities are new niches where life thrives. This complicates Derrida's "well-computed binarism," "in which the stuff of the world is 'rigorously divided into remedies and poisons, seeds of life and seeds of death, good and bad traces'" (in Clark 2002, p. 108). Both SARS and avian influenza – indeed, most diseases related to food – are Clark's "demon-seeds of the late modern bestiary" (2002, p. 108). Tim Luke (2000, p. 49) explains that commodities in this bestiary are:

> Endowed with this life of sorts, capital as commodified artifacts can act, becoming a host of artifactants whose alien will, intelligence and matter energize the "animated monster" of all fixed capital collectivized in every commercial society. Dead objects are hardly dead; they are essentially always extrusions undead subjects whom are or which are inseparable from the production of commodities.

These poisonous, animated, meat commodities contaminate both those that shape them and those that consume them. Chicken has begun to be associated with the biophysical processes and labor that brings the meat into freezer sections. Now the blood, feces, and the dirt on the blades across the world can be brought to mind in the very intimate act of eating.

Yet forgetting and displacement is central to consumption. As Robbins (1999, p. 413) states, "Meat's globally ubiquitous class-based appeal is a central dietary element of the alleged democracy brought by modernity and capitalism." In China, a new middle class asserts this modern democratic consumption. Rising urban wealth can be equated to the rise of meat consumption in the Guangdong population (Weiss and MacLean 2004; Zhan 2005). Presently, Zhan explains, in her recent trip to China she experienced "a post-SARS 'feeding frenzy' … people felt as if they had just been released from prison and returned to consumption with a vengeance" (Zhan 2005, pp. 34–5). The social and economic reasons of consumption, the taste of luxury and freshness entailed in civet cats, is central to the class-based signification of meat.

Consumption/Body

There is a fine line between flesh that is human and alive and the dead inert animal for consumption that is labeled meat (Probyn 1999, p. 221). The fine line intersects Callard's concern about the ubiquitous term "body": "I fear that this fascination [with the body] is allowing too many attachments, and rather too many promises of subversion and displacement, to be glued onto the overworked figure of this fantasised body" (Callard 1998, p. 399). This concern over the shortcut of the body is similar to Sontag's dangerous metaphor, a forgetting or erasure of long and hard work that made the concept politically and theoretically robust. The work around the body as the site of disease is not a short cut. Rather, disease is a complicated length-ier route, embroiling science and epidemiology, understanding the body as a porous biological entity. The body is not a trope but a carrier, a niche, a life, and a person with rights. Callard (1998, p. 395) importantly asks "What, to be blunt, does it actually mean to describe a body as hybridised or frag-mented?" The subtleties in food and food-borne disease are one way to answer this, and not subversively or metaphorically, but in terms of how the body in-corporates other materials of nature. The consumption of civet cats and poultry must be shared beyond Guangdong – a collective concern. This is in line with what Whatmore (1997, pp. 43–7) calls a "theory of the flesh" that allows the thickening of embodied, material, and discursive processes. Whatmore's project is to "flesh out" the material dimensions of the practices and technologies of connectivity. The politics and costs of this connectivity are best elucidated in disease. With disease there is the biological materiality, body integrity, the health of populations, but fear and myth. In elaborating one myth, Haraway says:

> [H]istory forces one to remember that the vampire is the figure of the Jew accused of the blood crime of polluting the wellsprings of European germ plasma and bringing both bodily plague and the national decay, or ... The vampires are the immigrants, the dislocated ones, accused of sucking the blood of the rightful possessors of the land ... (Haraway 1997, p. 215)

Blood plasma containing viruses being dislocated from the wild and then polluting the urban cores across the world – these fears have loud echoes. Yet Haraway does not have a monopoly on the vampire. As Marx writes: "Capital is dead labour, that, vampire-like, only lives by sucking living labour, and lives the more, the more labour it sucks" (in Godfrey et al. 2004, p. 26). In the history of capital as vampire, the sleeping victim could be seen as the laboring body.

The first documented SARS case was an animal handler, and with bird flu, the fear is that the laboring body is where the integrity of the human body will be compromised. As Harvey states, in his Marxist discussion of the body, "[c]apital ... frequently violates, disfigures, subdues, maims and destroys the integrity of the laboring body (even in ways that can be dangerous to the accumulation of capital) and does so on an uneven geographical basis" (Harvey 1998, p. 409). In the peri-urban industries, the working conditions for these chicken "custodians" need further investigation, especially in the uneven distribution of risk. Truly, "[h]ealthy bodies may be needed but deformities, pathologies, sickness are often produced" (Harvey 1998, p. 406). Harvey continues as follows: "The working body is more than just meat ... and laborers are more than just 'hands' ... The concept of the body is here in danger of losing its political purchase because it cannot provide a basis to define the *direction* as opposed to the locus of political action" (Harvey 1998, p. 414). Harvey reiterates that to focus on the effects on laboring bodies when inserted into the circulation of capital leads to different political projects. Disease and health could be seen as site for politics to be inserted with Harvey's use of the work of Butler (1993, p. 9), who says "a return to the notion of matter, not as a site or surface, but as a process of materialization that stabilizes over time to produce the effect of boundary, fixity, and surface we call matter" (Harvey 1998, p. 419). SARS showed that boundaries, surfaces, and matters are porous. Then what is in the process of materializing when bodies intermingle with animals under intense conditions of production? The transfer point at which the flows of capital and flows of blood materialize into disease could be seen in the city.

All Pooled Together ... Wet Markets

In the city, Clark states, there is the convergence of "the environmentalist belief in a nature which 'stays put' and the cosmopolitan celebration of culture free of groundedness and material responsibilities—[which] can be seen as derivatives of the same metropolitan detachment from the daily dynamics of bio-materiality" (Clark 2002, p. 117). The dynamics of bio-materiality – commodities being one dynamic – continuously flow into and pools together in the city. Instead of networks or chains that link food and disease together, perhaps we should be looking for "thickened connections" (Crang 1996, p. 57) where, like blood, relations congeal – scars stitch fleshy traffic together. First suggested by Thrift and Olds (1996), blood and flows are a metaphor for understanding the economy and the connections between cities. This insight can be extended for the human/non-human relationship. Castree (2001) invoked an affinity with the blood metaphor and the flows of materiality when he examined commodities and ANT. The ANT approach envisions a geographical imagination that is pluralized, multiperspectival, and reflexive; where multiple cultures, places, and ecologies, in Cook and Crang's words, "bleed into and mutually constitute one another" (in Castree 2001, p. 1520). This envisioning of the city works well with Marxist analysis of urban metabolism, illustrated through the example of wet markets.

Wet markets (or live animal markets) can be found in many countries throughout the world. There is usually carry-over of animals from one day to the next, and more expensive animals can stay from days to weeks; daily introduction of new animals provides ripe conditions for disease agents such as influenza (Webster 2004, p. 234). Tu et al., in their investigation of SARS antibodies in civet cats, concluded that the animal reservoir for the disease was in the wet markets due to multiple species in close proximity, not the farming practices (2004, p. 2246). The "wet" comes from the constant drenching of these stalls with water, which coincides with the fresh slaughter of live animals. This local freshness is where disease flourishes. This call and response of flows of blood and flows of water is indicative of the flux of biomaterials and market forces. Since the SARS outbreak some are calling for the global banning of wet markets. Yet as there are concerns of the legal repercussions of forcing thousands of business owners and workers out of business, and perhaps driving the wet markets underground, far from surveillance in that "wet markets serve as an early warning system" (Webster 2004, p. 236). In some cases, these monitoring systems and control of specific meat markets have been institutionalized. In Hong Kong after 1997's influenza outbreak, all aquatic birds were eliminated from the markets and now are sold chilled; a sample of each truckload of poultry is analyzed when entering Hong Kong (Webster 2004, p. 235). These wet markets are very local "hot zones," where social process, material metabolism, and spatial forms clot together, but when something goes wrong these clots can arrest the flow of people and commodities.

Wet markets are a useful illustration of Marxist understandings of urban metabolism, which, as a concept, is particularly open to relational or hybrid understandings of the city. Gandy explains that, "urban metabolism—with emphasis on phenomena such as commodity chains, the particulars of local context and the fluidity of urban form—are quite different from non-dialectical models of urban metabolism rooted in a homeostatic conception of the city as a self-regulating system" (Gandy 2004, p. 374). The SARS case should put at least one nail in the coffin of the homeostatic city – no city is self-regulating. In terms of wet markets, there are two sides to this illustration. The wetness is the cleansing in concert with the blood, the biology, flows of materiality, and the risks that ride those flows. On the market side of things, there are the forces of supply and demand; the political economy where commodities are acquired and exchanged – even cheap deals have hidden costs. It is the act of consumption – both in terms of monetary and brute physicality – that pools the flows in economy and biology. Marx took inspiration from von Liebig, who gave organisms a metabolic history-as-process that intermingled spaces of production and consumption in the city. Marx borrowed this metabolic interaction, the original German term being *stoffwechsel*, literally translated as "change of matter," which implies circulation, exchange, and transformation of material elements (Swyngedouw and Heynen 2003, p. 905). Commodities, disease, and money are all circulated in wet markets. As specific biological materials are transconfigured, new entities emerge from these processes – one being the SARS virus. The emergence of SARS from these wet markets brings home the implications of urban metabolism. Swyngedouw and Heynen clarify that "[n]ew socionatural forms are continuously produced as moments and things in this molecular metabolic process of accumulation" (2003, p. 905). As wet markets or urban poultry producers accumulate more and more animals; the biophysical intensifies and metabolizes new or transformed microbial agents.

But wet markets are also a pool for stereotypes. The international media linked what they termed the "age-old tradition" of eating wild animals with what Zhan calls "the deadly filthiness of such entanglements" (2005, p. 37). Zhan provides a Reuters report (2003, October 27) that should be repeated at length:

> Two little boys giggle as they play hide and seek among hundreds of filthy cages packed tight with civet cats, dogs, porcupines and squirrels … Amid the stench of death and decay, traders of exotic animals … haggle over prices with customers … Narrow passageways are strewn with animal dung, urine, entrails and grimy fodder … A few steps away, men with iron pipes clubbed a dog unconscious and slit its throat. Others squatted around another dead dog, plucking it clean of hair with their bare fingers. (Zhan 2005, p. 37)

The historical echoes of this act must be flagged. The first is the sensational quasi-reporting by Upton Sinclair's *The Jungle* (2003) that opened the doors of the Chicago stockyards of the early 1900s. Sinclair's widely read exposé spawned the Food and Drug Administration in the United States. The Orientalism and the racial qualities of the Reuters report can be seen in the disgust with certain practices and the "racial signification" of the accusation,[2] together with the sense of outrage – "you eat that, under these conditions, you put those children in danger." The last echo from history is the surveillance of "how the other half lives" by Victorian-era sanitary police – the monitoring of the "unwashed masses." Over SARS and avian influenza we see the resurgence of what Gandy (2004) calls the "bacteriological city" and the corresponding resurrection of a "hygienist city" or "antibiotic urbanism."

But the blame should not be placed on the butchers, or Guangdong, or even China, because, as Marx declares, out-sensationalizing Reuters, "Capital comes dripping from head to foot, from every pore, with blood and dirt" (Godfrey et al. 2004, p. 26).

Dripping Commodities in the City

As Castree suggests, "commodities are transgressive: they are both things and relations, particular and general, local and global, here and there. The capitalist commodity works in a space of flows and a web of interconnections where the 'insides' and the 'outsides' of places, peoples, and ecologies become ever harder to fathom" (2001, p. 1522). Yet in the flow of the wet market, the transgression is by little microorganisms and viruses that navigate these interconnections on the backs of commodities. Theory and metaphor should not contribute to symbolic injustice or racial stereotypes of wet markets, Guangdong, or China. Rather than blame the people of Guangdong as the problem, this chapter has looked to spread the responsibility. The risky, visceral component of meat is pandemic. Avian influenza shows these relationships are diffused. SARS-stock provided an example of how the porousness of the city bleeds into the markets of Guangdong and the cattle lots of Alberta. In the flow of materials through spatial arteries – that link the wild to livestock, the rural to the urban, the intestines of birds to the stomachs of humans – what should be clear is the heart that pumps these flows is the market. These dripping commodities must touch down, and this is where multiple processes such as ecology, culture, place, and politics bleed into one another.

What does this portend for the future? McMichael (2001) proposes that we are entering a new great historical transition; a resurgence of disease spurned by intensified human, animal, and environmental relations. But beyond environmental indicators, we should unpack the security, control, and stigma involved in the institutionalization of a global "sanitary utopia" (McMichael 2001, p. 114). For food, perhaps "careful consumption," raised by Crewe (2001), will rise to the surface. This may mean, according to Castree (2001) "getting with the fetish" in commodities. There is already a double fetish in the thing-like quality of social relations, and how we imagine and construct our connections to the risky geography of commodities. Yet perhaps a third fetish could be added; the older understanding of fetish where the commodity and the religious come crashing together. The WHO may be the new rabbis, with a new form of international halal. Will meat be ceremoniously drained of all blood, all impurities? With new rituals from science and the formalities in bureaucracy, the purifying of meat may mean the tracing and certifying of all the materials that make up our food. But as

Latour (1988, p. 35) reminds us, "Cholera is no respecter of Mecca, it enters the intestine of the hadji." Diseases have the acute ability to cross any border that we throw up.

NOTES

1 The terms "fleshy traffic" and "feverish borders," used here and in the chapter title, are taken from Whatmore (2004) and Stassart and Whatmore (2003), respectively.
2 See Timothy Choy's discussion of wet markets in San Francisco in Zhan (2005, p. 38).

Concluding Remarks

Roger Keil and S. Harris Ali

The most fundamental issue this book has sought to address was the question of how pathogens interact with biophysical, political, economic, and cultural factors to produce and eventually control a contemporary urban disease outbreak. The sheer quantity of variables involved, and the complexity of the interactions amongst them (operating at and across different scales – local, regional, national, and global), necessitated the need to find a more encompassing approach. Correspondingly, the analytical challenge was to develop an appropriate perspective through which we could approach this seemingly unwieldy problematic in a manageable way. A clue to a potentially suitable entry point came from our initial observations that SARS spread through a network of economically and cultural significant cities – that is, "global cities" that were linked together through the flows of people, information, capital, resources, technologies, and so on (Ali and Keil 2006). From here it was soon realized that perhaps the notion of *networks* itself could serve as central concept that would enable us to incorporate the myriad of factors implicated in the spread of SARS into our study, while at the same time allowing us to adequately capture the inherent complexity of an urban disease outbreak as an emergent phenomenon. In this light, one of the major objectives of this volume was to explicate the role of global networks (and networks more generally) in the contemporary *spread of infectious disease*. If networks were instrumental for the spread of disease, then important issues still remained for us as social scientists, specifically those concerning the *political and socio-cultural ramifications* of such networked spread.

We took up these questions by investigating the unique challenges that the spread of disease through the global cities network had for *urban health governance* and the *cultural politics* of these cities.

It is evident from many of the chapters in this book that both the microbial traffic and pathogen ecology of infectious diseases today are influenced by the nature of global cities and the networked connections amongst them. Attempts to characterize this connectivity and to analyze the implications of this for the spread and reaction to infectious diseases are challenging for several reasons. Perhaps the most significant of these reasons is the fact that the cities themselves are in a constant state of flux; thus the connections between cities are likewise always changing. Cities are in a constant process of internal change; thus, for example, Marcuse and Van Kempen note that "The center of cities decline or change form and functions, and new business districts spring up; immigrants cluster together and mix with others; ethnic and racial groups are segregated in ghettoes and slums; or they escape to more liveable neighbourhoods; new cultural enclaves are formed, while old ones disappear; new forms of cities are created at the edges of metropolitan areas; suburbanization never seems to end" (2000, p. 1). At the same time, the networked flows of people, resources, capital, and so on that connect the cities have intensified with globalization. That is, as Estair Van Wagner (Chapter 1), S. Harris Ali (Chapter 14), and Bruce Braun (Chapter 15) have noted, the city as a convergence site of many different flows has become an ever-changing and emergent nexus of forces. Each contributing flow has its own distinct "rhythm," and the convergence of the different flows results in the emergence of the city that takes the form of a dynamic, polyrhythmic, and porous entity (Smith 2003). When the fluid and networked character of our cities is taken into account, new questions concerning infectious disease arise. For example: How has institutional governance and regulation changed to meet the challenges of the globalized fluidity of global cities and their network connections? What new issues of urban vulnerability to disease and questions of public health "security" have arisen within this context? What new public health infrastructures are being put into place?[1] What are the new forms of inequality, the racialization of disease and citizenship rights that can be discerned under these circumstances? In fact, it could even be asked if we are indeed dealing with new issues or simply with old issues in new form. The contributions in this book have sought answers to these types of questions. In what follows, we discuss some of the general implications of these works for understanding the relationship of cities with infectious disease *vis-à-vis* networks, governance, and culture, as well as what the study of such relationships means for the field of urban studies more generally.

From the standpoint of the potential global threat of infectious disease spread, the work presented in this book suggests that we may have to rethink our common perception of what urban governance entails. That is, urban governance may soon have to be more centrally concerned with questions of widespread disease, life, and death (Agamben 2002) and the construction of new internal boundaries and regulations just at the time as globalization seems to suggest the breakdown of some traditional scalar incisions such as national borders. Thus, we now have to consider how the development of a post-Westphalian constellation places new demands on the governance of urban regions.[2] For example, how do disease and health issues impact the rearrangement of the governance of public/private space in cities? Clearly, the case studies reviewed in this book indicate that hospitals, quarantine, and cultural spaces were fundamentally reassessed in the aftermath of SARS, with the concomitant recalibration of their place in the order of public and private everyday lives and the official geographies of the city. As such, in light of SARS and other EIDs, more general questions arise. For example: What are acceptable uses of space by various bodies in cities? Or, how do everyday uses of city space, both private and public, intersect with the geographies of health and disease? Sometimes the physical geography of health care changed during SARS (in Beijing, for example, a new hospital was built to fight the disease); in other cases, the geography of hospital care is associated more closely with specific user groups (Chinese-Canadians; homeless people). Homes (in Toronto) or recreational spaces (in Hong Kong) are turned into quarantine areas, and culturally marked neighborhoods (e.g., Chinatown in Toronto) become signifiers of infected space. While purification and biopolitics were the characteristics associated with the hygienic city of the last century, we have now entered a phase in which the potential re-emergence of infectious disease at a mass scale forces us to rethink the relationship of our built environments, our institutional arrangements, and our practices as urban dwellers. This has to do as much with the changing nature of cities as basing points of the global economy – to use quite a conventional concept from global cities theory – as with the kinds of re-emerging diseases with which we now have to deal.

Policy-makers and planners have taken up the challenge presented to them by SARS and other EIDs. Reactions have spanned a broad spectrum from affirmative "new normalization" in the wake of 9/11 to critical assessments of progressive urban policy in a period of globally constituted medical emergencies. Matthew and McDonald have argued, for example, in the *Journal of the American Planning Association*, that: "it is important to ask what cities should do to prepare for a major disease event." They address this issue by posing a set of important technical questions:

Do urban health care systems have adequate surveillance and surge capacity? Have cities stockpiled appropriate medications and worked out effective quarantine, evacuation, distribution, and risk communication strategies? Are regional cooperation protocols in place? Is decision-making authority clearly established at the most desirable level? Are linkages between the private and public sectors, and across government agencies secure and have they been tested? And are lines of communication established to ensure access to information, including classified information, and other forms of assistance that may be required? (2006, p. 109)

In answering these questions, the authors employ "scale-free" network theory to advise American city leaders of the dangers of today's networked world: "Cities now connect to the world through multiple pathways, each made up of many links. City leaders and planners should not assume that external threats are being deterred or managed effectively at the federal level, as they were during the Cold War era. Instead, they should assess the vulnerabilities and resources of their particular communities, and plan security postures that complement or even act independently of national security policy" (2006, p. 112). Pointing out that the current infectious disease threats "fall outside the routine experiences of urban public health officials and doctors" (2006, p. 113), Matthew and Macdonald recommend that "planners seek out and work with both public and private sector groups with roles in disaster planning; design land and transportation planning information systems to aid an support decision makers during crises; encourage greater self-sufficiency in food production and consumption; assist in the design of humane, realistic evacuation strategies and routes; and consider the effects of their day-to-day recommendations to disease risk and response" (2006, pp. 113–15; see also Malizia 2006). It is against just such a backdrop that Ali et al. (2006) warn against security excesses in urban emergency planning and point explicitly to the "messiness of urban life" as a reminder of the challenges faced in the process of establishing a policy that respects civil rights and democratic process.

The analyses presented in this book have added two important dimensions to this type of work which we believe will increase our understanding of the role of urban health governance in the fight against EIDs. First, they highlight the point that the governance of cities today is unimaginable without the modern constitution of the "bacteriological city" at its base (Gandy 2005), which created and institutionalized managerial processes of technological, engineering, and scientific nature required to guarantee a modicum of public health; and to lay the foundation of an economic development and demographic growth ostensibly unencumbered by the incalculable onset of disease outbreaks, which had wreaked havoc upon urban populations and their economies until the twentieth century in Europe and North America. It is on the basis of this century-old history that we now need to rethink urban health governance. Second, it is necessary to extend our view beyond the national institutional level when looking at the governance of EIDs in cities, as extra-national organizations such as the US Centers for Disease Control (CDC) and supra-national organizations such as the World Health Organization (WHO) exert significant influence on urban health governance in any country, sometimes not even mediated through national policy or institutions as conventionally dictated by the scalar chain of command (Fidler 2004; Heymann 2005). Understanding these types of changing configurations in the exercise of political power will undoubtedly have a key role to play in analyzing how the public health security state establishes itself in a globalized world. This is seen, for example, in considering the relationship between the WHO and the City of Toronto. Some critics have argued that it was political economic pressures (and not health-based concerns) that persuaded federal and municipal officials to lobby for the lifting of the WHO travel advisory imposed on Toronto (Walkom 2003). In effect, the WHO travel alert essentially jeopardized the world city status of Toronto, and local political and economic elites stepped in to lift the stigma of the travel alert, to restore that status in the eyes of the world community. Such efforts, critics contend, led to a premature lessening of public health vigilance in regard to SARS in Toronto (Boyle 2003). On the other hand, others, such as the WHO director of communicable disease surveillance, have argued that the WHO travel advisory imposed on Toronto would ultimately harm the fight against SARS, as other world cities may become less forthcoming in reporting outbreaks (or be less open) because of the fear of economic consequences and stigma in the global city network (Galloway 2003). In any case, both positions illustrate how the health security state may be influenced/compromised in today's network of world cities. Furthermore, such shifts in public health governance have implications for the cultural politics of the city, particularly as influenced through biopolitical machinations that are in turn influenced by larger socio-political currents such as those associated with neoliberalization and the ideological thrust of post-9/11 "securitization."

Peterson and Lupton (1996) note that the governmentality that regulates disease has shifted from the collective to the individual. This is a major biopolitical shift, which is mostly played out at the level of urban governance. In the contemporary period, health and disease have been recast as individual responsibilities rather than social ones (Petersen and Lupton 1996; Sanford and Ali 2005). It is exactly this – neoliberal – governmentality of individualized notions of health and sickness that existed when SARS arrived. It is within this contextual framework that we have to understand the new thinking and agency around infectious disease in the city. It adds to the general shift in the current city from traditional notions of control in favor of a more broadly orchestrated mix of state and market interventions. Public health governance in the age of SARS has – at least potentially – moved to a bundle of strategies that fit well into the overall securitization of urban society: "The hygienist discourses of the past have been radically extended by new technologies of surveillance and control in order to construct the *cordons sanitaires* of the twenty-first century. New defensive structures have developed that combine long-standing mechanisms of social exclusion such as housing markets with enhanced forms of social control through a mix of architectural, ideological and intelligence-gathering processes" (Gandy 2005, p. 33).

The SARS outbreak response also occurred within the context of the "new normal" – a state of affairs based on an increased vigilance of, and attention to, matters of "security" in the post-9/11 era. The "security state" of the new normal has increased the range of its power to control its subjects in an ever-expanding field of human activity, including control through the monitoring and surveillance of email exchanges and website postings, telephone messages, the monitoring of public spaces through closed circuit television cameras, and so on. It could be said that with SARS, the global security state (in the form of the WHO) had extended its range into the field of health care as the movement of people, particularly air travelers but also those visiting and working in hospitals, became closely monitored and justified on the basis of "public health security." Similarly, at the local level, the degree to which the security state had expanded its power varied from global city to global city, as revealed with the very tight security and surveillance measures adopted in Singapore compared to Hong Kong and Toronto. Second, the emergence of an intensified security state was reinforced by broader neoliberal trends in governance, whereby the state has become "hollowed out" (Jessop 2000) – retreating from traditional spheres of governance by implementing policies of deregulation and downloading to private corporations, particularly in the healthcare sector. This has allowed market hegemony to enter into significant segments of the healthcare sectors – sectors that were previously the sole jurisdiction of governments. For example, in Singapore, the city-state government offloaded the responsibility for the surveillance and monitoring of quarantined individuals to a private security company.

Where the opening of borders had meant progress for the proponents of globalization, they now constituted a threat to communities that were vulnerable not just to financial disinvestment and de-industrialization, but also to new health threats. The perceptions of "others" as health threats was undoubtedly reinforced at a subtle and tacit level in the wake of the attacks of 9/11, and the "new normal." Under such social and political circumstances, infection may become the "metaphorical essence" of globalization (Sarasin 2006), in which the dark side of globalization rears its head in the form of the insidious threat based on the association of viral invaders as human invaders from outside, where the "other" is seen as a menacing threat – illustrated, for example, by the "racialization of disease" described by

Roger Keil and S. Harris Ali (Chapter 9) and Susan Craddock (Chapter 11). The racialization of disease and racial profiling are examples of other forms of inequality that may arise with the adoption of biosecurity measures, but it should also be noted that the differential adherence to and enforcement of biosecurity measures also have implications for the inequalities in global health, and that they bring to the fore the issue of what should be considered a "global good" (and by whom?).

Fidler (2004) argues that the control of SARS was a global good because it benefited more than one region or continent, but Guilloux (2006) questions the criteria used to make this assessment. Citing Fidler's own observations, Guilloux notes that although malaria affects hundreds of millions and kills over one million in the global South, this disease does not qualify as a global disease because the cross-border transmission is low, leaving us "wondering whether a disaster has to threaten rich people seriously, if it wants to be recognized as global" (2006, p. 62). The emphasis on the health problems of the wealthy, as opposed to the health of all, is reflected in the analysis by Matthew Gandy (Chapter 10). For example, Gandy notes that the developed world's (but particularly the American) preoccupation with bioterrorism threats, under the mantle of national biosecurity, has resulted in drastic reductions in research funding for other diseases, especially those affecting the global South, thus intensifying the global inequalities in health. A further example of this is given by Susan Craddock (Chapter 11), in her analysis of tuberculosis. Craddock notes that tuberculosis (like malaria) is not particularly feared in the global North (except perhaps in its antibiotic resistant form), because the disease is associated with largely disenfranchised groups, such as immigrants, the homeless, and the imprisoned, and as such, is relegated to the lowest levels in the hierarchy of public health concerns. Similarly, Victor Rodwin (Chapter 2) demonstrates that even *within* the largest global cities of the developed world, it is the poor and vulnerable subpopulations that are disproportionately affected by infectious disease – a situation that is significantly exacerbated because national health policies and systems tend to neglect the plight of these subpopulations.

In sum, it can be noted that, among other things, what the SARS outbreaks in global cities around the world have demonstrated is the extreme vulnerability of places in the global economy to rapid changes brought on by the acceleration of social and ecological relationships. Such an acceleration has occurred through increased technological connectivity and an extended interdependence of societies and economies around the world. At the same time, reaction and response to disease outbreaks in our "networked society" have provided us with an opportunity to understand the impacts that changing social and political currents such as neoliberalism and the "new normal" now have on our lives, as related to an almost countless number of public and private aspects of daily life, including issues involving governance, biosecurity, health policy, multiculturalism, inequality, our relations with animals, technology and the media, changing social norms related to hygiene, and so on. Consideration and further analysis of such issues will undoubtedly be of critical import in the future as an increasingly urbanized, yet globalized, world is forced to contend with the next EID threat, such as possibly the human-to-human transmission of avian flu.

NOTES

1 Defined as "the capacity of local officials to perform the core functions of public health": assessment, policy development, assurance (Rodwin and Gusmano 2002, p. 446 fn.).

2 " 'Westphalian' refers to the governance framework that defined international public health activities from the mid-nineteenth century," based on the political logic of sovereign nation-states that had come into existence after the Thirty Years War (Fidler 2003, pp. 485–6).

Bibliography

Abraham, T. (2004) *Twenty-First Century Plague: The Story of SARS.* Baltimore: Johns Hopkins University Press.

Abu-Lughod, J. (1999) *New York, Chicago, Los Angeles: America's Global Cities.* Minneapolis: Minnesota University Press.

Adam, B., U. Beck, and J. Van Loon. (2000) *The Risk Society and Beyond: Critical Issues for Social Theory.* London: Sage.

Affonso, D., G. Andrews, and L. Jeffs. (2004) "The Urban Geography of SARS: Paradoxes and Dilemmas in Toronto's Health Care." *Journal of Advanced Nursing* 45(6): 568–78.

Agamben, G. (1998) Homo sacer: *Sovereign Power and Bare Life*, translated by D. Heller Roazen. Stanford: Stanford University Press.

Agamben, G. (2002) Homo sacer: *die souveräne Macht und das nackte Leben.* Frankfurt am Main: Suhrkamp.

Akeroyd, A. (2004) "Coercion, Constraints, and 'Cultural Entrapments': A Further Look at Gendered and Occupational Factors Pertinent to the Transmission of HIV in Africa." In E. Kalipeni, S. Craddock, J.R. Oppong, and J. Ghosh, J. (eds.), *HIV and AIDS in Africa: Beyond Epidemiology.* Oxford: Blackwell, pp. 89–103.

Alagiri, P., T. Summers, and J. Kates. (2002) *Spending on HIV/AIDS in Resource-Poor Settings.* Henry J. Kaiser Family Foundation/Ford Foundation. Online at: http://www.kff.org/hivaids/loader.cfm?url=/commonspot/security/getfile.cfm&PageID=28514 (accessed November 14, 2004).

Alexy, B., B. Nichols, M.A. Heverly, and L. Garzon. (1997) "Prenatal Factors and Birth Outcomes in the Public Health Service: A Rural/Urban Comparison." *Research in Nursing & Health* 20: 61–70.

Ali, S.H. (2004) "A Socio-Ecological Autopsy of the *E. coli* O157:H7 Outbreak in Walkerton, Ontario, Canada." *Social Science and Medicine* 58(12): 2601–12.

Ali, S.H., and R. Keil. (2006) "Global Cities and the Spread of Infectious Disease: The Case of Severe Acute Respiratory Syndrome (SARS) in Toronto, Canada." *Urban Studies* 43(3): 491–509.

Ali, S.H., R. Keil, C. Major, and E. Van Wagner. (2006) "Pandemics, Place and Planning: Learning from SARS." *Plan Canada* 46(3): 34–6.

Allahwala, A. (2006) "Investigating Biopolitics: Promises and Limitations." *Capitalism, Nature, Socialism* 17(1): 50–7.

Alland, D., G. Kalkut, A. Moss, et al. (1994) "Transmission of Tuberculosis in New York City: An Analysis by DNA Fingerprinting and Conventional Epidemiologic Methods." *New England Journal of Medicine* 330(24): 1710–16.

Amin, A., and N. Thrift. (2002) *Cities: Reimagining the Urban.* Cambridge: Polity Press.

Anderson, K. (1992) *Vancouver's Chinatown: Racial Discourse in Canada, 1874–1980.* Kingston: McGill-Queen's University Press.

Anderson, W. (1996) "Immunities of Empire: Race, Disease, and the New Tropical Medicine, 1900–1920." *Bulletin of the History of Medicine* 70(1): 94–118.

Andrulis, D.P. (1997) "The Urban Health Penalty: New Dimensions and Directions in Inner-City Health Care." In *Inner City Health Care.* Philadelphia, PA: American College of Physicians.

Angell, M. (2004) *The Truth about Drug Companies: How They Deceive Us and What to Do About It.* New York: Random House.

Appadurai, A. (1996) *Modernity at Large: Cultural Dimensions of Globalization.* Minneapolis: University of Minnesota Press.

Appadurai, A. (2002) "Deep Democracy: Urban Governmentality and the Horizon of Politics." *Public Culture* 14: 21–47.

Apple Daily. (2003) "Infection Route of Life-Threatening Pneumonia," February 11, 2003 (in Chinese).

Arguin, P.M., A.W. Navin, S.F. Steele, L.H. Weld, and P.E. Kozarsky. (2004) "Health Communication during SARS (Preparedness and Response)." *Emerging Infectious Diseases* 10(2): 377–80.

Armstrong, P., and H. Armstrong. (2003) *Wasting Away: The Undermining of Canadian Health Care,* 2nd edn. Oxford: Oxford University Press.

Asian Pacific Post. (2003) "Killer Virus Also Causing Severe Acute Racism Syndrome." April 10. Online at: http://www.asianpacificpost.com (accessed April 28, 2005).

Atlas, R. (1999) "Combating the Threat of Biowarfare and Bioterrorism." *BioScience* 49: 465–77.

Attaran, A., K.I. Barnes, C. Curtis, et al. (2004) WHO, the Global Fund, and Medical Malpractice in Malaria Treatment." *The Lancet* 363: 237–40.

Baehr, P. (2006) "Susan Sontag, Battle Language and the Hong Kong SARS Outbreak of 2003." *Economy and Society* 35(1): 42–64.

Ballard, J.G. (2000) *Super-Cannes.* New York: Picador.

Banta, J.E. (2001) "Commentary: From International Health to Global Health." *Journal of Community Health* 26(2): 73–7.

Bardsley, M. (1999) *Health in Europe's Capitals.* Project Megapoles, Directorate of Public Health, East London and the City Health Authority, London.

Barnett, T. (2002) *AIDS in the 21st Century: Disease and Globalization*. London: Palgrave.

Barrett, R., C.W. Kuzawa, T. McDade, and G.J. Armelagos. (1998) "Emerging and Re-Emerging Infectious Diseases: The Third Epidemiologic Transition." *Annual Revirew of Anthropology* 27: 247–71.

Barss, P. (1992) "Epidemic Field Investigation as Applied to Allegations of Chemical, Biological, or Toxin Warfare." *Politics and the Life Sciences* 11(5).

Bashford, A. (2004) *Imperial Hygiene: A Critical History of Colonialism, Nationalism and Public Health*. London: Palgrave.

Basrur, S.V., B. Yaffe, and B. Henry. (2004) "SARS: A Local Public Health Perspective." *Canadian Journal of Public Health* 95(1): 22–4.

Bauman, Z. (2004) *Wasted Lives: Modernity and its Outcasts*. Cambridge: Polity Press.

Bayer, R., and A. Fairchild. (2002) "The Limits of Privacy: Surveillance and the Control of Disease." *Health Care Analysis* 10: 19–35.

Beaverstock, J.V., R.G. Smith, R.G., and P.J. Taylor. (2000) "World City Network: A New Metageography?" *Annals of the Association of American Geographers* (Millennial Issue) 90: 123–34.

Beck, U. (1992) *The Risk Society: Towards a New Modernity*. London: Sage.

Bein, A. (1964) "The Jewish Parasite: Notes on the Semantics of the Jewish Problem with Special Reference to Germany." *Yearbook of the Leo Baeck Institute* 9: 3–40.

Bell, D.J., S. Robertson, and P. Hunter. (2005) "Animal Origins of SARS Coronavirus: Possible Links with the International Trade in Small Carnivores." In A.R. McLean, R.M. May, J. Pattison, and R. Weiss (eds.), *SARS: A Case Study in Emerging Infections*. New York: Oxford University Press, pp. 51–60.

Bellamy, R., C. Ruewnde, T. Corrah, K. McAdam, H. Whittle, and A. Hill. (1998) "Variations in the NRAMP1 Gene and Susceptibility to Tuberculosis in West Africans." *New England Journal of Medicine* 338(10): 640–4.

Bellush, J., and D. Netzer. (1997) *Capital Divided*. London: London Research Centre.

Benbow, N., Y. Wang, and S. Whitman. (1998) *Big Cities Health Inventory, 1997: The Health of Urban USA*. Chicago: Department of Health.

Benitez, M.A. (2003) "Health Chief Admits SARS Flaws." *South China Morning Post*, August 23, 2003, EDT1.

Bergeron, S.L., and A.L. Sanchez. (2004) "Media Effects on Students during SARS Outbreak." *Emerging Infectious Diseases* 11(5): 732–4.

Berkowitz, B. (2006) "Christian Groups Find New Allies at USAID." *Inter Press Service News* Agency (January 17). Online at: http://www.ipsnews.net (accessed June 7, 2006).

Berry, B. (1961) *Central Place Studies*. Philadelphia, PA: Regional Science Research Institute.

Bestor, T. (1989) *Neighborhood Tokyo*. Stanford: Stanford University Press.

Bingham, N., and N. Thrift. (2000) "Some New Instructions for Travelers: The Geography of Bruno Latour and Michel Serres," In M. Crang and N. Thrift (eds.), *Thinking Space*. London: Routledge, pp. 281–301.

Birdlife International. (2006) "Birdlife International Statement on Avian Influenza." Online at: http://www.birdlife.org/action/science/species/avian_flu/.

Bloom, B. (2002) "Tuberculosis – The Global View." *New England Journal of Medicine* 346(19): 1434–5.

Board on International Health, Institute of Medicine. (1997) *America's Vital Interest in Global Health: Protecting Our People, Enhancing Our Economy, and Advancing Our International Interests.* Washington, DC: National Academies Press.

Body-Gendrot, S. (1996) "Paris: A 'Soft' Global City?" *New Community* 22: 595–605.

Bond, M. (1991) *Beyond the Chinese Face: Insights from Psychology.* Oxford: Oxford University Press.

Booker, M.K. (1994) *The Dystopian Impulse in Modern Literature: Fiction as Social Criticism.* Westport, CT: Greenwood.

Booth, C.M., and T.E. Stewart. (2005) "Severe Acute Respiratory Syndrome and Critical Care Medicine: The Toronto Experience." *Critical Care Medicine* 33(1) Supplement: S53–60.

Borgdorff, M.W., M.A. Behr, N.J.D. Nagelkerke, P.C. Hopewell, and P.M. Small. (2000) "Transmission of Tuberculosis in San Francisco and its Association with Immigration and Ethnicity." *International Journal of Tuberculosis and Lung Disease* 4(4): 287–94.

Boseley, S. (2004) "France Accuses US of Aids Blackmail." *The Guardian* (London), July 14.

Boseley, S. (2006a) "Aids Pandemic Spreading to Every Corner of the Globe, Says the UN." *The Guardian* (London), May 31.

Boseley, S. (2006b) "World Bank Accused of Deception over Malaria." *The Guardian* (London), June 3.

Boudreau, J.-A., R. Keil, and D. Young. (forthcoming) *Changing Toronto: Governing the In-Between the Global and the Local.* Toronto: Broadview Press.

Boudreau, J.-A., P. Hamel, B. Jouve, and R. Keil. (2006) "Comparing Metropolitan Governance: The Cases of Montreal and Toronto." *Progress in Planning* 66(1): 7–59.

Boudreau, J.-A., P. Hamel, B. Jouve, and R. Keil. (2007) "New State Spaces in Canada: Metropolitanization in Montreal and Toronto Compared." *Urban Geography* 28(1): 30–53.

Bournes, D.A., and M. Ferguson-Paré. (2005) "Persevering through a Difficult Time during the SARS Outbreak in Toronto." *Nursing Science Quarterly* 18(4): 324–33.

Boyd, W. (2001) "Making Meat: Science, Technology, and American Poultry Production." *Technology and Culture* 42: 631–64.

Boyd, W., and M. Watts. (1997) "Agro-Industrial Just-in-Time: The Chicken Industry and Postwar American Capitalism." In D. Goodman and M. Watts (eds.), *Globalising Food: Agrarian Questions and Global Restructuring.* New York: Routledge.

Boyle, T. (2003) "York Central Doctor Claims Province Eased up on SARS: Political Pressure Blamed as 'Guard Let Down.'" *The Toronto Star*, May 27, p. A6.

Braun, B. (2007) "Biopolitics and the Molecularization of Life." *Cultural Geographies* 14(1): 6–28.

Braun, L. (2002) "Race, Ethnicity, and Health: Can Genetics Explain Disparities?" *Perspectives in Biology and Medicine* 45(2): 159–74.

Breakwell, G.M., and J. Barnett. (2003) "Social Amplification of Risk and the Layering Method." In N.F. Pidgeon, R.E. Kasperson, and P. Slovic (eds.), *The Social Amplification of Risk.* Cambridge: Cambridge University Press, pp. 80–101.

Breiman, R.F., M.R. Evans, W. Preiser, J. Maquire, A. Schnur, A. Li, et al. (2003) "Role of China in the Quest to Define and Control SARS." In S. Knobler, A. Mahmoud, S. Lemon, et al. (eds.), *Learning from SARS: Preparing for the Next Outbreak*. Washington, DC: The National Academies Press.

Brenner, N. (2000) "The Urban Question as a Scale Question: Reflections on Henri Lefebvre, Urban Theory and Politics of Scale." *International Journal of Urban and Regional Research* 24(2): 361–73.

Brenner, N., and R. Keil (eds.). (2006) *The Global Cities Reader*. New York: Routledge.

Bridge, G., and A. Smith. (2003) "Intimate Encounters: Culture—Economy—Commodity." *Environment and Planning D: Society and Space* 21(3): 257–68.

BBC (British Broadcasting Corporation). (2003) "Text of Blair's Speech." Online at: http://news.bbc.co.uk/2/hi/uk_news/politics/3076253.stm

Brown, C. (2004a) "Emerging Zoonoses and Pathogens of Public Health Significance – An Overview." In B. Vallat and L. King (eds.), *Emerging Zoonoses and Pathogens of Public Health Concern. OIE Scientific and Technical Review* 23(2): 435–42.

Brown, S. (2004b) "The Economic Impact of SARS." In C. Loh and Civic Exchange (eds.), *At the Epicentre: Hong Kong and the SARS Outbreak*. Hong Kong: Hong Kong University Press, pp. 179–93.

Buehler, J.W., R. Berkelman, D. Hartley, and C. Peters. (1995) CISET (Committee on International Science, Engineering and Technology). *Global Microbial Threats in the 1990s: Report of the Committee on International Science, Engineering and Technology's Working Group on Emerging and Reemerging Infectious Diseases*. Washington, DC: National Science and Technology Council, 3 pp.

Buehler, J.W., R.L. Berkelman, D.M. Hartley, and C.J. Peters. (2003) "Syndromic Surveillance and Bioterrorism-Related Epidemics." *Emerging Infectious Diseases* 9: 1197–204.

Business Week. (2003) "One Scary Bug," April 14.

Butler, J. (1993) *Bodies that Matter: On the Discursive Limits of "Sex,"* New York: Routledge.

Cadot, E., V. Rodwin, A. and Spira. (2007) "In the Heat of the Summer: Lessons from the Heat Waves in Paris." *Journal of Urban Health* 84(4).

Callard, F.J. (1998) "The Body in Theory." *Environment and Planning D: Society and Space* 16: 387–400.

Callon, M. (1986) "Some Elements of a Sociology of Translation: Domestication of the Scallops and the Fishermen of St. Brieuc Bay." In J. Law (ed.), *Power, Action and Belief: A New Sociology of Knowledge?* London: Routledge & Kegan Paul, pp. 196–233.

Campbell, A. (2004) *The SARS Commission Interim Report: SARS and Public Health in Ontario*. Toronto: Commission to Investigate the Introduction and Spread of SARS in Ontario, April 15. Online at: http://www.health.gov.on.ca/english/public/pub/ministry_reports/campbell04/campbell04.pdf

Campbell, A. (2005) *Second Interim Report: SARS and Public Health Legislation*. Toronto: Commission to Investigate the Introduction and Spread of SARS in Ontario. Online at: http://www.health.gov.on.ca/english/public/pub/ministry_reports/campbell05/campbell05.pdf

Canadian Federation of Independent Business. (2005) *Post-SARS Recovery Survey Report: Results of CFIB Survey on SARS Impact and Recovery Measures.* Toronto: CFIB. Online at: http://www.cfib.ca/legis/ontario/pdf/5422.pdf

Castells, M. (2000) *The Rise of the Network Society,* 2nd edn. Oxford: Blackwell.

Castree, N. (2001) "Commodity Fetishism, Geographical Imaginations and Imaginative Geographies." *Environment and Planning A* 33: 1519–25.

Cavalli-Sforza, L.L., P. Menozzi, and A. Piazza. (1994) *The History of Human Genes.* Princeton, NJ: Princeton University Press.

CBC (Canadian Broadcasting Corporation). (2003a) "Concert Helps Raise Morale of SARS Workers." Online at: http://www.toronto.cbc.ca/regional/servlet/View?filename=to_stoneshealth20030731 (accessed July 31, 2006).

CBC (Canadian Broadcasting Corporation). (2003b) "In Depth SARS Benefit Concert: Toronto Rocked." Online at: http://www.cbc.ca/news/background/sarsbenefit/ (accessed July 31, 2006).

CBC (Canadian Broadcasting Corporation). (2003c) "SARS Not Under-Reported: Medical Officials." Online at: http://www.cbc.ca/story/news/national/2003/05/28/sars_underreport030528.html

CDC (Department of Health and Human Services, Centers for Disease Control and Prevention). (2003) "MMWR Weekly Update: Severe Acute Respiratory Syndrome – Worldwide and United States." Online at: http://www.cdc.gov/MMWR/preview/mmwrhtml/mm5228a4.htm (accessed October 25, 2006).

CDC (Department of Health and Human Services, Centers for Disease Control and Prevention). (2005) *Controlling Tuberculosis in the United States: Morbidity and Mortality Weekly Report,* November 4: 54.

Cervino, A.C., S. Lakiss, O. Sow, and A.V. Hill. (2000) "Allelic Association between the NRAMP1 Gene and Susceptibility to Tuberculosis in Guinea-Conakry." *Annals of Human Genetics* 64: 507–12.

Chan, C.L.W. (2003) "The Social Impact of SARS: Sustainable Action for the Rejuvenation of Society." In T. Koh, A. Plant, and E.H. Lee (eds.), *The New Global Threat: SARS and its Impacts.* Singapore: World Scientific, pp. 123–46.

Chaplin, S. (1999) "Cities, Sewers and Poverty: India's Politics of Sanitation." *Environment and Urbanization* 11(1): 145–58.

Cheng, P., D. Wong, L. Tong, S. Ip, A. Lo, C. Lau, et al. (2004) "Viral Shedding Patterns of Coronavirus in Patients with Probable Severe Acute Respiratory Syndrome." *The Lancet* 363(9422): 1699–700.

Chew, S.K. (2003) "Fighting SARS Together: The Singaporean Way," Paper presented at Seminar on SARS, Institute of Southeast Asian Studies, Singapore, 7 May.

Chin, D., K. Dereimer, P. Small, et al. (1998) "Differences in Contributing Factors to Tuberculosis Incidence in U.S.-Born and Foreign-Born Persons." *American Journal of Respiratory and Critical Care Medicine* 158(6): 1797–803.

Chou, C.M. (2003) "Each Hospital is Working on its Own, Health Care Workers and Citizens Lost their Lives." *Hong Kong Economic Times,* June 3. Online at: http://www.synergynet.org.hk/m3_303.htm (accessed March 18, 2005; in Chinese).

Chua, B.H. (1995) *Communitarian Ideology and Democracy in Singapore.* London: Routledge.

Clark, C. (2005) "Canadians Want Strict Security, Poll Finds." *The Globe and Mail*, August 11, A1–A5.

Clark, N. (2002) "The Demon-Seed: Bioinvasion as the Unsettling of Environmental Cosmopolitanism." *Theory, Culture & Society* 19(1–2): 101–25.

Cleaveland, S., M.K. Laurenson, and L.H. Taylor. (2001) "Disease of Humans and their Domestic Mammals: Pathogen Characteristics, Host Range and the Risk of Emergence." *Philosophical Transactions of the Royal Society, London B* 356: 991–9.

Collier, S.J., and A. Lakoff. (2006) "Vital Systems Security." In *Laboratory for the Anthropology of the Contemporary*. Online at: http://anthropos-lab.net/

Collins, R. (2004) *Interaction Ritual Chains*. Princeton, NJ: Princeton University Press.

Comoraw, A. (2000) "Less than Scary Health Scares: Killer Cranberries?" *US News and World Report*, November 13. Online at: http://www.usnews.com/usnews/health/articles/001113/archive_009807.htm

Congress of the United States. (2003) *Congressional Hearings before the US–China Economic and Security Commission: SARS in China. Implications for Information Control, Internet Censorship, and the Economy*. Washington, DC: US Government Printing Office. Online at: http://www.uscc.gov

Cook, I., and P. Crang. (1996) "The World on a Plate," *Journal of Material Culture* 1(2): 131–53.

Cooper, M. (2006) "Pre-Empting Emergence: The Biological Turn in the War on Terror." *Theory, Culture & Society* 23(4): 113–35.

Cossar, J.H. (1994) "Influence of Travel and Disease: An Historical Perspective." *Journal of Travel Medicine* 1(1): 36–9.

Cowley, G., et al. (1995) "Outbreak of Fear," *Newsweek* 52.

Craddock, S. (1995) "Sewers and Scapegoats: Spatial Metaphors of Smallpox in Nineteenth Century San Francisco." *Social Science & Medicine* 41: 957–68.

Craddock, S. (2000) *City of Plagues: Disease, Poverty, and Deviance in San Francisco*. Minneapolis: University of Minnesota Press.

Crang, P. (1996) "Displacement, Consumption, and Identity." *Environment and Planning A* 28: 47–67.

Crewe, L. (2001) "The Besieged Body: Geography of Retailing and Consumption." *Progress in Human Geography* 25(4): 629–40.

Cronon, W. (1994) "The Trouble with Wilderness, or, Getting Back to the Wrong Nature." In W. Cronon (ed.), *Uncommon Ground: Toward Reinventing Nature*. New York: W.W. Norton, pp. 69–90.

Crouse, T. (1972) *The Boys on the Bus: Riding with the Campaign Press Corps*. New York: Random House.

Cummins, L. (1920) "Tuberculosis in Primitive Tribes and its Bearing on the Tuberculosis of Civilized Communities." *International Journal of Public Health* 1: 137–71.

Cummins, L. (1929) "Virgin Soil – and After: A Working Conception of Tuberculosis in Children, Adolescents, and Aborigines." *British Medical Journal*, July 13: 39–41.

Curley, M., and N. Thomas. (2004) "Human Security and Public Health in Southeast Asia: The SARS Outbreak." *Australian Journal of International Affairs* 58(1).

Cussins, C. (2005) *Making Parents: The Ontological Choreography of Reproductive Technologies*. Cambridge, MA: The MIT Press.

D'Cunha, C. (2003) "The SARS Experience in Ontario, Canada," Presentation to Ontario SARS Commission ("Campbell Commission"), Toronto, September 29.

D'Cunha, C. (2004) "SARS: Lessons Learned from a Provincial Perspective." *Canadian Journal of Public Health* 95(1): 25–6.

Davis, M. (2004) "Planet of Slums: Urban Involution and the Informal Proletariat." *New Left Review* 26: 5–34.

Davis, M. (2005) *The Monster at Our Door: The Global Threat of Avian Flu.* New York: New Press.

Davis, M. (2006) *Planet of Slums.* London: Verso.

De Cock, K.M., D. Mbori-Ngacha, and E. Marum. (2002) "Shadow on the Continent: Public Health and HIV/AIDS in Africa in the 21st Century." *The Lancet* 360: 67–72.

De Hart, R. (2003) "Health Issues of Air Travel." *American Review of Public Health* 24: 133–51.

Deleuze, G. (1994) *Difference and Repetition.* New York: Columbia University Press.

Deleuze, G., and F. Guattari. (1987) *A Thousand Plateaus: Capitalism and Schizophrenia.* Minneapolis: University of Minnesota Press.

Delgado, C.L. (2003) "Rising Consumption of Meat and Milk in Developing Countries has Created a New Food Revolution." *Journal of Nutrition* 133 (11 Suppl. 2).

Delgado, J., A. Baena, S. Thim, and A. Goldfeld. (2002) "Ethnic-Specific Genetic Associations with Pulmonary Tuberculosis." *The Journal of Infectious Diseases* 186: 1463–8.

Demmler, G., and B. Ligon. (2003) "Severe Acute Respiratory Syndrome (SARS): A Review of the History, Epidemiology, Prevention, and Concerns for the Future." *Seminars in Pediatric Infectious Diseases* 14(3): 240–4.

Derudder, B. (2003) "Beyond the State: Mapping the Semi-Periphery through Urban Networks." *Capitalism, Nature, Socialism* 14: 91–119.

Derudder, B., and P.J. Taylor (2005) "The Cliquishness of World Cities." *Global Networks* 5(1): 71–91.

Derudder, B., P.J. Taylor, F. Witlox, and G. Catalano. (2003) "Hierarchical Tendencies and Regional Patterns in the World City Network: A Global Urban Analysis of 234 Cities." *Regional Studies* 37: 875–86.

Dillon, M. (2003) "Virtual Disorder: A Life Science of (Dis)order." *Millennium: Journal of International Studies* 32(3): 531–58.

Dodge, M., and R. Kitchin. (2004) "Flying through Code/Space: The Real Virtuality of Air Travel." *Environment and Planning A* 36: 195–211.

DOE (Department of the Environment) and Government Office for London. (1996) *Four World Cities: A Comparative Study of London, Paris, New York, and Tokyo.* London: Llewelvn-Davies, UCL Bartlett school of Planning, and Comedia.

Dorling, D. (2004) "Healthy Places, Healthy Spaces." *British Medical Bulletin* 69: 101–14.

Drache, D. (2004) *The Global Cultural Commons after Cancun: Identity, Diversity and Citizenship.* Toronto: Robarts Centre for Canadian Studies. Online at: http://www.yorku.ca/ drache/academic/papers/wto_identity.pdf

Draus, P. (2004) *Consumed in the City: Observing Tuberculosis at Century's End.* Philadelphia, PA: Temple University Press.

Driedger, L. (2003) "Changing Boundaries: Sorting Space, Class, Ethnicity and Race in Ontario." *Canadian Review of Sociology and Anthropology* 40: 593–621.

Dubos, R., and J. Dubos. (1952) *The White Plague: Tuberculosis, Man, and Society*. New Brunswick: Rutgers University Press.

Duckett, J. (2003) "To Control SARS, Fix Mainland Health Systems' Weak Links." *South China Morning Post*, News 1.

Durkheim, E. (1995) *The Elementary Forms of Religious Life*, translated and with an Introduction by Karen E. Fields. New York: The Free Press.

Duster, T. (2003) *Backdoor to Eugenics*, 2nd edn. New York: Routledge.

Dwosh, H.A., H.H.L. Hong, D. Austgarden, S. Herman, and R. Schabas. (2003) "Identification and Containment of an Outbreak of SARS in a Community Hospital." *Canadian Medical Association Journal* 168(11).

Dyck, I., and R. Kearns. (1995) "Transforming the Relations of Research: Towards Culturally Safe Geographies of Health and Healing." *Health and Place* 1(3): 137–47.

Dyer, G. (2006) "Waiting for the Pandemic." *The Walrus* 3(1): 44–54.

Eastwood, J.B., et al. (2005) "Loss of Health Professionals from Sub-Saharan Africa: The Pivotal Role of the UK." *The Lancet* 365: 1893–900.

EMRO-WHO (Eastern Mediterranean Regional Office – World Health Organization). (2005) "Avian Influenza." *Press Release no. 15, Cairo*. Online at: www.emro.who.int/pressreleases/2005/no15.htm

Evandrou, M. (2006) "Inequalities among Older People in London: The Challenge of Diversity." In V. Rodwin and M. Gusmano (eds.), *Growing Older in World Cities: New York, London, Paris and Tokyo*. New York: Vanderbilt University Press.

Evans, R. (1988) "Epidemics and Revolutions: Cholera in Nineteenth-Century Europe." *Past and Present* 120: 123–46.

Farmer, P. (1996) "Social Inequalities and Emerging Infectious Diseases." *Emerging Infectious Diseases* 2(4): 259–69.

Farmer, P. (1999) *Infections and Inequalities: the Modern Plagues*. Berkeley, CA: University of California Press.

Farmer, P., and E. Nardell. (1998) "Editorial: Nihilism and Pragmatism in Tuberculosis Control." *American Journal of Public Health* 88(7): 1014–15.

Featherstone, M. (1990) "Global Culture: An Introduction." In M. Featherstone (ed.), *Global Culture*. London: Sage.

Feldmann, H., et al. (2002) "Emerging and Re-Emerging Infectious Diseases." *Medical Microbiology and Immunology* 191(2): 63–74.

Ferns, C. (1999) *Narrating Utopia: Ideology, Gender, Form in Utopian Literature*. Liverpool: Liverpool University Press.

Fidler, D.P. (2003) "SARS: Political Pathology of the First Post-Westphalian Pathogen." *The Journal of Law, Medicine & Ethics* 31(4): 485–505.

Fidler, D.P. (2004) *SARS, Governance and the Globalization of Disease*. New York: Palgrave Macmillan.

Fine, B., and E. Leopold. (1993) *The World of Consumption*. London: Routledge.

Fischer, B., and B. Poland. (1998) "Exclusion 'Risk' and Social Control: Reflections on Community Policing and Public Health." *Geoforum* 29(2): 187–97.

Fitness, J., S. Floyd, D.K. Warndorff, L. Sichali, L.M. Waungulu, A.C. Crampin, P.E.M. Fine, and A.V.S. Hill. (2004) "Large-Scale Candidate Gene Study of Leprosy Susceptibility in the Karonga District of Northern Malawi." *The American Journal of Tropical Medicine and Hygiene* 71(3): 330–40.

Fitzpatrick, K., and M. LaGory. (2000) *Unhealthy Places: The Ecology of Risk in the Urban Landscape.* London: Routledge.

Focas, C. (1998) *The Four World Cities Transport Study: London, New York, Paris, Tokyo.* London: London Research Centre/The Stationery Office. Online at: http://www.london.research.gov.uk

Foucault, M. (1965) *Madness and Civilization. A History of Insanity in the Age of Reason,* translated by R. Howard. New York: Pantheon.

Foucault, M. (1996) *Les Mots et les Choses (Order of Things).* Paris: Gallimard.

Foucault, M. (1972 [1969]) *Archaeology of Knowledge,* translated by A.M. Sheridan Smith. New York: Pantheon.

Foucault, M. (1973) *The Birth of the Clinic: An Archaeology of Medical Perception.* New York: Vintage.

Foucault, M. (1977) *Discipline and Punish. The Birth of the Prison,* translated by A. Sheridan. New York: Pantheon.

Foucault, M. (1978) *The History of Sexuality: Volume 1,* translated by R. Hurley. New York: Random House.

Foucault, M. (1979) *Discipline and Punish.* London: Peregrine Books.

Foucault, M. (1980) "Questions on Geography." In C. Gordon (ed.), *Power/Knowledge. Selected Interviews and Other Writings 1972–1977.* New York: Pantheon, pp. 64–5.

Foucault, M. (1984a) "Nietzsche, Genealogy, History." In P. Rabinow (ed.), *The Foucault Reader.* London: Penguin.

Foucault, M. (1984b) "Space, Knowledge, Power: Interview with Paul Rabinow." In P. Rabinow (ed.), *The Foucault Reader.* New York, Pantheon, pp. 239–56.

Foucault, M. (1990) *The History of Sexuality, An Introduction.* New York: Pantheon.

Foucault, M. (1991) "Governmentality." In G. Burchell, C. Gordon, and P. Miller (eds.), *The Foucault Effect: Studies in Governmentality.* London: Harvester, pp. 87–104.

Foucault, M. (1994) "La vérité et les formes juridiques." In M. Foucault, *Dits et Ecrits 1954–1988: Volume 2.* Paris: Gallimard, pp. 538–645.

Foucault, M. (1999) *In Verteidigung der Gesellschaft.* Frankfurt am Main: Suhrkamp.

Foucault, M. (2003) *Society Must Be Defended: Lectures at the College de France, 1975–1976.* New York: Picador.

Foucault, M. (2004a) "Je suis un artificier." In R.P. Droit (ed.), *Michel Foucault, Entretiens.* Paris: Odile Jacob.

Foucault, M. (2004b) *Society Must Be Defended: Lectures at the College de France, 1975–1976.* London: Penguin.

Foucault, M. (2006) *Geschichte der Gouvernementalität 1: Sicherheit, Territorium und Bevölkerung.* Frankfurt am Main: Suhrkamp.

Fredriksson-Bass, J., and A. Kanabus. (2006) *HIV and AIDS in India.* Online at: http://www.avert.org/aidsindia.htm (accessed June 7, 2006).

Freudenberg, N. (2000) "Health Promotion in the City: A Review of Current Practice and Future Prospects in the United States." *Annual Review of Public Health* 21: 473–503.

Friedmann, J. (1986) "The World City Hypothesis." *Development and Change* 17: 69–83. Reprinted in P. Knox and P. Taylor (eds.). (1995) *World Cities in a World-System.* New York: Cambridge University Press, pp. 318–31.

Friedmann, J., and G. Wolff. (1982) "World City Formation: An Agenda for Research and Action." *International Journal of Urban and Regional Research* 3: 309–44.

Gagneux, S., et al. (2006) "Variable Host–Pathogen Compatibility in *Mycobacterium tuberculosis.*" *Proceedings of the National Academy of Sciences of the United States of America* 103(8): 2869–73.

Galabuzi, G.-E. (2004) "Social Exclusion." In D. Raphael (ed.), *Social Determinants of Health.* Toronto: Canadian Scholars' Press, pp. 235–52.

Galloway, G. (2003) "WHO Concedes Advisory Damaged Toronto." *The Globe and Mail,* May 1, pp. 1–2.

Gandy, M. (1999) "The Paris Sewers and the Rationalization of Urban Space." *Transactions of the Institute of British Geographers* 24: 23–44.

Gandy, M. (2002) *Concrete and Clay: Reworking Nature in New York City.* Cambridge, MA: The MIT Press.

Gandy, M. (2004) "Rethinking Urban Metabolism: Water, Space and the Modern City." *City* 8(3): 371–87.

Gandy, M. (2005) "Cyborg Urbanization: Complexity and Monstrosity in the Contemporary City." *International Journal of Urban and Regional Research* 29(1): 26–49.

Gandy, M. (2006a) "Planning, Anti-Planning and the Infrastructure Crisis Facing Metropolitan Lagos." *Urban Studies* 43: 71–96.

Gandy, M. (2006b) "Zones of Indistinction: Some Thoughts on the Bio-Politics of Urban Space." *Cultural Geographies* 13: 497–516.

Gandy, M. (2006c) "The Bacteriological City and its Discontents." *Historical Geography* 34: 14–25.

Gandy, M., and A. Zumla (eds.). (2003) *The Return of the White Plague: Global Poverty and the "New" Tuberculosis.* London: Verso.

Gao, P.S., S. Fujishima, X.Q. Mao, et al. (2000) "Genetic Variants of NRAMP1 and Active Tuberculosis in Japanese Populations." *Clinical Genetics* 58: 74–6.

Garrett, L. (1994) "Commentary: Human Movements and Behavioral Factors in the Emergence of Diseases." *Annals of the New York Academy of Science* 740: 312–18.

Garrett, L. (1996) "The Return of Infectious Disease." *Foreign Affairs* 75(1): 66–79.

Garrett, L. (2000) *Betrayal of Trust: The Collapse of Global Public Health.* New York: Hyperion.

GaWC (Globalization and World Cities). (2004) "Global and World Cities." Online at: http://www.lboro.ac.uk/gawc (accessed April 1, 2008).

Geiter, L. (ed.). (2001) "Ending Neglect: The Elimination of Tuberculosis in the United States." Institute of Medicine, Committee on the Elimination of Tuberculosis in the United States. Washington, DC: National Academies Press.

Gertel, J., and S. Samir. (2000) "Cairo: Urban Agriculture and 'Visions' for a Modern City." In N. Bakker, M. Dubbeling, S. Gundel, U. Sabel-Koschella, and H. de Zeeuw (eds.), *Growing Cities, Growing Food: Urban Agriculture on the Policy Agenda. A Reader on Urban Agriculture.* Feldafing, Germany: German Foundation for International Development (DSE).

Gibson, K., and R. Jean-Louis. (2003) "SARSstock: Musicians Rock to Heal Toronto." *CNN Headline News*, September 29.

Giddens, A. (1990) *The Consequences of Modernity*. Stanford: Stanford University Press.

Gillmor, D. (2004) "Coming Soon." *Toronto Life*, February, pp. 60–5.

Glass, R.I. (2004) "Perceived Threats and Real Killers." *Science* 304(5673): 927.

Gleeson, B. (1996) "A Geography for Disabled People." *Transactions of the Institute of British Geographers* 21(2): 387–96.

Glyn, A. (2005) "Imbalances of the Global Economy." *New Left Review* 34: 5–37.

Godfrey, R., J. Gavin, and J. Campbell. (2004) "Sucking, Bleeding, Breaking: On the Dialectics of Vampirism, Capital, and Time." *Culture and Organization* 10(1): 25–36.

Goffman, E. (1967a [1955]) "On Face-Work: An Analysis of Ritual Elements in Social Interaction." In E. Goffman (ed.), *Interaction Ritual. Essays on Face-to-Face Behavior*. New York: Pantheon, pp. 5–45.

Goffman, E. (1967b [1956]) "The Nature of Deference and Demeanor." In E. Goffman (ed.), *Interaction Ritual. Essays on Face-to-Face Behavior*. New York: Pantheon, pp. 47–95.

Goffman, E. (1974 [1959]) *The Presentation of Self in Everyday Life*. London: Penguin.

Goodman, D. (1999) "Agro-Food Studies in the 'Age of Ecology': Nature, Corporeality, Bio-Politics." *European Society for Rural Sociology* 39(1).

Goonewardena, K., and S. Kipfer. (2005) "Spaces of Difference: Reflections from Toronto on Multiculturalism, Bourgeois Urbanism and the Possibility of Radical Urban Politics." *International Journal of Urban and Regional Research* 29(3): 670–8.

Gopalakrishna, G., P. Choo, Y.S. Leo, B.K. Tay, Y.T. Lim, A.S. Khan, and C.C. Tan. (2004) "SARS Transmission and Hospital Containment." *Emerging Infectious Disease* 10(3): 395–400.

Gordon, D. (1999) "Confrontations with the Plague in Eighteenth-Century France." In A. Johns (ed.), *Dreadful Visitations: Confronting Natural Catastrophe in the Age of Enlightenment*. London: Routledge, pp. 3–29.

Gould, P. (1999) *Becoming a Geographer*. Syracuse: Syracuse University Press.

Gostin, L.O. (2001) "Health Information: Reconciling Personal Privacy with the Public Good of Human Health." *Health Care Analysis* 9: 321–35.

Gostin, L.O., R. Bayer, and A. Fairchild. (2003) "Ethical and Legal Challenges Posed by Severe Acute Respiratory Syndrome: Implications for the Control of Severe Infectious Disease Threats." *Journal of the American Medical Association* 290(24): 3229–37.

Gottmann, J. (1979) "World Cities and their Present Problems." In G. Wynne (ed.), *Survival Strategies: Paris and New York*. New Brunswick, NJ: Transaction.

Gradmann, C. (2000) "Invisible Enemies: Bacteriology and Language of Politics in Imperial Germany." *Science in Context* 13(1): 9–30.

Graham, D.T., and N. Poku. (1998) "Population Movements: Health and Security." In N. Poku and D.T. Graham (eds.), *Redefining Security: Population Movements and National Security*. Westport, CT: Praeger, pp. 203–34.

Grain. (2006a) "Fowl Play: The Poultry Industry's Central Role in the Bird Flu Crisis." Online at: http://www.grain.org/briefings/?id=194

Grain. (2006b) "The Top-Down Global Response to Bird Flu." *Against the Grain.* Online at: http://www.grain.org/articles/?id=12

Greenwood, C.M.T., T.M. Fujiwara, L.J. Boothroyd, et al. (2000) "Linkage of Tuberculosis of Chromosome 2q35 Loci, Including *NRAMP1*, in a Large Aboriginal Canadian Family." *The American Journal of Human Genetics* 67(2): 405–16.

Guan and Sheng 2003, from Chapter 14.

Guan, Y., B.J. Zheng, Y.Q. He, et al. (2003) "Isolation and Characterization of Viruses Related to the SARS Coronavirus from Animals in Southern China." *Science* 302: 276–8.

Guilloux, A. (2006) "SARS, Governance and the Globalization of Disease – Book Review of David P. Fidler." *China Perspectives*, January–February.

Gusmano, M., V. Rodwin, and D. Weisz. (2006) "A New Way to Compare Health Systems: Avoidable Hospital Condition in Manhattan and Paris." *Health Affairs* 25(2): 510–20.

Gwyn, R. (2002) *Communicating Health and Illness.* London: Sage.

H5N1, News and Resources about Avian Flu. (2006) "Hungarians Resist Bird Flu Blame." Online at: http://crofsblogs.typepad.com/h5n1/.

Habermas, J. (1989) *The Structural Transformation of the Public Sphere: An Inquiry into a Category of Bourgeois Society.* Cambridge: Polity Press.

Hajer, M. (2003) "Policy without Polity? Policy Analysis and the Institutional Void." *Policy Sciences* 36: 175–95.

Hall, P. (1984) *The World Cities*, 3rd edn. New York: St Martin's Press.

Hall, S. (1991a) "Old and New Identities, Old and New Ethnicities." In A.D. King (ed.), *Culture, Globalization and the World System.* Basingstoke: Macmillan Education, pp. 41–68.

Hall, S. (1991b) "The Local and the Global: Globalization and Ethnicity." In A.D. King (ed.), *Culture, Globalization and the World System.* Basingstoke: Macmillan Education, pp. 19–40.

Hannigan, J. (2006) *Environmental Sociology: A Social Constructionist Perspective*, 2nd edn. New York: Routledge.

Haraway, D. (1991) *Simians, Cyborgs, and Women: The Reinvention of Nature.* London: Free Association Books.

Haraway, D. (1997) *Modest*Witness@Second*Millennium.FemaleMan*Meets*OncoMouse: Feminism and Technoscience.* New York: Routledge.

Harrison, M., and M. Worboys. (1997) "A Disease of Civilization: Tuberculosis in Britain, Africa and India, 1900–39." In L. Marks and M. Worboys (eds.), *Migrants, Minorities, and Health: Historical and Contemporary Studies.* New York: Routledge, pp. 932124.

Harvey, D. (1998) "The Body as an Accumulation Strategy." *Environment and Planning D: Society and Space* 16: 401–21.

Harvey, D. (2005) *A Brief History of Neoliberalism.* Oxford: Oxford University Press.

Hatfield, E., J. Cacioppo, and R. Rapson. (1994) *Emotional Contagion.* Cambridge: Cambridge University Press.

Hawryluck, L., W.L. Gold, S. Robinson, et al. (2004) "SARS Control and Psychological Effects of Quarantine, Toronto, Canada." *Emerging Infectious Diseases* 10(7), July.

Heath, D., R. Rapp, and K.S. Taussig. (2004) "Genetic Citizenship." In D. Nugent and J. Vincent (eds.), *A Companion to the Anthropology of Politics*. Oxford: Blackwell.

Held, D., A. McGrew, D. Goldblatt, and J. Perraton. (2002) "Rethinking Globalization." In D. Held and A. McGrew (eds.), *The Global Transformations Reader: An Introduction to the Globalization Debate*, 2nd edn, Oxford: Blackwell, Ch. 3.

Herman, E.S., and N. Chomsky. (2002) *Manufacturing Consent: The Political Economy of the Mass Media*, 2nd edn. New York: Pantheon.

Hertzler, J.O. (1965) *The History of Utopian Thought*. New York: Cooper Square, pp. 48–50.

Heymann, D. (2004) "From Smallpox to SARS and Polio: What Has the World Learned?" Paper delivered at the "Controlling the Risk: Science to Combat Global Infectious Diseases" Conference, Toronto, November 9–10.

Heymann, D.L. (2005) "The International Response to the Outbreak of SARS, 2003." In A.R. McLean, R.M. May, J. Pattison, and R.A. Weiss (eds.), *SARS: A Case Study in Emerging Infections*. Oxford: Oxford University Press, pp. 61–80.

Heymann, D., and G. Rodier. (2004) "Global Surveillance, National Surveillance, and SARS." *Emerging Infectious Diseases* 10(2): 173–5.

Heymann, D., M.K. Kindhauser, and G. Rodier. (2005) "Coordinating the Global Response." In *SARS: How a Global Epidemic Was Stopped*. Geneva: World Health Organization.

HHS (Department of Health and Human Services). (2004) *Pandemic Influenza Response and Preparedness Plan*. US Department of Health and Human Services. Online at: http://www.hhs.gov/nvpo/pandemicplan

Hinchliffe, S. (1999) "Cities and Natures: Intimate Strangers." In J. Allen, D. Massey, and M. Pryke, *Unsettling Cities*. London: Routledge, pp. 138–66.

Hinchliffe, S. (2001) "Indeterminacy In-Decisions – Science, Policy and Politics in the BSE (Bovine Spongiform Encephalopathy) Crisis." *Transactions of the Institute of British Geographers* 26(2): 182–204.

Hinchliffe, S. (2007) *Spaces for Nature*. London: Sage.

Hinchliffe, S., and S. Whatmore. (2006) "Living Cities: Towards a Politics of Conviviality." *Science as Culture* 15(2): 123–38.

Hinchliffe, S., M. Kearnes, M. Degen, and S. Whatmore. (2007) "Ecologies and Economies of Action – Sustainability, Calculations, and Other Things." *Environment and Planning A* 39(2): 260–82.

Ho, K.L. (2003) "SARS Policy-Making and Lesson-Drawing." In T. Koh, A. Plant, and E.H. Lee (eds.), *The New Global Threat: Severe Acute Respiratory Syndrome and its Impacts*. Singapore: World Scientific, pp. 195–208.

Hon, K., A. Li, F. Cheng, T. Leung, and P. Ng. (2003) "Personal View of SARS: Confusing Definition, Confusing Diagnoses" [correspondence]. *The Lancet* 361: 1984–5.

Hong Kong Business Journal. (2003) "Focus of *Business Journal*." February 12, 2003 (in Chinese).

Hooker, C. (2006) "Drawing the Lines." In A. Bashford (ed.), *Medicine at the Border: Disease, Globalization and security*. London: Palgrave Macmillan.

Horton, R. (1998) "The Infected Metropolis." *The Lancet* 347(8995): 134–5.

Hospital Authority of Hong Kong. (2002) "Annual Report 2001–2002." Online at: http://www.ha.org.hk/hesd/v2/AHA/ANR0102/9-21.pdf (accessed March 21, 2005).

Hospital Authority of Hong Kong Review Panel. (2003) *Report of the Hospital Authority Review Panel on the SARS Outbreak.* September. Hong Kong: Hospital Authority. Online at: http://www.anthropos-lab.net/publications/index.html

Huang, Y., and C.M. Leung. (2005) "Western-Led Press Coverage of Mainland China and Vietnam during the SARS Crisis: Reassessing the Concept of 'Media Representation of the Other,'" *Asian Journal of Communication* 15(3): 302–18.

HUD (Housing and Urban Development). (1998) *The State of the Nation's Cities.* Washington, DC: Department of Housing and Urban Development.

Ingram, A. (2005) "The New Geopolitics of Disease: Between Global Health and Global Security." *Geopolitics* 10: 522–45.

Institute of Medicine (IOM). (1992) *Emerging Infections: Microbial Threats to Health in the United States.* Washington, DC: National Academies Press.

Isin, E.F., and M. Siemiatycki. (2002) "Making Space for Mosques: Struggles for Urban Citizenship in Diasporic Toronto." In S.H. Razack (ed.), *Race, Space, and the Law: Unmapping a White Settler Society.* Toronto: Between the Lines, pp. 185–209.

Jacmenovic, M. (2005) "Southern China Is Not the Only Source for Volatile Live Animal Markets." Online at: http://www.hsus.org/wildlife/issues_facing_wildlife (accessed April 28, 2005).

Jacobs, L. (2005) *Rights and Quarantine During the SARS Public Health: Legal Consciousness in Hong Kong, Shanghai and Toronto.* Unpublished manuscript, York University, Toronto.

Jansen, S. (2003) *"Schädlinge": Geschichte eines wissenschaftlichen und politischen Konstrukts, 1840–1920.* Princeton, NJ: Princeton University Press.

Janz, C.P. (1981) *Friedrich Nietzsche. Biographie.* Munich: Deutscher Taschenbuch Verlag.

Jessop, B. (2000) "The Crisis of the National Spatio-Temporal Fix and the Tendential Ecological Dominance of Globalizing Capital." *International Journal of Urban and Regional Research* 24: 323–60.

Jensen, M. (2006) "Environment, Mobility, and the Acceleration of Time: A Sociological Analysis of Transport Flows in Modern Life." In G. Spaargaren, A.P. Mol, and F.H. Buttel (eds.), *Governing Environmental Flows: Global Challenges to Social Theory.* Cambridge, MA: The MIT Press, pp. 327–50.

Jones, C., and R. Porter (eds.). (1994) *Reassessing Foucault: Power, Medicine and the Body.* London: Routledge.

Kaika, M. (2005) *City of Flows: Modernity, Nature and the City.* London: Routledge.

Kaika, M., and E. Swyngedouw. (2000) "Fetishizing the Modern City: the Phantasmagoria of Urban Technological Networks." *International Journal of Urban and Regional Research* 24(1): 120–38.

Kalipeni, E., S. Craddock, J.R. Oppong, and J. Ghosh, J. (eds.) (2004) *HIV and AIDS in Africa: Beyond Epidemiology.* Oxford: Blackwell.

Kasperson, R., O. Renn, P. Slovic, H. Brown, J. Emel, R. Goble, et al. (1988) "The Social Amplification of Risk: A Conceptual Framework." *Risk Analysis* 8: 178–87.

Kaufman, F. (2005) "The Secret Ingredient: Keeping the World Kosher." *Harpers*, 1.

Kearns, G. (1991) "Cholera, Nuisances and Environmental Management in Islington, 1830–55." *Medical History* 11: 94–125.

Kearns, R.A. (1994) "Putting Health and Health Care into Place: An Invitation Accepted and Declined." *Professional Geographer* 46: 111–15.

Keil, R. (1998a) "Globalization Makes States: Perspectives of Local Governance in the Age of the Global City." *Review of International Political Economy* 5: 616–46.

Keil, R. (1998b) *Los Angeles: Globalization, Urbanization and Social Struggles.* Chichester: John Wiley & Sons.

Keil, R., and S.H. Ali. (2007) "Governing the Sick City: Urban Governance in the Age of Emerging Infectious Disease." *Antipode* 9: 846–73.

Keller, R. (2007) "Geographies of Power, Legacies of Mistrust: Colonial Medicine in the Global Present." In S. Craddock and J. Gunn (eds.), *Epidemics, History, and the Present.* Special issue of *Historical Geography*.

Kim, J., A. Shakow, K. Mate, C. Vanderwarker, R. Gupta, and P. Farmer. (2005) "Limited Good and Limited Vision: Multidrug-Resistant Tuberculosis and Global Health Policy." *Social Science and Medicine* 61: 847–59.

King, L.J. (1984) *Central Place Theory.* Beverly Hills, CA: Sage.

King, N.B. (2002) "Security, Disease, Commerce: Ideologies of Postcolonial Global Health." *Social Studies of Science* 32(5/6): 763–80.

King, N.B. (2003) "Immigration, Race and Geographies of Difference in the Tuberculosis Pandemic." In M. Gandy and A. Zumla (eds.), *The Return of the White Plague: Global Poverty and the "New" Tuberculosis.* London: Verso, pp. 39–54.

King, N.B. (2004) "The Scale Politics of Emerging Diseases." *Osiris* 19: 62–76.

Kipfer, S., and R. Keil. (2002) "Toronto, Inc.? Planning the Competitive City in Toronto." *Antipode* 34: 227–64.

Kiple, K.F. (ed.). (2003) *The Cambridge Historical Dictionary of Disease.* Cambridge: Cambridge University Press.

Kirsch, S., and D. Mitchell. (2004) "The Nature of Things: Dead Labor, Nonhuman Actors, and the Persistence of Marxism." *Antipode* 36(4): 687–705.

Klein, I. (1986) "Urban Development and Death: Bombay City, 1870–1914." *Modern Asian Studies* 20: 725–54.

Klein, I. (1994) "Imperialism, Ecology and Disease: Cholera in India, 1850–1950." *Indian Economic and Social History* 31: 491–518.

Klein, N. (2003) "Bush's Aids 'Gift' Has Been Seized by Industry Giants." *The Guardian* (London), October 13.

Kleinman, A., and J.L. Watson. (2006) *SARS in China.* Stanford: Stanford University Press.

Knobler, S., Mahmoud, A., Lemon, S., & Pray, L., (eds.) (2006), "The Impact of Globalization on Infectious Disease Emergence and Control." In *Forum on Microbial Threats, Board on Global Health, Institute of Medicine.* Washington, DC: National Academies Press.

Knobler, S., Mahmoud, A., Lemon, et al. (eds.). (2004) *Learning from SARS: Preparing for the Next Disease Outbreak, Institute of Medicine.* Washington, DC: National Academies Press.

Knox, P., and P. Taylor (eds.). (1995) *World Cities in a World-System.* Cambridge: Cambridge University Press.

Koh, T., A. Plant, and E.H. Lee (eds.). (2003) *The New Global Threat: Severe Acute Respiratory Syndrome and its Impacts.* Singapore: World Scientific.

Kohlmorgen, L. (2004) "Global health governance und UN AIDS: Elemente eines globalen Integrationsmodus." *Peripherie: Zeitschrift für Politik und Ökonomie in der Dritten Welt* 93/94: 139–65.

KPMG. (2003) *Tourism Expenditures in Major Canadian Markets: Where We've Been, Where We're Going, and Why.* KPMG and the Hotel Association of Canada, Toronto. Online at: http://www.kpmg.ca/en/news/documents/TourismExpenditures.pdf

Krause, R. (1993) "Foreword." In S. Morse (ed.), *Emerging Viruses.* New York: Oxford University Press.

Kraut, A. (1994) *Silent Travelers: Germs, Genes, and the "Immigrant Menace,"* New York: Basic Books.

Krieger, N. (1994) "Epidemiology and the Web of Causation: Has Anyone Seen the Spider? *Social Science & Medicine* 39: 887–903.

Krieger, N. (2001) "Theories for Social Epidemiology in the 21st Century: An Ecosocial Perspective." *International Journal of Epidemiology* 30: 668–77.

Lancet, The. (2006) "Avian Influenza Goes Global, but Don't Blame the Birds." Editorial. *The Lancet Infectious Diseases* 6(4): 185.

Latham, A., and D. McCormack. (2004) "Moving Cities: Rethinking the Materialities of Urban Geographies." *Progress in Human Geography* 28(6): 701–24.

Latour, B. (1987) *Science In Action: How to Follow Scientists an Engineers through Society.* Cambridge, MA: Harvard University Press.

Latour, B. (1988) *The Pasteurization of France.* Cambridge, MA: Harvard University Press.

Latour, B. (1993) *We Have Never Been Modern.* Cambridge, MA: Harvard University Press.

Latour, B. (2005) *Reassembling the Social: An Introduction to Actor-Network-Theory.* New York: Oxford University Press.

Lau, S., P. Woo, K. Li, et al. (2005) "Severe Acute Respiratory Syndrome Coronavirus-Like Virus in Chinese Horseshoe Bats." *Proceedings of the National Academy of Sciences of the United States* 102(39): 14040–5.

Law, J. (1987) "Technology and Heterogeneous Engineering: The Case of Portuguese Expansion," In W.E. Bijker, et al. (eds.), *The Social Construction of Technological Systems: New Directions in the Sociology and History of Technology.* Cambridge, MA: The MIT Press, pp. 109–34.

Law, J. (1994) *Organizing Modernity.* Oxford: Blackwell.

Law, J. (1999) "ANT and After." In J. Law and J. Hassard (eds.), *Actor Network Theory and After.* Oxford/Keele: Blackwell/Sociological Review, pp. 15–25.

Law, J. (2004) *After Method: Mess in Social Science Research.* London: Routledge.

Law, J., and J. Urry. (2004) "Enacting the Social." *Economy and Society* 33(3): 390–410.

Lee, J.W., and W.J. McGibbin. (2004) "Estimating the Global Economic Costs of SARS." In S. Knobler, A. Mahmoud, S. Lemon, et al. (eds.), *Learning from SARS: Preparing for the Next Disease Outbreak*. Washington, DC: Institute of Medicine of the National Academies Press, pp. 234–46.

LegCo (Legislative Council of Hong Kong). (2004) *Report on "Legislative Council Select Committee to Inquire into the Handling of the Severe Acute Respiratory Syndrome Outbreak by the Government and the Hospital Authority."* Hong Kong: Legislative Council.

Leifer, M. (1998) "Singapore in Regional and Global Context: Sustaining Exceptionalism." In H.Y. Lee and A. Mahizhnan (eds.), *Singapore: Re-Engineering Success*. Singapore: SIPS and Oxford University Press, pp. 19–30.

Leila, R. (2006a) "Poultry Industry Collapses." *Al-Ahram Weekly*, Cairo.

Leila, R. (2006b) "Wrong Vaccine Spread Virus." *Al-Ahram Weekly*, Cairo.

Leiss, W. (2001) *In the Chamber of Risks: Understanding Risk Controversies*. Montreal: McGill-Queens University Press.

Lemke, T. (2003) "Rechtssubjekt oder Biomasse? Reflexionen zum Verhältnis von Rassismus und Exklusion." *Stingelin*, pp. 160–83.

Lerner, B. (1998) *Contagion and Confinement: Controlling Tuberculosis along the Skid Road*. Baltimore: Johns Hopkins University Press.

Leslie, D., and S. Reimer. (1999) "Spatializing Commodity Chains." *Progress in Human Geography* 23(3): 401–20.

Leu, S.Y. (2003) "One Year On, the Spectre of SARS Has Returned." *South China Morning Post*, EdT5.

Leung, C., and J. Guan. (2004) *Yellow Peril Revisited: Impact of SARS on the Chinese and Southeast Asian Canadian Communities*. Toronto: The Chinese Canadian National Council.

Leung, P.C., and E.E. Ooi. (eds.). (2003) *SARS War: Combating the Disease*. Singapore: World Scientific.

Lewington, J., and J. Rusk. (2003) "The SARS Scare: Lastman's Outrage." *Globe and Mail*, April 24, p. A8.

Lewontin, R., and R. Levins. (2003) "The Return of Old Diseases and the Appearance of New Ones." In M. Gandy and A. Zumla (eds.), *The Return of the White Plague: Global Poverty and the "New" Tuberculosis*. London: Verso, pp. 1–6.

Ley, D. (2004) "Transnational Spaces and Everyday Lives." *Transactions of the Institute of British Geographers* 29: 151–64.

Li, W. (1998) "Anatomy of a New Ethnic Settlement: The Chinese Ethnoburb in Los Angeles." *Urban Studies* 35: 479–501.

Liff, J.M., W.C. Chow, and R.S. Greenberg. (1991) "Rural–Urban Differences in Stage at Diagnosis: Possible Relationship to Cancer Screening." *Cancer*, March 1.

Lim, S., T. Closson, G. Howard, and M. Gardam. (2004) "Collateral Damage: The Unforeseen Effects of Emergency Outbreak Policies." *The Lancet Infectious Diseases* 4, November: 697–703.

Lim, V.K.G. (2003) "War with SARS: An Empirical Study of Knowledge of SARS Transmission and Effects of SARS on Work and the Organization." *Singapore Medical Journal* 44(9): 457–63.

Lin, J. (1998) *Reconstructing Chinatown: Ethnic Enclave, Global Change*. Minneapolis: University of Minnesota Press.

Lines, J., et al. (1994) "Trends, Priorities, and Policy Directions in the Control of Vector-Borne Diseases in Urban Environments." *Health Policy and Planning* 9: 113–29.

Lippmann, W. (1925) *The Phantom Public.* New York: Harcourt, Brace.

Loh, C., and Civic Exchange (eds.). (2004) *At the Epicentre: Hong Kong and the SARS Outbreak.* Hong Kong: Hong Kong University Press.

Loh, C., and J. Welker. (2004) "SARS and the Hong Kong Community." In C. Loh and Civic Exchange (eds.), *At the Epicentre: Hong Kong and the SARS Outbreak.* Hong Kong: Hong Kong University Press, pp. 215–34.

Loh, C., V. Galbraith, and W. Chiu. (2004) "The Media and SARS." In C. Loh and Civic Exchange (eds.), *At the Epicentre: Hong Kong and the SARS Outbreak.* Hong Kong: Hong Kong University Press.

Lombardo, J., H. Burkom, E. Elbert, et al. (2003) "A Systems Overview of the Electronic Surveillance System for the Early Notification of Community-Based Epidemics (ESSENCE II)." *Journal of Urban Health* 80: 32–42.

Lorne, F.T. (2003) "Will SARS Result in Financial Crisis? Differentiating Real Transient and Permanent Economic Effects of a Health Crisis." In T. Koh, A. Plant, and E.H. Lee (eds.), *The New Global Threat: Severe Acute Respiratory Syndrome and its Impacts.* Singapore: World Scientific, pp. 165–72.

Louria, D.B. (2000) "Emerging and Re-Emerging Infections: The Societal Determinants." *Futures* 32: 581–94.

Luk, T.Q. (2003) "The Mystery of Atypical Pneumonia in China." *Apple Daily*, April 2, 2003, E13 (in Chinese).

Luke, T.W. (2000) "Cyborg Enchantments: Commodity Fetishism and Human/ Machine Interactions." *Strategies* 13(1).

Lulka, D. (2004) "Stabilizing the Herd: Fixing the Identity of Nonhumans." *Environment and Planning D: Society and Space* 22: 439–63.

Ma, R. (2005) "Media, Crisis, and SARS: An Introduction." *Asian Journal of Communication* 15(3): 241–6.

MacAskill, E. (2006) "US Blocking International Deal on Fighting Aids." *The Guardian* (London), June 2.

MacKinnon, I. (2007) "Urbanisation in Asia Blamed for Lethal Epidemic of Dengue Fever." *The Guardian* (London), August 1.

Magnusson, W. (1996) "The Global City as World Order." In *The Search for Political Space.* Toronto: University of Toronto Press, pp. 287–91.

Mainous, A.G. III, and F.P. Kohrs. (1995) "A Comparison of Health Status between Rural and Urban Adults." *Journal of Community Health* 20(5): 423–31.

Malizia, E.E. (2006) "Planning and Public Health: Research Options for an Emerging Field." *Journal of Planning Education and Research* 25: 428–32.

Manheim, J.B. (1998) "The News Shapers: Strategic Communication as a Third Force in News Making." In D. Graber, D. McQuail, and P. Norris (eds.), *The Politics of News: The News of Politics.* Washington, DC: CQ Press.

Mannheim, K. (1936) *Ideology and Utopia: An Introduction to the Sociology of Knowledge.* London: Kegan Paul.

Manning, N. (2002) "Actor Networks, Policy Networks and Personality Disorder." *Sociology of Health and Illness* 24(5): 644–66.

Marcuse, P., and R. Van Kempen (eds.). (2000) *Globalizing Cities: An International and Comparative Perspective*. Oxford: Blackwell.

Marginson, S., and E. Sawir. (2005) "Interrogating Global Flows in Higher Education." *Globalization, Societies and Education* 3(3): 281–309.

Markel, H. (1999) *Quarantine! East European Jewish Immigrants and the New York City Epidemics of 1892*. Baltimore: The Johns Hopkins University Press.

Martin, E. (1994) *Flexible Bodies: The Role of Immunity in American Culture from the Days of Polio to the Age of AIDS*. Boston: Beacon Press.

Mason, P., P. Grabowski, and W. Du. (2005) "Severe Acute Respiratory Syndrome, Tourism and the Media." *International Journal of Tourism Research* 7: 11–21.

Massumi, B. (2002) *Parables for the Virtual: Movement, Affect, Sensation*. Durham, NC: Duke University Press.

Matthew, R., and B. McDonald. (2006) "Cities under Siege: Urban Planning and the Threat of Infectious Disease." *Journal of the American Planning Association* 72(1): 109–17.

Mayer, J.D. (2000) "Geography, Ecology and Emerging Infectious Diseases." *Social Science and Medicine* 90: 937–52.

Mayer, J.D. (2006) "Appendix C: Changing Vector Ecologies: Political Geographic Perspectives." In S. Knobler, A. Mahmoud, S. Lemon, and L. Pray (eds.), *The Impact of Globalization on Infectious Disease Emergence and Control: Exploring the Consequences and Opportunities Workshop Summary*. Washington, DC: The National Academies Press, pp. 197–205.

McBride, D. (1991) *From TB to AIDS: Epidemics among Urban Blacks since 1900*. Albany: State University of New York Press.

McCombs, M.E., and D.L. Shaw. (1972) "The Agenda-Setting Function of the Mass Media." *Public Opinion Quarterly* 36(2): 176–85.

McCombs, M.E. (1993) "The Evolution of Agenda-Setting Research: Twenty-Five Years in the Marketplace of Ideas." *Journal of Communication* 43(2): 58–67.

McMichael, A.J. (1993) *Planetary Overload: Global Environmental Change and the Health of the Human Species*. Cambridge: Cambridge University Press.

McMichael, A.J. (2001) "Human Culture, Ecological Change, and Infectious Disease: Are We Experiencing History's Fourth Great Transition?" *Ecosystem Health* 7(2): 107–15.

McNeill, W.H. (1976) *Plagues and Peoples*. Oxford: Blackwell.

Mediacorp Channel 5 (2003a) *True Courage Episode 1: The Victims* (aired June 3, 8.30 p.m.).

Mediacorp Channel 5 (2003b) *True Courage Episode 2: The Nurses* (aired June 10, 8.30 p.m.).

Meltzer, M. (2004) "Multiple Contact Dates and SARS Incubation Periods." *Emerging Infectious Diseases* 10(2): 207–9.

Meyers, L.A., B. Pourbohloul, M.E.J. Neman, D.M. Skowronski, and R.C. Brunham. (2005) "Network Theory and SARS: Predicting Outbreak Diversity." *Journal of Theoretical Biology* 232: 71–81.

Miller, D. (1999) "Risk, Science and Policy: Definitional Struggles, Information Management, the Media and BSE." *Social Science and Medicine* 49(9): 1239–55.

Mingpao. (2003) "Sackings Point to Determination." April 22, 2003, E04 (in Chinese).

Ministry of Finance, Singapore Government. (2003) "Annual Budget Statement." Online at: http://www.mof.gov.sg/budget_2003/debate_speech/ (accessed February 20, 2004).

Ministry of Information and the Arts, Singapore Government. (1998/99) *Arts, Cultural and Music Scenes*. Singapore: MITA Publications.

Mitchell, T. (2002) *Rule of Experts: Egypt, Techno-Politics, Modernity*. Berkeley, CA: University of California Press.

Mol, A. (1999) "Ontological Politics: A Word and Some Questions." In J. Law and J. Hassard (eds.), *Actor Network Theory and After*. Oxford/Keele: Blackwell/ Sociological Review, pp. 74–89.

Mol, A. (2002) *The Body Multiple: Ontology in Medical Practice*. Durham, NC: Duke University Press.

Mol, A. (2008) *The Logic of Care: Health and the Problem of Patient Choice*. London: Routledge.

Mol, A., and G. Spaargaren. (2006) "Toward a Sociology of Environmental Flows: A New Agenda for Twenty-First-Century Environmental Sociology." In G. Spaargaren, A. Mol, and F. Buttel (eds.), *Governing Environmental Flows: Global Challenges to Social Theory*. Cambridge, MA: The MIT Press, pp. 39–82.

Monke, J. (2004) "Avian Influenza: Multiple Strains Cause Different Effects Worldwide." In *CRS Report for Congress*. Online at: http://www.RS21747.ncseonline.org/ nle/crsreports/04May/RS21747.pdf (accessed April 3, 2006).

Moon, G. (1990) "Conceptions of Space and Community in British Health Policy." *Social Science & Medicine* 30: 165–71.

Moore, B. (2000) *Moral Purity and Persecution in History*. Princeton, NJ: Princeton University Press.

Morse, S.S. (1992) "Epidemiologic Surveillance for Investigating Chemical Biological Warfare and for Improving Human Health." *Politics and the Life Sciences* 11: 29.

Moy, P. (2003) "Officials Have Failed to Keep Us Updated, Say Doctors." *South China Morning Post*, April 1, 2003, NEWS3.

Murdie, R.A., and C. Teixeira. (2000) "The City as Social Space." In T. Bunting and P. Filion (eds.), *Canadian Cities in Transition. The Twenty-First Century*, 2nd edn. Don Mills: Oxford University Press, pp. 198–223.

Murdoch, J. (1997a) "Inhuman/Nonhuman/Human: Actor-Network Theory and the Prospects for a Nondualistic and Symmetrical Perspective on Nature and Society." *Environment and Planning D: Society and Space* 15(6): 731–56.

Murdoch, J. (1997b) "Towards a Geography of Heterogeneous Associations." *Progress in Human Geography* 21(3): 321–37.

Murdoch, J. (1998) "The Spaces of Actor-Network Theory." *Geoforum* 29(4): 357–74.

Murphy, R. (2004) "Disaster of Sustainability: The Dance of Human Agents with Nature's Actants." *The Canadian Review of Sociology and Anthropology* 41(3): 249–66.

NACSPH (National Advisory Committee on SARS and Public Health). (2003) *Learning from SARS: Renewal of Public Health in Canada*. Ottawa: Health Canada.

Naimark, N.M. (2001) *Fires of Hatred: Ethnic Cleansing in Twentieth-Century Europe*. Cambridge, MA: Harvard University Press.

NAPH (National Association of Public Hospitals). (1995) *Urban Social Health*. Washington, DC: National Association of Public Hospitals.

National Advisory Committee. (2003) *Renewal of Public Health in Canada: Learning from SARS*. National Advisory Committee on SARS and Public Health, Ottawa. Online at: http://www.phac-aspc.gc.ca/publicat/sars-sras/pdf/sars-e.pdf

National Intelligence Council. (2000) *The Global Infectious Disease Threat and its Implications for the United States.* Online at: http://www.cia.gov/cia/reports/nie/report/nie99-17d.html

Naylor, C.D., C. Chantler, and S. Griffiths. (2004) "Learning from SARS in Hong Kong and Toronto." *Journal of the American Medical Association* 291(20): 2483–7.

Naylor, D., S. Basrur, M.G. Bergeron, R.C. Brunham et al. (2003) *Learning from SARS: Renewal of Public Health in Canada.* Report of the National Advisory Committee on SARS and Public Health. Ottawa: Health Canada.

Neuberg, L., and V. Rodwin. (2002) "Infant Mortality in Four World Cities: New York, London, Paris and Tokyo." *Indicators – The Journal of Social Health* 2(1), Winter.

Neustadt, R.E., and H.V. Fineberg. (1983) *The Epidemic that Never Was: Policy-Making and the Swine Flu Scare.* New York: Vintage.

Newman, J. (2006) "Canada Cracks Down on Rising Violence." *The Christian Science Monitor*, May 26. Online at: http://www.csmonitor.com/2006/0526/p07s02-woam.html (accessed June 5, 2006).

Ng, M.K. (2005) "Planning Culture in Two Transitional Chinese Cities: Hong Kong and Shenzhen." In B. Sanyal (ed.), *Comparative Planning Cultures.* New York: Routledge.

Ng, M.K. (2006) "World-City Formation under an Executive-Led Government: The Politics of Harbour Reclamation In Hong Kong." In M.K. Ng (guest editor), *Special Issue on Planning Asian World Cities in an Age of Globalization, Town Planning Review* 77(3): 311–37.

Ngok, M. (2003) "SARS and the HKSAR Governing Crisis." In T. Koh, A. Plant, and E.H. Lee (eds.), *The New Global Threat: Severe Acute Respiratory Syndrome and its Impacts.* Singapore: World Scientific, pp. 107–24.

Nolte, E., and M. McKee. (2004) *Does Health Care Save Lives? Avoidable Mortality Revisited.* London: Nuffield Trust.

Olds, K., and H. Yeung. (2004) "Pathways to Global City Formation: A View from the Developmental City-State of Singapore." *Review of International Political Economy* 11(3): 489–521.

Omi, S. (2005) "Overview." In *SARS: How a Global Epidemic Was Stopped.* Geneva: World Health Organization.

Osborne, T. (1996) "Security and Vitality: Drains, Liberalism and Power in the 19th Century." In A. Barry, T. Osborne, and N. Rose (eds.), *Foucault and Political Reason: Liberalism, Neo-Liberalism and the Rationalities of Government.* London: UCL Press, pp. 99–121.

Osterholm, M.T. (1997) "Cyclosporiasis and Raspberries – Lessons for the Future." *New England Journal of Medicine* 336(22): 1597–9.

Osterholm, M.T. (1999a) "Emerging Diseases: An Outdated Concept?" *First Annual William J. Bicknell Lecture.* Boston University School of Public Health.

Osterholm, M.T. (1999b) "Lessons Learned Again: Cyclosporiasis and Raspberries." *Annals of Internal Medicine* 130(3): 233–4.

Osterholm, M.T. (2000) "The Changing Epidemiology of Food-Borne Disease." *International Journal of Clinical Practice* 115: 60–4.

Ow, C.H. (1984) "Singapore: Past, Present and Future." In P.S. You and C.Y. Lim (eds.), *Singapore: Twenty-Five Years of Development*. Singapore: Nan Yang Xing Zhou Lianhe Zaobao, pp. 366–85.

Parr, H. (2002) "Medical Geography: Diagnosing the Body in Medical and Health Geography 1999–2000." *Progress in Human Geography* 26(2): 240–51.

Parker, S. (2004) *Urban Theory and the Urban Experience: Encountering the City*. London: Routledge.

Patton, C. (2002) *Globalizing AIDS*. Minneapolis: University of Minnesota Press.

Pavlin, J. (1999) "Epidemiology of Bioterrorism." *Emerging Infectious Diseases* 5: 528–30.

Peck, J. (2007) "Liberating the City: Between New York and New Orleans." *Urban Geography* 27(8): 681–713.

Peiris, Malik, and Yi Guan. (2005) "Confronting SARS: A View from Hong Kong." In A.R. McLean, R.M. May, J. Pattison, and R.A. Weiss (eds.), *SARS: A Case Study in Emerging Infections*. New York: Oxford University Press.

Peluso, N., and M. Watts (eds.). (2001) *Violent Environments*. Ithaca, NY: Cornell University Press.

Petersen, A., and R. Bunton (eds.). (1997) *Foucault, Health and Medicine*. London: Routledge.

Petersen, A., and D. Lupton. (1996) *The New Public Health: Health and Self in the Age of Risk*. London: Sage.

Philo, C. (1995) "Animals, Geography and the City: Notes on Inclusions and Exclusions." *Environment and Planning D: Society and Space* 13: 655–81.

Philo, C., and C. Wilbert (eds.). (2000) *Animal Spaces, Beastly Places*. London: Routledge.

Pidgeon, N., R. Kasperson, and P. Slovic (eds.). (2003) *The Social Amplification of Risk*. Cambridge: Cambridge University Press.

Pirages, D., and P. Runci. (2000) "Ecological Interdependence and the Spread of Infectious Diseases." In M. Cusimano (ed.), *Beyond Sovereignty: Issues for a Global Agenda*. New York: St. Martins Press.

PKF Consulting. (2004) *The Impacts of the Iraq War and SARS*. Toronto: PKF Consulting, the Ontario Ministry of Tourism and Recreation and Canadian Tourism Commission. Online at: http://www.tourism.gov.on.ca/english/tourdiv/research/studies/pkf_execsum1_june2003_e.pdf

Porter, M. (1995) "The Competitive Advantage of the Inner City." *Harvard Business Review* 73: 55–72.

Powell, D., and W. Leiss. (1997) *Mad Cows and Mother's Milk: The Perils of Poor Risk Communication*. Montreal: McGill-Queens University Press.

Probyn, E. (1999) "Beyond Food/Sex: Eating and an Ethics of Existence." *Theory, Culture & Society* 16(2): 215–18.

Public Health Agency of Canada. (2006) *Canadian Pandemic Influenza Plan for the Health Sector*. Ottawa: Public Health Agency of Canada. Online at: http://www.phac-aspc.gc.ca/cpip-pclcpi/index.html

Quah, S.R., and H.P. Lee. (2004) "Crisis Prevention and Management during SARS Outbreak, Singapore." *Emerging Infectious Diseases* 10(2): 364–8.

Ramesh, R. (2006a) "Drug Firms Seek to Stop Generic HIV Treatment." *The Guardian* (London), May 11.

Ramesh, R. (2006b) "HIV Infections Fall by a Third in Southern India." *The Guardian* (London), March 31.

Rao, G. (2002) "The Political Economy of Multiculturalism: Nation, Identity, Nationalism and the State." Paper presented at the Annual Conference of the Canadian Political Science Association, Toronto, Ontario, May 30.

Rasromani, W.K. (2006) "Poultry Company to Expand Slaughtering Capacity by more than Three Times with New Facility." *Daily Star Egypt*, Cairo.

Ratzan, S. (1998) *The Mad Cow Crisis: Health and the Public Good*. London: UCL Press.

Razack, S.H. (2002a) "Introduction: When Place Becomes Race." In S.H. Razack (ed.), *Race, Space, and the Law: Unmapping a White Settler Society*. Toronto: Between the Lines, pp. 1–20.

Razack, S.H. (ed.). (2002b) *Race, Space, and the Law: Unmapping a White Settler Society*. Toronto: Between the Lines.

Reardon, J. (2005) *Race to the Finish: Identity and Governance in an Age of Genomics*. Princeton, NJ: Princeton University Press.

Redfield, P. (2000) *Space in the Tropics: From Convicts to Rockets in French Guiana*. Berkeley, CA: University of California Press.

Reuters. (2003) "Bloody Animal Trade Thrives in Post-SARS China." Online at: http://www.healthypages.net/news.asp?newsid=3788 (accessed October 5, 2006).

Reynolds, B. (2005) *Crisis Risk and Emergency Communication: By Leaders for Leaders*. Atlanta: Centers for Disease Control and Prevention. Online at: http://www.cdc.gov/ communication/emergency/leaders.pdf

Reynolds, G. (2004) "The Flu Hunters." *The New York Times Magazine*, November 7, 36–43, 52, 68, 92–3.

Riley, J.C. (1987) *The Eighteenth-Century Campaign to Avoid Disease*. London: Palgrave Macmillan.

Robbins, P. (1999) "Meat Matters: Cultural Politics along the Commodity Chain in India." *Ecumene* 6(4).

Robinson, J. (2002) "Global and World Cities: A View from Off the Map." *International Journal of Urban and Regional Research* 26: 531–54.

Rodwin, V.G., and M. Gusmano. (2002) "The World Cities Project: Rationale, Organization, and Design for Comparison of Megacity Health Systems." *Journal of Urban Health: Bulletin of the New York Academy of Medicine* 79(4): 445–63.

Rodwin, V.G., and M. Gusmano (eds.). (2006) *Growing Older in World Cities: New York, London, Paris and Tokyo*. New York: Vanderbilt University Press.

Rodwin, V.G., and L. Neuberg. (2005) "Infant Mortality and Income in 4 World Cities: New York, London, Paris and Tokyo." *American Journal of Public Health* 95: 86–90.

Roper, W., et al. (1992) "Strengthening the Public Health System." *Public Health Reports* 107(6).

Rosa, H. (2003) "Social Acceleration: Ethical and Political Consequences of a Desynchronized High-Speed Society." *Constellations* 10(1): 3–33.

Rose, N. (2006) *The Politics of Life Itself: Biomedicine, Power and Subjectivity in the 21st Century*. Princeton, NJ: Princeton University Press.

Rose, N., and C. Novas. (2004) "Biological Citizenship." In A. Ong and S. Collier (eds.), *Global Assemblages: Technology, Politics, and Ethics as Anthropological Problems.* Oxford: Blackwell.

Rosner, D., and G. Markowitz. (2002) "Industry Challenges to the Principle of Prevention in Public Health: The Precautionary Principle in Historical Perspective.". *Public Health Reports* 117(6): 501–12.

Russell, E. (1996) " 'Speaking of Annihilation': Mobilizing for War against Human and Insect Enemies 1914–1945." *The Journal of American History* 82(4): 1505–29.

Ryu, S., Y.K. Park, G.H. Bai, et al. (2000) "3'UTR Polymorphisms in the NRAMP1 Gene are Associated with Susceptibility to Tuberculosis in Koreans." *International Journal of Tuberculosis and Lung Diseases* 4: 577–80.

Samers, M. (2002) "Immigration and the Global City Hypothesis: Towards an Alternative Research Agenda." *International Journal of Urban and Regional Research* 26(2): 389–402.

Sanford, S., and S.H. Ali. (2005) "The New Public Health Hegemony: Response to Severe Acute Respiratory Syndrome in Toronto." *Social Theory and Health* 3: 105–25.

Sarasin, P. (2001) *Reizbare Maschinen. Eine Geschichte des Körpers 1765–1914.* Frankfurt am Main: Suhrkamp.

Sarasin, P. (2003) "Zweierlei Rassismus? Die Selektion des Fremden als Problem in Michel Foucaults Verbindung von Biopolitik und Rassismus." *Stingelin*, pp. 55–79.

Sarasin, P. (2004) *Anthrax.* Frankfurt am Main: Suhrkamp.

Sarasin, P. (2006) *Anthrax: Bioterror as Fact and Fantasy.* Cambridge, MA: Harvard University Press.

SARPN (Southern African Regional Poverty Network). (2006) *The Johannesburg Position on HIV/AIDS and Women's and Girl's Rights in Africa.* Online at: htpp://www. sarpn.org.za/documents/d0002000/index.php (accessed June 8, 2007).

SARS Expert Committee. (2003) *SARS in Hong Kong: From Experience to Action.* Hong Kong: SARS Expert Committee. Online at: http://www.sars-expertcom.gov.hk/eindex.html

Sassen, S. (1998) *Globalization and its Discontents. Essays on the New Mobility of People and Money.* New York: The New Press.

Sassen, S. (2000) *Cities in a World Economy*, 2nd edn. Thousand Oaks, CA: Pine Forge Press.

Sassen, S. (2002) *The Global City: New York, London, Tokyo*, 2nd edn. Princeton, NJ: Princeton University Press (first published 1991).

Sawicki, J. (1991) *Disciplining Foucault: Feminism, Power, and the Body.* New York: Routledge.

Schabas, R. (2003) "Prudence, Not Panic." *Canadian Medical Association Journal* 168: 1432–4.

Scott, A.J. (ed.). (2001) *Global City-Regions: Trends, Theory, Policy.* Oxford: Oxford University Press.

Seigworth, G. (2000) "Banality for Cultural Studies." *Cultural Studies* 14(2): 227–68.

Serres, M., and B. Latour. (1995) *Conversations on Science, Culture and Time.* Ann Arbor: University of Minnesota Press.

Shatkin, G. (1998) "'Fourth World' Cities in the Global Economy: The Case of Phnom Penh, Cambodia." *International Journal of Urban and Regional Research* 22: 378–93.

Sheard, S., and H. Power (eds.). (2000) *Body and City: Histories of Urban Public Health.* Aldershot: Ashgate.

Shek, G.C. (2002) "Economy and Investment – My Views on Medical Services." *Hong Kong Economic Times,* July 13. Online at: http://libwisesearch.wisers.net/ wisesearch/tool.do?_ (accessed on March 18, 2005).

Sheller, M. (2004) "Mobile Publics: Beyond the Network Perspective." *Environment and Planning D: Society and Space* 22: 39–52.

Short, J.R. (2004) "Black Holes and Loose Connections in the Global Urban Network." *The Professional Geographer* 56: 295–302.

Short, J.R., et al. (1996) "The Dirty Little Secret of World Cities Research: Data Problems in Comparative Analysis." *International Journal of Urban and Regional Research* 20: 697–717.

Sigal, L.V. (1973) *Reporters and Officials.* Lexington, MA: D.C. Heath.

Simmel, G. (1950 [1908]) *The Sociology of Georg Simmel,* translated, edited and with an Introduction by Kurt H. Wolff. New York: The Free Press.

Simon, D. (1995) "The World City Hypothesis: Reflections from the Periphery." In P. Knox and P. Taylor (eds.), *World Cities in a World-System.* Cambridge: Cambridge University Press, pp. 132–55.

Sinclair, U. (2003) *The Jungle.* New York: W.W. Norton.

Skinner, H. (2003) *The Fog of SARS. Understanding Public Response.* Presentation to the Learning from SARS symposium, September 17, 2003, University of Toronto. Online at: http://www.phs.utoronto.ca/sars2003/Skinner%20SARS.pdf

Skouby, S.O. (1998) "Oral Contraceptives and Venous Thrombosis: End of the Debate?" *European Journal of Contraception and Reproductive Health Care* 3(2): 59–64.

Slackman, M. (2006) "Bird Flu or Not, Egyptians Keep their Ducks." *International Herald Tribune,* May 31.

Slingenbergh, J. et al. (2004) "Ecological Sources of Zoonotic Diseases." In B. Vallat and L. King (eds.), *Emerging Zoonoses and Pathogens of Public Health Concern. OIE Scientific and Technical Review* 23(2): 467–84.

Slovic, P. (ed.). (2000) *The Perception of Risk.* New York: Monarch Books.

Small, P., P. Hopewell, S. Singh, et al. (1994) "The Epidemiology of Tuberculosis in San Francisco: A Population-Based Study Using Conventional and Molecular Methods." *New England Journal of Medicine* 330(24): 1703–9.

Smith, D., and M. Timberlake. (2002) "Hierarchies of Dominance among World Cities: A Network Approach." In S. Sassen (ed.), *Global Networks, Linked Cities.* New York: Routledge, pp. 117–44.

Smith, M.P. (2001) *Transnational Urbanism: Locating Globalization.* Oxford: Blackwell.

Smith, R.G. (2003a) "World City Actor-Networks," *Progress in Human Geography* 27: 25–44.

Smith, R.G. (2003b) "World City Topologies." *Progress in Human Geography* 27(5): 561–82.

Snider, P.B. (1967) "'Mr. Gates' Revisited: A 1966 Version of the 1949 Case Study." *Journalism Quarterly* 44(3): 419–27.

Sontag, S. (1990) *Illness as Metaphor and, AIDS and its Metaphors.* New York: Doubleday.

Sooksom, R. (2006) "Not in Our Backyard." *The Walrus* 3(1): 46–50.

Spaargaren, G., A. Mol, and F.H. Buttel. (2006) *Governing Environmental Flows: Global Challenges to Social Theory.* Cambridge, MA: The MIT Press.

Spiess, L. (2003) "SARS, Censorship, and the Battle for China's Future." *The Walrus* 1: 59–67.

Spinoza, B. (1994) [1677]: *Ethics,* translated by E. Curley. Princeton, NJ: Princeton University Press.

Spitzer, W.O. (1999) "The Aftermath of a Pill Scare: Regression to Reassurance." *Human Reproduction Update* 5(6): 736–45.

St. John, R.K., A. King, D. de Jong, M. Bodie-Collings, S.G. Squires, and T.W.S. Tam. (2005) "Border Screening for SARS." *Emerging Infectious Diseases* 11(1): 6–10.

Stares, P., and M. Yacoubian. (2005) "Terrorism as Virus." *The Washington Post,* August 23, p. A15.

Stassart, P., and S. Whatmore. (2003) "Metabolising Risk: Food Scares and the Un/re-Making of Belgian Beef." *Environment and Planning A* 35(3): 449–62.

Statistics Canada. (2005) "Population by Mother tongue, by Census Metropolitan Areas, Toronto." Online at: http://www40.statcan.ca/l01/cst01/demo12c.htm (accessed February 21, 2006).

Statistics Canada. (2005) *Population Projection Projections of Visible Minority Groups, Canada, Provinces, Regions 2001–2017.* Ottawa: Statistics Canada.

Statistics Singapore. (2004a) "Key Statistics." Online at: http://www.singstat.gov. sg/keystats/annual/indicators.html (accessed February 13, 2004).

Statistics Singapore. (2004b) "Singapore Economy." Online at: http://www.singstat. gov.sg/keystats/economy.html#overview (accessed February 13, 2004).

Stead, W.W., J.W. Senner, W.T. Reddick, and J.P. Lofgren. (1990) "Racial Differences in Susceptibility to Infection by *Mycobacterium tuberculosis.*" *New England Journal of Medicine* 322(7): 422–7.

Stern, A.M. (1999) "Buildings, Boundaries, and Blood: Medicalization and Nation-Building on the U.S.–Mexico Border, 1910–1930." *Hispanic American Historical Review* 79(1): 41–81.

Stohr, K. (2003) "A Multicentre Collaboration to Investigate the Cause of Severe Acute Respiratory Syndrome." *The Lancet* 361: 1730–3.

Straits Times, The (2003a) "Battling a National Crisis." April 25.

Straits Times, The (2003b) "Do Your Part. Stop Selfish Behaviour." May 3.

Straits Times, The (2003c) "Forum." May 6.

Straits Times, The (2003d) "SARS Bug Can Survive for Days: WHO." May 5.

Straits Times, The (2003e) "SARS Fears Spark Protest in Taiwan." April 29.

Straits Times, The (2003f) "SARS: Shaming Isn't the Name of the Game." May 21.

Straits Times, The (2003g) "SIA Lines Up Action Plan to Battle Crisis." April 30.

Straits Times, The (2003h) "Singapore Hot Anti-SARS Export: Thermal Scanners." April 30.

Straits Times, The (2003i) "Singapore 'Made Right Decisions.'" May 6.

Straits Times, The (2003j) "Peasants Riot against Quarantine Centers in 2 Chinese Provinces." May 6.

Straits Times, The (2003k) "People Stared and Pointed at Her." April 29.

Straits Times, The (2003l) "Think about Families of Health Care Workers Too." May 5.

Straits Times, The (2003m) "WHO Praises Singapore's Moves to Fight Virus." May 1.

Streats. (2003) "Globalisation's dark side," April 8.

Sulston, J. (2003) "The Rich World's Patents Abandon the Poor to Die." *The Guardian* (London), February 18.

Sung, Y.W., and F. Cheung. (2003) "Catching SARS in the HKSAR: Fallout on Economy and Community." In T. Koh, A. Plant, and E.H. Lee (eds.), *The New Global Threat: Severe Acute Respiratory Syndrome and its Impacts.* Singapore: World Scientific, pp. 147–63.

Susser, I., and Z. Stein. (2004) "Culture, Sexuality and Women's Agency in the Prevention of HIV/AIDS in Southern Africa." In E. Kalipeni, S. Craddock, J.R. Oppong, and J. Ghosh (eds.), *HIV and AIDS in Africa: Beyond Epidemiology.* Oxford: Blackwell, pp. 133–43.

Svoboda, T., B. Henry, L. Shulman, et al. (2004) "Public Health Measures to Control the Spread of the Severe Acute Respiratory Syndrome during the Outbreak in Toronto." *New England Journal of Medicine* 350(23): 2352–61.

Swain, J., V. Finkelstein, S. French, and M. Oliver (eds.). (1994) *Disabling Barriers, Enabling Environments.* London: Sage.

Swyngedouw, E., and N. Heynen. (2003) "Urban Political Ecology, Justice and the Politics of Scale." *Antipode* 35(5).

Szreter, S. (1997) "Economic Growth, Disruption, Deprivation, Disease and Death: On the Importance of the Politics of Public Health for Development." *Population and Development Review* 23: 693–728.

Szreter, S., and G. Mooney. (1998) "Urbanization, Mortality, and the Standard of Living Debate: New Estimates of the Expectation of Life at Birth in Nineteenth-Century British Cities." *Economic History Review* LI: 84–112.

Taber, J. (2003) "Ontario Seeks Federal Disaster Relief." *Globe and Mail*, April 23, p. A1.

Takano, T. (1991) *Steps Toward Healthy City Tokyo.* Promotion Committee for Healthy City Tokyo, Department of Public Health and Environmental Science, Tokyo Medical and Dental University, May.

Takeuchi, S., T. Takano, and K. Nakamura. (1995) "Health and Its Determining Factors in the Tokyo Megacity." *Health Policy* 33(1).

Tambyah, P.A. (2003) "The Infection Control Response to SARS in Hospitals and Institutions." In T. Koh, A. Plant, and E.H. Lee (eds.), *The New Global Threat: Severe Acute Respiratory Syndrome and its Impacts.* Singapore: World Scientific, pp. 243–72.

Taylor, P.J. (2004) *World City Network: A Global Urban Analysis.* London: Routledge.

Temkin, O. (1977) "An Historical Analysis of the Concept of Infection." In O. Temkin (ed.), *The Double Face of Janus and Other Essays in the History of Medicine.* Baltimore: Johns Hopkins University Press, pp. 456–71.

Teo, P., B.S.A. Yeoh, G.L. Ooi, and K.P.Y. Lai. (2004) *Changing Landscapes of Singapore.* Singapore: McGraw-Hill.

Thacker, E. (2005a) "Living Dead Networks." *FibreCulture Journal* 4. Online at: http://journal.fibreculture.org/issue4/issue4_thacker.html

Thacker, E. (2005b) "Nomos, Nosos and Bios." In *Culture Machine.* Online at: http://culturemachine.tees.ac.uk/frm_f1.htm

Thompson, G.F. (2004) "Is All the World a Complex Network?" *Economy and Society* 33(3): 411–24.

Thomson, E., and C.H. Yow. (2004) "The Hong Kong SAR Government, Civil Society and SARS." In J. Wong and Y. Zhen (eds.), *The SARS Epidemic: Challenges to China's Crisis Management.* Singapore: World Scientific, pp. 199–220.

Thrift, N. (1996) *Spatial Formations.* London: Sage.

Thrift, N. (2000a) "Actor-Network Theory." In R.J. Johnston, D. Gregory, G. Pratt, and M. Watts (eds.), *Dictionary of Human Geography*, 4th edn. Oxford: Blackwell.

Thrift, N. (2000b) "Afterwords." *Environment and Planning D* 18: 213–56.

Thrift, N. (2006) "From Born to Made: Technology, Biology and Space." *Transactions of the Institute of British Geographers* 30: 463–76.

Thrift, N., and K. Olds. (1996) "Refiguring the Economic in Economic Geography." *Progress in Human Geography* 20(3): 311–37.

Tian, Y., and C.M. Stewart. (2005) "Framing the SARS Crisis: A Computer-Assisted Text Analysis of CNN and BBC Online News Reports of SARS." *Asian Journal of Communication* 15(3): 289–301.

Today (2003) "Crunch Time." April 21.

Todd, G. (1995) "'Going Global' in the Semi-Periphery: World Cities as Political Projects. The Case of Toronto." In P. Knox and P. Taylor (eds.), *World Cities in a World- System.* New York: Cambridge University Press, pp. 192–214.

Tu, C., G. Crameri, X. Kong, et al. (2004) "Antibodies to SARS Coronavirus in Civets." *Emerging Infectious Diseases* 10(12).

Tulchinsky, T.H., and E.A. Varavikova. (1996) "Addressing the Epidemiologic Transition in the Former Soviet Union: Strategies for Health System and Public Health Reform in Russia." *American Journal of Public Health* 86: 313–23.

UNAIDS (The Joint United Nations Programme on HIV/AIDS). (2006) *Report on the Global AIDS Epidemic.* New York: UNAIDS. Online at: http://data.unaids.org/pub/Global Report/2006 (accessed June 8, 2007).

UN-HABITAT (United Nations Human Settlements Programme). (2003) *The Challenge of Slums: Global Report on Human Settlements 2003.* London: Earthscan.

UN-HABITAT (United Nations Human Settlements Programme). (2006) "Urbanization: Facts and Figures." Online at: http://www.unhabitat.org/mediacentre/backgrounders.asp (accessed June 20, 2006).

United Nations Population Fund. (2007) "UNFPA State of World Population 2007: Unleashing the Potential of Urban Growth." Online at: http://www.unfpa.org/swp/2007/english/introduction.html (accessed April 1, 2008).

United States House of Representatives. (2006a) *A Failure of Initiative: Final Report of the Select Bipartisan Committee to Investigate the Preparation for and Response to Hurricane Katrina.* Washington, DC: US House of Representatives.

United States House of Representatives. (2006b) *Requests for Fiscal Year 2006 Supplemental Appropriations for the Departments of Defense, Justice, and Homeland Security.* House Document 109-111, 109th Congress, 2nd session.

United States, Committee on Labor and Human Resources. (1995) "Committee on Labor and Human Resources, Hearing on Emerging Infections, October 18, 1995." Online at: http://thomas.loc.gov/cgi-bin/query/R?r104:FLD001:D01219

Urry, J. (2004a) "Connections." *Environment and Planning D* 22: 22–37.

Urry, J. (2004b) "The Complexities of the Global." *Theory, Culture & Society* 22(5): 235–54.

Urry, J. (2005) "Mobile Sociology." *British Journal of Sociology* 51(1): 185–203.

Vasagar, J., and J. Borger. (2005) "Bush Accused of AIDS Damage to Africa." *The Guardian* (London), August 30.

Vidler, A. (1992) *The Architectural Uncanny: Essays in the Modern Unhomely*. Cambridge, MA: The MIT Press.

Villeneuve, P., and A.-M. Seguin. (2000) "Power and Decision-Making in the City: Political Perspectives." In T. Bunting and P. Filion (eds.), *Canadian Cities in Transition*, 2nd edn. Oxford: Oxford University Press, pp. 544–64.

Virchow, R. (1848/1985) *Collected Essays on Public Health and Epidemiology*. Cambridge: Science History Publications.

Vlahov, D., and S. Galea. (2002) "Urbanization, Urbanicity and Health." *Journal of Urban Health* 79(4): s1–2.

Wagner, M.M., J.M. Robinson, F.-C.Tsui, et al. (2003) "Design of a National Retail Data Monitor for Public Health Surveillance." *Journal of the American Medical Informatics Association* 10: 409–18.

Walker, D. (2004) *For the Public's Health: A Plan of Action*. Final Report of the Ontario Expert Panel on SARS and Infectious Disease Control (chaired by Dr David Walker, Dean, Faculty of Health Sciences and Director of School of Medicine, Queen's University), April 16. Toronto: Government of Ontario.

Walkom, T. (2003) "The Harsh Reality of SARS: The Main Problem with this Disease is not Its Effect on the Tourist Trade. It is the Effect on Human Health. SARS Kills." *The Toronto Star*, April 29, p. A23.

Wallace, D., and R. Wallace. (2003) "The Recent Tuberculosis Epidemic in New York City: Warning from the De-Developing World." In M. Gandy and A. Zumla (eds.), *The Return of the White Plague: Global Poverty and the "New" Tuberculosis*. London: Verso.

Wallace, R., and D. Wallace. (1997) "The Destruction of US Minority Urban Communities and the Resurgence of Tuberculosis: Ecosystem Dynamics and the White Plague in the Developing World." *Environment and Planning A* 29: 269–91.

Wallace, R., et al. (1995) "The Spatiotemporal Dynamics of AIDS and TB in the New York Metropolitan Region from a Sociogeographic Perspective: Understanding the Linkages of Central City and Suburbs." *Environment and Planning A* 27: 1085–108.

Wallisa, P., and B. Nerlich. (2005) "Disease Metaphors in New Epidemics: The UK Media Framing of the 2003 SARS Epidemic." *Social Science and Medicine* 60: 2629–39.

Wang, M., and A. Jolly. (2004) "Changing Virulence of the SARS Virus: The Epidemiological Evidence." *Bulletin of the World Health Organization* 82(7): 547–52.

Washer, P. (2004) "Representations of SARS in the British Newspapers." *Social Science and Medicine* 59: 2561–71.

Watkins, K. (2006) "We Cannot Tolerate Children Dying for a Glass of Water." *The Guardian* (London), March 8.

Weber, S. (2005) *Targets of Opportunity: On the Militarization of Thinking.* New York: Fordham University Press.

Webster, R.G. (2004) "Wet Markets: A Continuing Source of Severe Acute Respiratory Syndrome and Influenza?" *The Lancet* 363: 234–36.

Weindling, P. (1999) "A Virulent Strain: German Bacteriology as Scientific Racism, 1890–1920." In B. Harris and E. Waltraud (eds.), *Race, Science and Medicine, 1700–1960.* London: Routledge, pp. 218–34.

Weindling, P. (2000) *Epidemics and Genocide in Eastern Europe, 1890–1945.* Oxford: Oxford University Press.

Weisz, D., and M.K. Gusmano. (2004) "Gender Disparities in the Treatment of Coronary Artery Disease for Older Persons: A Comparative Analysis of National and City-Level Data." *Gender Medicine* 1(1): 29–40.

Weiss, R., and A. McLean. (2004) "What Have We Learnt from SARS?" *Philosophical Transactions of the Royal Society, London B* 359: 1137–40.

Weiss, R., and A. McMichael. (2004) "Social and Environmental Risk Factors in the Emergence of Infectious Diseases." *Nature Medicine* 10(12): S70–6.

Weisz, D., M. Gusmano, V. Rodwin, L. and Neuberg. (2007) "Population Health and the Health System: A Comparative Analysis of Avoidable Mortality in Three Nations and their World Cities." *European Journal of Public Health* 1(7).

Wekerle, G., and P. Jackson (2005) "Urbanizing the Security Agenda." *City: Analysis of Urban Trends, Culture, Theory, Policy, Action* 9(1): 33–49.

Whatmore, S. (1997) "Dissecting the Autonomous Self—Hybrid Cartographies for a Relational Ethics." *Environment and Planning D: Society and Space* 15: 37–53.

Whatmore, S. (2004) "Humanism's Excess: Some Thoughts on the 'Post-Human/ist Agenda." *Environment and Planning A* 36: 1341–63.

Wheelis, M. (1992) "Strengthening Biological Weapons Control through Global Epidemiological Surveillance." *Politics and the Life Sciences* 11: 181.

White, D.M. (1950) "The 'Gatekeeper': A Case Study in the Selection of News." *Journalism Quarterly* 27(4): 383–90.

White, L.T. III. (2003) "SARS Anti-Populism and Elite Lies: Temporary Disorders in China." In T. Koh, A. Plant, and E.H. Lee. (eds.), *The New Global Threat: Severe Acute Respiratory Syndrome and its Impacts.* Singapore: World Scientific, pp. 31–68.

White House, The. (2002) "The National Security Strategy of the United States of America, September 2002." Online at: http://www.whitehouse.gov/nsc/nss.pdf

Wilbert, C. (2006) "Profit, Plague and Poultry: The Intra-Active Worlds of Highly Pathogenic Avian Flu." *Radical Philosophy* 139: 2–8.

Wilkins, L. (2005) "Plagues, Pestilence and Pathogens: The Ethical Implications of News Reporting of a World Health Crisis." *Asian Journal of Communication* 15(3): 247–54.

Williams, R. (1973) *The Country and the City.* New York: Oxford University Press.

Williams, S. (2001) "From Smart Bombs to Smart Bugs: Thinking the Unthinkable in Medical Sociology and Beyond." *Sociological Research Online* 6(4).

Wilson, M. (1995) "Travel and the Emergence of Infectious Diseases." *Emerging Infectious Diseases* 1(2): 39–46.

Wilson, M.L. (2001) "Ecology and Infectious Disease." In J.L. Aron and J.A. Patz (eds.), *Ecosystem Change and Public Health: A Global Perspective.* Baltimore: The Johns Hopkins University Press, pp. 283–326.

Wilson, N., G. Thomson, and O. Mansoor. (2004) "Print Media Response to SARS in New Zealand." *Emerging Infectious Diseases* 10(8): 1461–5.

Wolch, J., and J. Emel. (1998) *Animal Geographies: Place, Politics and Identity in the Nature–Culture Borderlands.* New York: Verso.

Wolch, J. (1996) "Zoopolis." *Capitalism, Nature, Socialism* 7: 21–48.

Wood, P., and L. Gilbert. (2005) "Multiculturalism in Canada: Accidental Discourse, Alternative Vision, Urban Practice." *International Journal of Urban and Regional Research* 29(3): 679–91.

WHO (World Health Organization). (1948) "Constitution," 45th edn (2006). Online at: http://www.who.int/governance/eb/who_constitution_en.pdf

WHO (World Health Organization). (1986) *Ottawa Charter for Health Promotion.* Geneva: World Health Organization.

WHO (World Health Organization). (1998) *Health 21 – Health for All in the 21st Century: An Introduction.* European Health for all Series No. 5. Copenhagen: World Health Organization Regional Office for Europe.

WHO (World Health Organization) Communicable Disease Surveillance and Response. (2003a) *Severe Acute Respiratory Syndrome (SARS): Status of the Outbreak and Lessons for the Immediate Future.* Geneva: World Health Organization.

WHO (World Health Organization). (2003b) *Summary of Probable SARS Cases with Onset of Illness from 1 November 2002 to 31 July 2003.* Geneva: WHO. Online at: http://www.who.int./csr/ sars/country/table2004_04_21/en/index.html

WHO (World Health Organization). (2003c) "Summary Table of SARS Cases by Country, November 2002–7 August 2003." Online at: http://www.who.int/esr/ sars/country/2003_08_15/en/print.html (accessed July 15, 2004).

WHO (World Health Organization). (2003d) *Treating 3 Million by 2005: Making it Happen.* The WHO strategy. Geneva: World Health Organization. Online at: http://www.who.int/3by5/publications/documents/isbn9241591129/en (accessed November 8, 2004).

WHO (World Health Organization). (2003e) "Update 95 – SARS: Chronology of a Serial Killer." Online at: http://www.who.int/csr/don/2003_07_04/en/print. html (accessed March 2003).

WHO (World Health Organization). (2005) *Estimating the Impact of the Next Influenza Pandemic: Enhancing Preparedness.* Geneva: WHO. Online at: http://www.who.int/ csr/disease/influenza/preparedness2004_12_08/en

WHO (World Health Organization). (2006a) *Avian Influenza Fact Sheet February 2006.* Online at: http://www.who.int/mediacentre/factsheets/avian_influenza/en/print. html

WHO (World Health Organization). (2006b) *Questions and Answers on Avian Influenza.* Geneva: World Health Organization.

WHO (World Health Organization). (2006c) "Tuberculosis Fact Sheet." Online at: http://www.who.int/mediacentre/factsheets/fs104/en/index.html

World Travel & Tourism Council. (2003) *SARS has a Massive Impact on Travel and Tourism in Affected Destinations.* Online at: http://www.wttc.org/newsll.htm (accessed August 2, 2004).

WTO (World Trade Organization). (2001) *Declaration on the TRIPS agreement and Public Health, Adopted on 14 November 2001.* Online at: http://www.wto.org/english/ thewto_e/minist_e/min01_e/mindecl_trips_e.htm (accessed November 8, 2004).

Yeoh, B.S.A., and T.C. Chang. (2001) "Globalizing Singapore: Debating Transnational Flows in the City." *Urban Studies* 38(7): 1025–44.

Yu, D., et al. (2003) "Prevalence of IgG Antibody to SARS-Associated Coronavirus in Animal Traders – Guangdong Province, China, 2003." In *Morbidity & Mortality Weekly Report* 52(41) (October 17): 986–7.

Zackowitz, M.G. (2006) "Bird Flu Takes Wing." *National Geographic* 29(3): 24.

Zelicoff, A., J. Brillman, J., D.W. Forslund, et al. (2001) "The Rapid Syndrome Validation Project (RSVP)." *Proceedings of the American Medical Informatics Association Symposium* 2001: 771–5.

Zhan, M. (2005) "Civet Cats, Fried Grasshoppers, and David Beckham's Pajamas: Unruly Bodies after SARS." *American Anthropologist* 107(1): 31–42.

Zheng, B., et al. (2004) "SARS Related Virus Predating SARS Outbreak, Hong Kong." *Emerging Infectious Diseases* 10(2): 176–8.

Zheng, Y., and L.F. Lye. (2003) "SARS and China's Political System." In T. Koh, A. Plant and E.H. Lee. (eds.), *The New Global Threat: Severe Acute Respiratory Syndrome and Its Impacts.* Singapore: World Scientific, pp. 45–75.

Zhong, N., and G. Zeng. (2005) "Management and Prevention of SARS in China." In A.R. McLean, R.M. May, J. Pattison, and R.A. Weiss (eds.), *SARS: A Case Study in Emerging Infections.* New York: Oxford University Press.

Zhong, N. (2004) "Management and Prevention of SARS in China." *Philosophical Transactions of the Royal Society, London* 359: 1115–16.

Zukin, S. (1991) *Landscapes of Power: From Detroit to Disney World.* Los Angeles: University of California Press.

Index